Gluten-Free, Hassle Free

Gluten-Free, Hassle Free

A SIMPLE, SANE, DIETITIAN-APPROVED
PROGRAM FOR EATING YOUR WAY
BACK TO HEALTH

SECOND EDITION

Marlisa Brown, MS, RD, CDE, CDN

Illustrations by Kenneth Brown and William Cypser
Cartoon content by Marlisa Brown

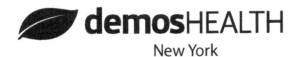

demosHEALTH

New York

Visit our website at www.demoshealth.com

ISBN: 978-1-936303-58-8
e-book ISBN: 978-1-61705-196-8

Acquisitions Editor: Julia Pastore
Compositor: diacriTech

Medical information provided by Demos Health, in the absence of a visit with a health care professional, must be considered as an educational service only. This book is not designed to replace a physician's independent judgment about the appropriateness or risks of a procedure or therapy for a given patient. Our purpose is to provide you with information that will help you make your own health care decisions.

The information and opinions provided here are believed to be accurate and sound, based on the best judgment available to the authors, editors, and publisher, but readers who fail to consult appropriate health authorities assume the risk of injuries. The publisher is not responsible for errors or omissions. The editors and publisher welcome any reader to report to the publisher any discrepancies or inaccuracies noticed. The author does not intend for this information to serve as a substitute for medical advice; health concerns should be treated under the supervision of a doctor. In addition, every effort was made to check the gluten-free status of the foods listed, however manufacturers are often changing formulas, so always double-check the gluten-free status of your foods.

Library of Congress Cataloging-in-Publication Data

Brown, Marlisa.
  Gluten-free, hassle free : a simple, sane, dietitian-approved program for eating your way back to health / Marlisa Brown, MS, RD, CDE, CDN ; Illustrations by Kenneth Brown and William Cypser; Cartoon content by Marlisa Brown.
    pages cm
  Includes bibliographical references and index.
  ISBN 978-1-936303-58-8 (alk. paper)
1. Gluten-free diet—Recipes. 2. Celiac disease—Diet therapy—Recipes.
3. Gluten-free diet. I. Title.
  RM237.86.B759 2014
  641.3—dc23

                    2013034849

Special discounts on bulk quantities of Demos Health books are available to corporations, professional associations, pharmaceutical companies, health care organizations, and other qualifying groups. For details, please contact:

Special Sales Department
Demos Medical Publishing, LLC
11 West 42nd Street, 15th Floor
New York, NY 10036
Phone: 800-532-8663 or 212-683-0072
Fax: 212-941-7842
E-mail: specialsales@demosmedpub.com

Printed in the United States of America by Bradford and Bigelow.
17 / 5 4 3 2

IN LOVING MEMORY OF MY PARENTS,
ANN AND STUART BROWN, FOREVER CHERISHED

Contents

Foreword

In August 2006, when I started Allergicgirl.com, my blog about eating out in New York City with serious food allergies and dairy and wheat intolerances, I thought, *I'm alone*. But I was wrong. I quickly discovered a growing community of allergic girls and guys, celiac chicks and dudes, gluten-free men and women who were all trying to do the same thing: eat safely with joy.

I made it my personal mission to help others like me find that joy.

A licensed social worker since 2000, I established my food allergy coaching practice, Allergic Girl Resources, Inc., in 2007 to work one-on-one with clients with dietary restrictions who want to overcome fear and anxiety and find a way back to loving and enjoying food. And in 2008, I launched my Worry-Free Dinners program to bridge the gap between restaurants that want to serve the food-restricted community and food-restricted diners who want to reclaim positive and enjoyable dining-out experiences.

But how do you regain the intoxicating mix of food and joy after the doctor tells you that you can no longer eat certain foods lest you suffer dire consequences?

You may feel waves of sadness, frustration, confusion, denial, anxiety, depression, and anger. Yet you may feel some relief that symptoms that have gone unchecked or unexplained now have a name, a diagnosis. Whether it is a food allergy, food intolerance, celiac disease, or nonceliac gluten sensitivity, a diagnosis will help you regain some sense of control over your health. However, one of the hallmarks of a diagnosis of a dietary restriction is that you can't eat certain things—ever.

But what *can* you eat? And where do you find reliable information about how to create quick, easy daily meals and snacks that will make you feel better, not worse?

A crucial path back to loving food again after you're diagnosed is to see a registered dietitian, especially one who is knowledgeable about your dietary restriction diagnosis and needs. I met Marlisa Brown—a compassionate registered dietitian with thirty years of experience and a chef with her own set of dietary restrictions—in 2007 at the International Foodservice and Restaurant Show. She was giving a talk about food allergies and food service, using her mango allergy as an example. She had yet to discover what she now knows: that she had an undiagnosed lifelong non-celiac gluten sensitivity.

Marlisa has written a book to help herself, her mother (who had celiac disease), and you get back on that path to loving food again. With easy-to-create menu ideas and suggestions, tons of gluten-free recipes, smart grain substitutions, safe gluten-free resources, and a massive list of naturally gluten-free foods, you'll be surprised how much food there is to choose from.

With Marlisa as your guide, enjoy all of the delicious gluten-free meals ahead!

Sloane Miller, MFA, MSW, LMSW
President, Allergic Girl Resources, Inc.
allergicgirl@gmail.com
allergicgirl.blogspot.com/
worryfreedinners.blogspot.com/
allergicgirlresources.com/
twitter.com/@allergicgirl

It's Much Easier Than You Think

You're probably reading this book because you or someone you know has celiac disease or a non-celiac gluten sensitivity. By picking up this book, you've taken the first step to making gluten-free living easy and uncomplicated.

Gluten is often the hidden culprit at the root of many health problems. However, going gluten free and eating your way back to health doesn't have to be painful or difficult. Millions of people of all ages and backgrounds share the challenges of living gluten free. This book contains everything you need, including tips, strategies, recipes, and shortcuts to make your journey easier.

When people first learn (or suspect) that they can't eat gluten, they often feel angry, frustrated, and confused—and with good reason. They suddenly have to make huge, unexpected changes in what and how they eat. To most people, the whole prospect can seem overwhelming.

When I first began investigating gluten-free diets many years ago, I discovered layer upon layer of confusing (and sometimes contradictory) information on the subject. It took me some time to sort through it all and separate what was true from what was speculation, and what was somebody's best guess. My training made it easier for me to make sense of it all, but I saw how the details and contradictions could leave many people feeling lost. Plus, new research on celiac disease and gluten is continually being released, making it even more difficult for most to keep up with the newest information.

Even so, living without gluten doesn't have to be difficult or complex for you.

Part of my job as a registered dietitian and nutritional consultant is to make things simple and understandable for my patients. Over the past 20 years, so many people have come to me with gluten-related health problems, including my own mother. I still remember her reaction when she called me and said, "I just need to know what has gluten in it, can't you just tell me what I can and can't eat!" I tried to explain to her that it was more than a list of what she could and couldn't eat, but she was just frustrated and aggravated by that answer. "My own daughter the dietitian can't just tell me what to eat?"

I've also faced the same situation even more personally. For years I suffered from recurring stomach problems, but tests for everything always came back negative. I was eventually given a diagnosis of irritable bowel syndrome. But after my mother tested positive for celiac, I decided that celiac disease might also be my problem, since it runs in families. I needed to find a solution, so as an experiment, I tried a gluten-free diet. Within a few days, my stomach pains began to disappear. What do you know! I went back on a gluten-containing diet and went in for more gastrointestinal tests, just to be sure. It turns out I did not have celiac disease, but since I improved on a gluten-free diet I have been diagnosed with non-celiac gluten sensitivity.

I've been a foodie from birth. I was a chef before I became a dietitian. I love everything about food—cooking it, growing it, tasting it, and reading about it. So I knew I had to find ways to make the necessary dietary changes while still being able to enjoy the arts of cooking and eating. I also travel a lot and find myself dining out frequently.

In short, I know how you feel, and I understand the difficulties of living gluten free. This book is an uncomplicated, easy-to-follow way to make gluten-free eating work for anyone who likes to eat: for you, me, other chefs, other foodies, and anyone who needs to live gluten free.

Right now you're probably feeling stressed out, because you need to relearn how to shop, how to cook, and how to eat in restaurants. You also have to deal with your family, coworkers, friends, and acquaintances. They may not understand your diet, and they may not want to understand it—they may even think you're weird, neurotic, or just being difficult. This book will help you set them straight.

Maybe you've already looked at some of the other books on gluten-free cooking, eating, and living that have been so loaded with technical and scientific detail that you feel even more confused. You shouldn't need a PhD in nutrition in order to make the changes that will help you get and stay healthy. Gluten free *can* be hassle free.

As a registered dietitian and president of Total Wellness, Inc., a New York–based health consulting company, I have found that when people come to me for help, they don't want a long lecture or a longer list of things that they can't and shouldn't do. Instead, they want to know what they *can* do. They want someone who can lay things out for them and give them a step-by-step plan that lets them live their lives the way they're used to living them.

Everything about *Gluten-Free, Hassle Free* is designed to make gluten-free living as simple, doable, worry-free, and easy to understand as possible. From "Safe Supermarket Shopping" to "Gluten-Free at the Deli Counter and in Fast Food Restaurants" to "Making Social Events Easier for Everyone" to "Stocking a Gluten-Free Kitchen," each section of this book is practical, down to earth, and easy to follow. You can quickly find what you need, immediately put it into practice, and instantly begin improving your life. You'll also find a wealth of shortcuts, recipes, meal plans, tips, and special tools—each of which can save you time, trouble, headaches, and heartache.

Over the past 20 years, I've helped thousands of people dramatically improve their health through an easy step-by-step process. Many of these people have celiac disease or non-celiac gluten sensitivity. They come to my office looking for simple solutions; they leave not only with those solutions, but also with relief and hope.

I'm glad you're here. Your healthier, happier life begins right now.

Marlisa Brown

Acknowledgments

There are so many people who made this book possible whom I would like to thank: my husband Russell for endless gluten-free tastings, my family for their support, my brother Kenneth Brown for his creative Dee cartoon character, my brother David for helping me to explore content in difficult gluten-free situations, and my agent Stephany Evans for her encouragement from the very beginning of this project. In addition, special thanks go to registered dietitians, Catherine Brittan, Jacqueline Gutierrez, and Jodi Wright for their hard work on all aspects of this book, and to Sloane Miller for her special contributions. I would also like to thank my sisters-in-law (Rosemarie Kass, Barbara Schimmenti, and Eileen Ciaccio) for experimenting with gluten-free holiday meals, and my niece Janice Ciaccio and her mother Chris Howard for their culinary tips. Also, thanks to Michelle Moreau, a culinary nutritionist who reviewed recipes for me, and to my soul sister Constance Brown-Riggs for her continued encouragement during the development of this book. I also received a great deal of support from the nutrition department at CW Post, especially Sandy Sarcona. A special thanks to Ryan Whitcomb for his continued input, Dahlia Alese and Barbara Bonavoglia for their recipes, and Shelley Case, RD, and Carol Fenster for their work with celiac disease and gluten-free cooking as well as their creative feedback on this project. Thanks also go to my friends at the Gluten-Intolerance group of Long Island, Christopher M Singlemann, certified executive chef from the Watermill Caterers, and Vincent Barbieri, owner–operator of Café Formagio in Carle Place for their recipes.

In addition, I would like to thank the following researchers for their information and support: Dr. Peter Green, Dr. Ben Lebwohl, Dr. Armin Alaedini, and Suzanne Simpson, RD, from Columbia University, Dr. Chawla, Stony Brook Hospital, and Dr. Alessio Fasano, Center for Celiac Research at Massachusetts General Hospital, Anne Lee, RD, from Dr. Schär and Pam Cureton, RD, from the Center for Celiac Research for their tips and support.

Special thanks to:

- Catherine Brittan, MS, RD, LD
- Jodi Wright, MS, RD, CDN
- Jacqueline Gutierrez, MS, MSEd, RD, CDN
- Randy Yaskal at The Center for International Studies and Foreign Languages, Translatethisdocument.com

Gluten-Free, Hassle Free

STEP 1: GETTING STARTED

Is Your Diet Putting Your Health at Risk?

Finding Out If You Have Celiac Disease or Non-Celiac Gluten Sensitivity

Are You at Risk?

When it comes to our health, most of us usually accept our daily aches and pains as normal. We tend to distance ourselves from the thought that our health could decline until one day it does, and then we are forced to accept it.

None of us can predict the health challenges we'll encounter in our lifetime, but your body often does give clues. All you need to do is pay attention and know what to look for. In the case of celiac disease, sometimes just shortened to celiac, the symptoms show up in many different ways. The more you know about celiac disease and non-celiac gluten sensitivity, the easier it will be to get diagnosed.

What Is Celiac Disease?

Celiac disease is thought to have been around for thousands of years, and it may have started back when people began cultivating food and we switched to a diet that included wheat. After thousands of years, science has just begun to understand how to diagnose and treat celiac disease as well as the risks associated with it. It wasn't that long ago that celiac disease was considered a rare European disease and doctors in the United States thought the risk of celiac disease was reduced when people migrated to America. Recent research has discovered that celiac disease can affect as many as 1 in 133 in North America alone— approximately 3 million people. Celiac disease is an inherited disorder and if you have celiac disease there is a higher liklihood that some of your immediate family members may also have it. Celiac disease affects about 1 percent of the population in the world, including in Africa, Asia, and South America, and as many as 83 percent of the people living with celiac disease may go undiagnosed. Recent research has shown that the prevalence has been increasing, and in the past 50 years the number of people developing celiac disease worldwide has increased four to five times. Researchers have been speculating as to why this has occurred but the reason still remains unknown.

If you were asking yourself what is celiac disease, simply put, celiac disease is a reaction to the protein gluten (pronounced glOO-ten). Gluten is actually a mix of proteins, specifically gliadin and glutenin, found in wheat, rye, and barley. When you eat these starches, or when they are added to your food or medications, you are consuming gluten. Similarly, when people suffer from food allergies or sensitivities, they too are reacting to the proteins in those foods; therefore, for these individuals those proteins should be avoided. Celiac disease is not considered an allergy, but it is rather a sensitivity to the gluten found in those grains. This sensitivity will cause an autoimmune response any time that the protein gluten is ingested.

It used to be thought that celiac disease was a gastrointestinal problem because many who suffered with celiac disease also experienced gastrointestinal symptoms, but now we know that only a percentage of those with celiac disease will experience these symptoms. Today we have learned that celiac disease is an autoimmune disease that can cause a multitude of different symptoms that will vary from person to person. Therefore, for those with celiac disease, gluten must be avoided at all times to stop this autoimmune response. Depending on who you speak to, celiac disease may be referred to as a gluten sensitivity or as a gluten intolerance, but no matter how you say it, if the diagnosis is celiac disease, gluten can never be consumed again.

In addition to being found naturally in grains, gluten is also added to many foods, medications, and supplements. You may ask, why add gluten to food? Well, gluten is the "glue" that holds the ingredients together, giving breads and other foods that crispy, light texture that we all enjoy.

Since celiac disease is aggravated by the gluten found in the foods we eat, it often affects the digestive system, which is the root of its

WHAT IS GLUTEN?

"We know that gluten is a combination of several complex proteins that are not easily digested by humans. For most people, this incomplete breakdown of gluten peptides doesn't cause a problem and the gluten fragments pass without trouble through the digestive tract. For certain people with the genetic susceptibility to gluten-related disorders, the undigested gluten can create problems. When gluten is ingested and reaches the small intestine, it can trigger an immune response leading to increased intestinal permeability and, ultimately, to inflammation in genetically susceptible individuals."

—Dr. Alessio Fasano, Director of the Center for
Celiac Research at Mass achusetts General Hospital

absorption into the body, but as stated previously, it is an autoimmune disease not a gastrointestinal disease. Celiac usually presents itself in the small intestine, a 22-foot-long organ covered with tiny finger-like projections called villi. It is through the villi that our bodies absorb nutrients. Celiac disease will cause a flattening of the villi, making it difficult for our gastrointestinal tract to function normally. It is often difficult to diagnose celiac disease because the symptoms are varied, and since the villi get flattened in patchy segments it is easy to miss, especially if the exact section is not biopsied during testing.

Celiac disease affects each person differently: Some may have stomach pains or be depressed and tired all the time, others may feel sick only once in a while, and still others may feel just fine. However, no matter what the symptoms are, consuming gluten causes damage. Celiac disease can develop at any age, from infancy to adulthood, so it is difficult to know when to look for it. And because it can show up in many ways, your doctor may attempt to test or treat you for other ailments, such as Crohn's disease, chronic fatigue, irritable bowel syndrome, thyroid disorder, osteoporosis, diverticulitis, or rheumatoid arthritis—anything and everything but celiac disease. Because there are no "typical" symptoms of celiac disease, it is usually not the first thing doctors think of. It's no wonder that so many who have celiac disease still remain undiagnosed. It has been shown that most people with celiac disease can spend an average of about 11 years going to doctors and specialists before they figure out what the cause of their problems is. Numerous studies have shown that many people diagnosed with other diseases, such as irritable bowel syndrome, could actually be suffering with undiagnosed celiac disease.

How do we get celiac disease? We don't know how, but we now know that it runs in families (about 99 percent of people who have celiac disease will have at least one or both of the genetic markers HL DQ-2 or HL DQ-8) and if you have a first-degree relative (sibling or parent) with celiac disease, you will have a much higher chance of also having celiac disease. That is why if someone in your family has celiac disease, it is important that you be screened for it as well.

The following checklists will help you evaluate your risk and focus on prevention of secondary symptoms from earlier diagnoses. If you have already been diagnosed with celiac disease or suffer from a non-celiac gluten sensitivity, proceed directly to chapter 2, "Learning the Basics."

Recognizing Symptoms of Celiac Disease

Section A

Put a check next to any of the health problems below that you have:

———— Anemia
———— Behavioral changes
———— Bloating, gas, or abdominal pain
———— Bones that break easily
———— Bone or joint pain
———— Bruising
———— Chronic fatigue
———— Delayed growth as a child
———— Dental enamel problems
———— Depression or irritability
———— Diarrhea or constipation
———— Discolored teeth or enamel problems
———— Dry eyes
———— Edema (swelling, especially found in hands and feet)
———— Epstein–Barr
———— Failure to thrive (in children)
———— Fatigue
———— Frequent bowel movements
———— Frequent infections
———— Frequent illness

———— Hard-to-flush stools

———— Inability to lose weight

———— Indigestion

———— Infertility

———— Irritability

———— Joint pain

———— Lactose intolerance

———— Learning difficulties

———— Memory problems

———— Menstrual problems

———— Migraines

———— Mouth sores and ulcers (canker sores)

———— Nutritional deficiencies (such as iron, calcium, or vitamins A, D, E, and K)

———— Reflux (heartburn)

———— Seizures

———— Short stature

———— Skin problems and rashes

———— Tingling or numbness in hands and feet

———— Unexplained weight gain

———— Unexplained weight loss

Count how many items you have checked in Section A:

If you have checked two or more of the items in this section, and the source of these symptoms has not been identified, you should consider being screened for celiac disease.

Not everyone who has celiac disease will have symptoms!

Section B

Please check any of the following health problems with which you have been diagnosed:

———— Addison's disease

———— ADHD

———— Alopecia areata

——————   Anemia
——————   Autism
——————   Autoimmune disorders
——————   Central and peripheral nervous system disorders
——————   Dermatitis herpetiformis
——————   Down syndrome
——————   Family history of celiac disease (any relative with celiac disease)
——————   Gastrointestinal malignancies
——————   Hepatitis
——————   IBS (irritable bowel syndrome)
——————   Inflammatory bowel disease (ulcerative colitis, Crohn's disease)
——————   Intestinal lymphomas
——————   IgA deficiency
——————   Infertility
——————   Intestinal cancer
——————   Juvenile idiopathic arthritis
——————   Lymphoma
——————   Myasthenia gravis
——————   Non-Hodgkin's lymphoma
——————   Osteoporosis
——————   Pancreatic insufficiency
——————   Peripheral neuropathy
——————   Primary biliary cirrhosis
——————   Psoriasis
——————   Recurrent aphthous ulcerations
——————   Rheumatoid arthritis
——————   Sarcoidosis
——————   Scleroderma
——————   Selective IgA deficiency
——————   Sjögren's disease
——————   Systemic lupus erythematosus
——————   Thyroid disease
——————   Turner syndrome
——————   Type 1 diabetes (DM1) (in you or any of your first-degree relatives)
——————   Williams syndrome

Count how many items you have checked in section B.

If you have checked one or more of the items in this section, and any items in section A, consider being screened for celiac disease (especially if you have a family history).

You may think, "These lists are so long—they can't all be linked to celiac disease, can they?" But since celiac disease affects your immune system with gluten attacking through your gastrointestinal system, the symptoms will be different for each individual based on his or her genetic differences. This autoimmune attack can contribute to illness and the development of many disease states. How you are affected depends on your body's weak spots, which will influence where your immune system decides to attack.

For instance, it has long been known that there is a relationship between type 1 diabetes (which is caused by an immune system attack of the beta cells in the pancreas) and celiac disease. Is it possible that in some individuals gluten could be the trigger for this attack athough this has not been established? More recently, scientists have been looking at the chromosomal abnormalities that are similar among those with type 1 diabetes and those with celiac disease. Research is ongoing, and currently the American Diabetes Association's "Standards of Care" recommends that anyone with type 1 diabetes should be screened annually for celiac disease, and their first-degree relatives should be screened as well. We don't have all of the answers yet about the relationship between celiac disease and type 1 diabetes or the other disorders listed in the previous list, but one way to determine your potential risk for celiac disease is to take a look at the specific diseases that are most commonly associated with it and evaluate your symptoms and your family history. Future research will hopefully be able to teach us more about these connections.

Useful and Not-So-Useful Medical Tests

It is estimated that 1 in 100 people worldwide suffers from celiac disease. The easiest way to screen for celiac disease is with blood tests. Unfortunately, none of the tests alone are 100 percent accurate, nor can they be used to rule out celiac or to diagnose you. But they can help indicate your potential risk. In order to be screened for celiac disease it is important to make sure that you are still eating gluten, otherwise your test results may not be accurate. If you are already following a gluten-free diet, you must start eating gluten for several months prior to being tested for celiac disease.

**When Screening for Celiac Disease, These Blood Tests
Should Be Ordered:**

1. **IgA-tissue transglutaminase antibody (tTG):** If this test is positive, it is likely that you could have celiac disease, but it is not

conclusive in itself. If you are IgA deficient the accuracy of this test may be affected.

2. **IgA gliadin antibodies (AGA):** These tests are the older gliadin tests and are not as accurate as the newer tests, but they are still sometimes ordered.

3. **IgA endomysial antibodies (EMA):** This test, which is very specific for celiac disease, has mostly been replaced by the IgA anti-tTG test. It is expensive and rarely ordered.

4. **Deaminated gliadin peptide antibodies (DGP):** This test is a new version of the older AGA tests, and its accuracy is higher than that of the original tests. This is the best test to run when someone also has an IgA deficiency (see note below).

* Please note that when being screened for celiac disease it is also important to have a total serum IgA test, which is used to identify an IgA deficiency. Some of the screenings rely on the IgA to identify celiac disease; IgA deficiencies are common with celiac disease, and if you have an IgA deficiency the results of celiac screening may not be accurate; the DGP test can be helpful when this is the case.

Genetic Tests

About 99 percent of patients who have celiac disease also have one or both of the genes HLA-DQ2 and HLA-DQ8. Thus, if you come back negative on the previously listed blood tests but have symptoms of celiac disease and are positive on either the HL-DQ2 or HL-DQ8 tests, you still could have celiac disease. If you do not have the genetic markers it is unlikely that you could have celiac disease.

* Please note, your doctor can order these tests for you, or DNA testing is also available from Kimball Genetics, 101 University Blvd., Suite #350, Denver CO 80206, (800) 320-1807, www.kimballgenetics.com; and also from Prometheus Labs, www.prometheuslabs.com.

Interpreting the Results

- If you are positive on any one of the blood tests, talk to your doctor about additional diagnostic testing.

- If you are negative on the blood screening tests but have checked several items in section A or B and no other cause of your illness has been found, talk to your doctor about being tested further for celiac disease.

- If you are negative on the blood screening tests but have checked off anything in section A or B and have a relative who is suffering from celiac disease, talk to your doctor about further celiac testing.

- If you are either positive or negative on the blood tests and do not want to go for diagnostic tests right away, you can do a simple DNA test, as noted above. This test—which is sometimes covered by insurance—will isolate whether or not you have the gene or DNA that is found in 99 percent of those who develop celiac disease. If you do not have this genetic marker, it is very unlikely that you have celiac disease. If this test is positive you should talk to your doctor about testing further.

Diagnostic Tests

If you are positive on any of the blood tests, make sure you follow up by having an endoscopy of the small intestine (it is important that this is done with biopsies taken from the duodenum or jejunum areas). This is the only way to accurately diagnose celiac disease. Blood tests are a good screening tool, but they cannot currently be used alone to diagnose celiac disease. The endoscopic procedure is used to identify any flattened villi in the small intestine, which is what is indicated when someone has celiac disease. Villi are finger-like projections on the lining of your intestines that are responsible for nutrient absorption. An endoscopy, along with a biopsy, is the only way to get a conclusive diagnosis for celiac disease.

When you have an endoscopic procedure the doctor needs to take a minimum of 4 to 6 samples taken throughout the duodenum/duodenum bulb, which is essential since celiac disease can be patchy and can easily be missed during testing. Taking a number of samples from various locations will give you a better chance of being properly diagnosed; there is actually a linear relationship between the number of samples taken and the number of people who are correctly diagnosed with celiac disease. The endoscopic procedure is a relatively quick, painless procedure that is done while you are under anesthesia.

Try to find a specialist or gastroenterologist who works often with patients who have celiac disease. A gastroenterologist is a doctor who specializes in treatment and diagnosis of gastrointestinal problems. Some doctors work more extensively with celiac patients than others and are more likely to take sufficient samples, improving the chance of an accurate diagnosis.

Often, when a diagnosis of celiac disease is missed, it is due to either an insufficient number of samples taken or a misinterpretation of the test results. Sometimes an adequate number of samples are taken but the pathologist interpreting the results may not be a gastrointestinal expert, resulting in something being overlooked or missed. Years ago it was thought that the villi needed to be completely flattened to obtain a diagnosis; it is now known that this is not the case. The diagnosis criteria for identifying celiac disease is now done based on Marsh standards: Marsh 0 is normal; Marsh 1 and 2 are usually not celiac disease; and Marsh 3a, b, and c could all be indicative of celiac disease even though villi are not completely flattened in a and b. An inexperienced pathologist or one trained years ago may not be looking at the biopsy results based on the newest standards.

If a diagnosis of celiac is not found but an individual is suffering from gastrointestinal issues, it is important to have a full range of tests done to rule out any other illness. If nothing is found, consider being retested for celiac disease or consider looking into other possibilities such as non-celiac gluten sensitivity and other food intolerances.

In some cases it may not be possible to do a traditional endoscopy, such as with a patient who is a hemophiliac and at risk of bleeding during the procedure. In these cases a capsule endoscopy may be ordered, but again the skill of the pathologist is key in getting an accurate diagnosis. If you suspect that there is a misdiagnosis you could ask for copies of the biopsy slides so you can bring your results to a celiac research center for cofirmation of your results.

In Europe, they sometimes diagnose children without an endoscopic procedure when the following apply: they must have symptoms of celiac disease; positive findings from their blood work many times higher than the normal range; one or more of the genetic markers; and must respond favorably to a gluten-free diet. However, high readings on blood values is unusual, and this diagnostic approach is mostly being used in Europe, often because parents are hesitant to schedule their children for endoscopic testing. In the United States this testing method is not yet recognized as appropriate for diagnosing children, though some doctors have adopted the European model. The endoscopic test with biopsies is still the gold standard for diagnosing celiac disease.

Another Sign of Celiac Disease

A skin disorder called **dermatitis herpetiformis (DH)**, a prickly, itchy skin rash usually found on elbows, knees, and buttocks is closely associated with celiac disease. If you have dermatitis herpetiformis and it has been biopsied and shown to be positive for DH, no further testing is needed to confirm the diagnosis of celiac disease. A gluten-free diet should be implemented even if medications are being used as part of the treatment.

Celiac Sprue vs. Refractory Sprue

A very small percentage of people with celiac disease will not experience improved health even after six months to a year on a strict gluten-free diet. Although there are several possible reasons for a lack of response to a gluten-free diet, these individuals may have developed a rare disorder known as refractory sprue. Celiac disease research centers would be the best equipped to appropriately identify someone who is truly suffering from refractory sprue, which is especially important to diagnose given the risk of long term complications. Treatment options will vary depending on if it is type 1 or type 2 refractory sprue and how long the disease has progressed. These options may include a combination of therapies such as steroids and immune-suppressive drugs, along with a gluten-free diet.

Refractory sprue is thought to be a malignant condition, and people with this condition are often malnourished and have weakened immune systems. Close monitoring by a physician familiar with this disorder is necessary, since in many cases malabsorption and malnutrition progress despite treatment, and nutrition may have to be delivered via alternate routes, such as TPN (total parental nutrition)—IV feeding that bypasses the gastrointestinal tract completely and delivers nutrients directly into the bloodstream. This is why discovering and monitoring refractory sprue as soon as possible is essential.

It is unknown why refractory sprue develops. One theory is that since it is usually only found in older adults, it may have developed due to celiac disease having been present and untreated for many years. Left unchecked and untreated, refractory sprue can lead to many complications as well as higher risk for certain types of cancer. It is thought that something as simple as following a gluten-free diet early after diagnosis may reduce the risk of this condition developing. However, more research needs to be done to fully understand the causes and treatments of this condition.

Misdiagnosis and Multiple Conditions

Although celiac disease is usually the cause of flattened villi, it is not the only possible reason that villi can be flattened. For example, some blood pressure medications and autoimmune suppressant drugs may sometimes produce flattened villi as a side effect, though this is uncommon. If you have had no symptoms of celiac disease, had normal findings on the blood work, and are taking medications that could have affected your villi, you could be evaluated at a celiac research center to reconfirm your diagnosis of celiac disease. There are several other possible disorders that could also flatten villi, but they, too, are uncommon.

If you have had symptoms of celiac disease and a positive diagnosis but are not responding favorably to a gluten-free diet, first check with a registered dietitian who is an expert with gluten-free diets to make sure you are compliant with a gluten-free diet and are not making any errors. If your compliance is good, have a gastroenterologist evaluate you to see if there could be a secondary cause of the continued symptoms, such as SIBO (small intestinal bacterial overgrowth), FODMAPs, lactose intolerance, gastric motility issues, or parasites. If no other cause of your symptoms is found you should follow-up at a celiac research center to reconfirm your diagnosis and see if there are other possible reasons for your continued symptoms.

Non-Celiac Gluten Sensitivity

It is possible to pass screening and diagnostic tests and still be at risk for celiac disease, but if you do not have symptoms the risk is minimal. If you do have symptoms, and were positive on the genetic panel, consider being retested for celiac disease. If you have symptoms and do not wish to have repeat testing done, and no other medical explanation is found, consider experimenting with a test diet as you could have a non-celiac gluten sensitivity.

Non-celiac gluten sensitivity is an intolerance to the protein gluten that is not caused by celiac disease. Ingestion of gluten causes an immune response and usually gastrointestinal symptoms. It is unknown at present if it is also the cause of autoimmune issues. The diagnosis of non-celiac gluten sensitivity at this time is a diagnosis by elimination: rule out celiac disease or other health problems; rule out a wheat allergy; implement a gluten-free diet; and if a person responds favorably to a gluten-free diet then a diagnosis of non-celiac gluten sensitivity is found. This criteria was presented by Dr. Alessio Fasano, Professor Carlo Catassi, Dr. Anna Sapone, and Professor David Sanders in 2011.

Researchers are currently exploring biomarkers that could be used to help diagnose non-celiac gluten sensitivity, but at this time the only protocol is diagnosis by elimination.

Estimates on the number of those with non-celiac gluten sensitivity have varied; some specialists estimate it at 5 to 6 percent of the population. The number of those with celiac disease is thought to be 1 percent of the population, and the number of those with wheat allergies is not universally defined. Additional research is needed to obtain accurate estimates of all these disorders.

It is important to work with your doctor and registered dietitian when treating non-celiac gluten sensitivity. It is especially important to rule out the possibility of other sensitivities such as FODMAPs, which can sometimes be mistaken as non-celiac gluten sensitivity. In order to simply implement a gluten-free diet, try the easy-start meal plan found in chapter 2, implementation of the gluten-free diet should provide a rapid improvement to symptoms of non-celiac gluten sensitivity. At this time there is no cure for celiac disease or non-celiac gluten sensitivity; the only treatment is to follow a gluten-free diet.

Although it's understandable that anyone would want to start feeling better right away, it's generally not recommended to start the gluten-free diet if you are still being tested for celiac disease because if you are following a gluten-free diet it may interfere with your diagnosis, since your villi will begin to heal and your blood work will return to normal. Also, if you start the diet without being diagnosed, you may not be as committed to following the diet 100 percent of the time and your family members would not be alerted to be screened as well.

TIP   If you believe you may have a non-celiac gluten sensitivity and are thinking of starting a gluten-free diet, speak with your doctor first. It is important to rule out the possibility of other serious health problems that may be causing your symptoms.

Gluten Allergies

If you go to an allergist and get tested for an allergy to wheat, rye, or barley, this is not the same thing as being tested for celiac disease or non-celiac gluten sensitivity. However, if you come up positive when you have these tests, you could have an allergy. Wheat allergies are more common than rye or barely allergies. If you are highly allergic you would most likely already know this due to the extreme reactions, but a less severe allergy may have many different types of symptoms that are easier to miss. If you suspect an allergy it is best to be tested by a board certified allergy specialist, since some tests can indicate false positive results and a specialist is more likely to make an appropriate diagnosis. Prior to considering non-celiac gluten sensitivities it is important to rule out wheat or gluten allergies. If you have a wheat, rye, or barley allergy the treatment is the same as that for celiac disease and non-celiac gluten sensitivity—removal of the problem foods 100 percent of the time.

 WHEN WORKING WITH YOUR DOCTOR

Since celiac disease and non-celiac gluten sensitivity are often missed, it can sometimes be difficult to get medical professionals to agree that you may need to be retested. When advocating for your health, remember the following:

You have the right . . .
- To be heard
- To have all your questions answered
- To be retested if you do not have any diagnosis that explains your symptoms
- To a second opinion
- To see a specialist (such as a gastroenterologist who specializes in celiac disease)
- To be taken seriously—just because they haven't found the root of your illness doesn't mean it is all in your head
- To bring copies of your test results to a celiac research center
- If diagnosed, to see a registered dietitian who specializes in celiac disease

If You Have Celiac Disease or Non-Celiac Gluten Sensitivity

If you have celiac disease, following a gluten-free diet works by allowing those villi covering your small intestine to heal and return to normal so that you can once again absorb all the nutrients from food. This, in turn, allows your immune system to heal as well. Many people who start the diet after discovering that they have celiac disease will begin to feel better within a few days. However, for the villi to fully heal it may take several years for adults and about six months for children. The longer you take to be diagnosed the longer it may take for your villi to heal. You should also note that the gluten-free diet needs to be continued for life if you are to continue to maintain normal villi.

If you have non-celiac gluten sensitivity, your villi are not affected; only symptoms are used to evaluate a favorable response. Usually, implementation of a gluten-free diet provides immediate relief from symptoms.

Today, there is a huge amount of research being done for both celiac disease and non-celiac gluten sensitivity, and information is changing practically daily. Scientists are looking for different ways to treat celiac disease. One approach is to develop medications or shots to help the body handle the gluten protein so that if a small amount of gluten is ingested accidently, the response will not be as severe. Unfortunately these trials will not yet allow for the free consumption of gluten, and it may be some time, if ever, before this will be an option. There is no magic bullet. If you are diagnosed with celiac disease or non-celiac gluten sensitivity, following a gluten-free diet must be taken seriously. It is a lifelong commitment that takes dedication.

You may have already spent years feeling terrible and becoming frustrated because you have been going to doctor after doctor feeling as if no one is helping. Initially, you may feel overwhelmed when you realize all the changes you will need to make to follow a gluten-free lifestyle. But there are many ways to get support and help, and any change in lifestyle always feels overwhelming at first. In chapter 2, you will find an easy-start plan to begin following a gluten-free diet. It is also important to find a registered dietitian who specializes in celiac disease to answer any questions and to help you problem-solve any issues.

If you're a parent who has a child with celiac disease, it may be difficult to explain why he or she can no longer have their favorite foods. You may feel uncomfortable about asking your friends or family to make special dishes for you or asking about all the ingredients in the recipes. Going on vacation can be challenging, since all food is usually eaten out. You may also sometimes feel it is just easier to stay home! But don't give up. These are manageable situations and I have provided solutions for these issues throughout this book.

The good news is that today there is much more information available to help you follow a gluten-free lifestyle, including organizations, websites, and support groups. Supermarkets are starting to carry more gluten-free foods, and more and more companies are producing and selling thousands of gluten-free foods on the Internet. There is much greater awareness of celiac disease and non-celiac gluten sensitivity—even many restaurants now have gluten-free options listed on their menus, although some are not as educated as they should be to offer safe choices. Using the tips and meal plans found later in this book can make it easier for you to live gluten free while having a lot more options. Receiving a diagnosis of celiac disease can be difficult, but with patience and education you can lead a normal, happy, and healthier life.

Can Eating Less Gluten Improve Everyone's Health?

There are times you might consider a gluten-free diet even if you are sure you don't have celiac disease or a non-celiac gluten sensitivity. For example, if you are suffering from another health problem, especially a gastrointestinal problem such as inflammatory bowel disease, a large protein like gluten that is hard to digest may make you feel unwell. In addition, many parents of autistic children report an improvement in their child's behavior when they put their child on a gluten-free diet, and there is current research being done in this area. (Read more about autism and a gluten-free diet in chapter 17.)

Why is gluten causing so many problems today? Perhaps because it is a large protein that is difficult to digest, or maybe because we are adding gluten to so many foods. There is so much more to learn, but it is important to note that following a gluten-free diet can help a lot of people, as long as it is done in a healthful way.

Some people follow a gluten-free diet because it is the most recent diet craze; unfortunately, this confuses many people because they see some following the diets casually while others are stating they need to follow it strictly. This can make it difficult for restaurants and friends who may not always believe that for those with celiac disease or non-celiac gluten-sensitivity even a crumb can make someone ill.

Following a Gluten-Free Diet and Having Stomach Problems

Not everyone who has a gluten-related disorder will suffer from stomach problems. However, for those who do, issues can include bloating, pain, heartburn, constipation, diarrhea, gas, and more. If you are following a gluten-free diet but still experiencing stomach problems, you may be accidently contaminating your food with gluten. Consult with a registered dietitian to rule this out. If you are found to be 100 percent compliant and not responding you may have refractory sprue (mentioned earlier in this chapter), and this should be evaluated at a research center with the resources to provide an accurate diagnosis.

There also could be a secondary problem on top of celiac disease or non-celiac gluten sensitivity. If you have been diagnosed with celiac disease or identified with non-celiac gluten sensitivity, you probably already have had an endoscopy. This test can identify if there are any problems with possible reflux or ulcerations. If a colonoscopy had previously been done, then diseases such as ulcerative colitis, Crohn's disease, and diverticular disease may have already been discovered or ruled out. If a sonogram was done, it may have discovered problems such as gallstones, blockages in the ducts, and kidney stones. You may also have had a CT scan, which again probably would have isolated these types of problems.

But what if these conditions have been ruled out and you are still experiencing stomach problems? Ask your gastroenterologist if he or she has:

- Tested you for parasites.

- Tested you for fructose and lactose issues.

- Tested you for small intestinal bacterial overgrowth (SIBO).

- Tested you for gastroparesis (delayed gastric emptying).

If all these items have been ruled out you still might

- Have other food sensitivities or intolerances. A registered dietitian who specializes in these areas can help you identify these.

- Have sensitivity to FODMAPs (dietary intolerance to specific classes of carbohydrates, common for those who have IBS-type symptoms). A registered dietitian who specializes in this area can help you.

- Have a mild food allergy. A board-certified allergist can help determine possible food allergies. It is best to go to a specialist because many tests can result in false positive results.

- Benefit from probiotics and additional dietary interventions.

The most important thing for you to know is that there are many things that can cause similar symptoms. Don't just give up and decide that you will always suffer. Often, with the right tests and follow-up, you can resolve many issues. If you feel your doctor has given up on you, get a second opinion. You have the right to do whatever it takes to be well.

Quick Tips for Diagnosing Celiac Disease: What You Need to Know

About Getting Diagnosed

- Start by reviewing the list of possible symptoms that can be found with celiac disease.

- Get one of the blood tests described earlier in this chapter (especially IgA tTG, DGP, and total IgA). Remember, for the blood tests to be accurate you must be eating gluten as part of your regular diet.

- If your blood test is positive, follow up with an endoscopic procedure by a gastroenterologist who sees a lot of celiac patients. Blood testing is just a screening method. Only an endoscopic procedure with a positive biopsy can diagnose celiac disease. You cannot be diagnosed from blood tests alone.

- Request that your doctor takes at least four to six samples in the duodenal portion of your small intestine when the endoscopy is done. This gives you the best chance of being diagnosed accurately.

- Remember that celiac disease can be easily missed. A negative test result does not conclusively rule out celiac disease.

About Treatment

- Eliminating gluten from your diet is the only treatment if you are diagnosed with celiac disease.

- Research is ongoing, but currently there are no pills or enzymes that can allow you to consume gluten freely as part of your diet. Gluten must be avoided 100% of the time.

Quick Tips on Non-Celiac Gluten Sensitivity: What You Need to Know

About Getting Diagnosed

- Non-celiac gluten sensitivity is not celiac disease. It is a sensitivity to the protein gluten, and it can sometimes be mistaken for a diagnosis of FODMAPs.

- Many people with non-celiac gluten sensitivity will have gastro-intestinal problems following the consumption of any gluten.

- There are currently no tests for diagnosing non-celiac gluten sensitivity.

- To diagnose non-celiac gluten sensitivity you need to rule out celiac disease, wheat allergies, and any other health problems. If a person responds favorably to a gluten-free diet, then a diagnosis of non-celiac gluten sensitivity is found.

About Treatment

- Currently, the only treatment for non-celiac gluten sensitivity is removal of gluten from your diet. It is unknown if non-celiac gluten sensitivity improves over time or if it is more severe in some then in others. Currently, it is also unknown if it is an autoimmune disorder or if there are long term complications. Research is ongoing and more will be known over time.

> There are no pills, shots, or other therapies currently available to treat celiac disease or non-celiac gluten sensitivity. The only treatment at this time is 100 percent removal of gluten from your diet.

Learning the Basics and Getting Started Living Gluten Free

What Does Gluten-Free Living Really Mean?

The doctor walks in, reporting that the results of your tests have arrived, and it is good news. They have finally identified what has been making you so ill, and it is something that is easy to treat: the root of all your ailments is that you have celiac disease, which, put simply, means that you have a problem digesting the gluten found in food and it triggers an autoimmune response in your body. All you need to do is stop eating gluten. In a sigh of relief you burst out, "Thank God! Thank you so much—I was so worried. Now, tell me again, what did you say . . . gloo what?"

The doctor repeats, "Gluten—you can't eat gluten. Just stop eating gluten and you will feel like yourself again." He hands you some papers and says, "Here is a list of foods that may contain gluten."

What a relief—it's not as serious as you had feared. It is as if someone removed a huge weight from your shoulders: all you need to do is change your diet. This is something you can live with. You glance down at the list of foods the doctor gave you. Everything on the "do not eat" side are the foods that you do eat. Hardly any of the foods you normally eat are on the list noted as safe. If hardly anything is safe, how can you eat at all? Can having a problem with one little thing like gluten affect everything? *A million questions come to mind, but who can you ask? The doctor didn't give you any instructions except to follow this list,* but surely there has to be bigger list of foods you can eat, a list of gluten-free foods? You arrive home hungry after fasting for your tests, you open the fridge and stare blankly—what can you eat?

In theory, you're right that there must be a bigger list. But finding a list of foods that are gluten free is not as easy as it should be because gluten is often hidden within many foods. Gluten is used as filler and a flavoring agent and is often mixed into food during the production process due to cross-contamination. So you can't even always know what is okay to eat and what is not. Each label must be checked and analyzed. But don't despair; help is on the way!

D's Dieting Dilemmas

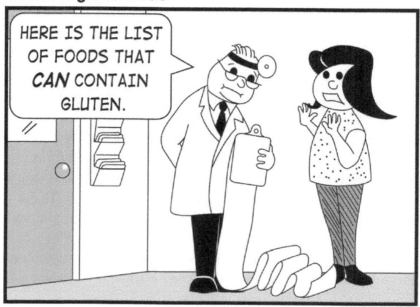

By M. Brown, Ken Brown, and Will Cypser ©

TIP   Getting started is easy as long as you have the right tools.

Getting Started

All you need to know is what to look for on labels, what to ask when calling companies about their products, what to look for when dining out, and how to substitute alternate grains and seasonings in your recipes when needed. As with anything new, acquiring these skills takes a little time. It may seem like a lot of work, but making these changes will be well worth the improvements you'll experience in your health and in your life.

Whether you are a great cook or buy all your meals on the run, the tools for success are the same:

- **Prepare your kitchen.** In order to prevent cross-contamination:

    - Buy condiments in squeeze bottles or buy separate spreadable products and mark them as gluten free.
    - Use separate utensils for serving gluten free foods.
    - Don't use a toaster that has been used with gluten-containing foods.
    - Have separate cooking pans for gluten-free foods.
    - Wipe down cooking surfaces before preparing foods.
    - Safely mark and separate all gluten-free products.

- **Shopping:** Buy gluten-free products, and use them in place of your regular breads, bagels, cereals, pizzas, and pastas. Find out which stores in your area carry gluten-free choices, and where these foods and ingredients can be ordered online. There is a large listing of companies that carry gluten-free choices in chapter 10.

- **Labels:** Start looking at food labels. Gluten may lurk where you least expect it. Ingredients that could contain wheat gluten may include seasonings, modified food starch, and hydrolyzed vegetable protein. Common ingredients that may contain barley gluten include malt, beer, and flavorings. For more information and details on what to look out for when reading labels, see chapter 6.

- **Dining Out:** Locate restaurants that have gluten-free menus or those that understand your dietary restrictions and are willing to work with you on making substitutions. This will make your dining experience much more enjoyable. In our resource section, I have included a list of restaurants that have already started listing gluten-free choices on their menus. Some restaurants have much more extensive gluten-free choices, so make sure you contact them and review their menu prior to dining out. The biggest difficulty with most restaurants is the hidden gluten due to cross-contamination, or a lack of understanding of what gluten free really means.

- **Events:** Trying to explain your restrictions to a busy waitstaff at a crowded noisy function can be uncomfortable. To be sure safe choices will be available when you will be dining at preset functions, such as weddings, large meetings, and conventions, call catering halls ahead of time. It is best to try to speak to the chef if possible. Banquet managers generally say yes to everything without first checking with the chef to see what can be done with certainty. By calling in advance, you will know which places can accommodate you, when you need to bring food with you, and where to find the best gluten-free cuisine.

- **Gluten-Free Cooking:** Start developing a list of great gluten-free recipe favorites. I have included many delicious recipes in this book in chapters 4 and 11, as well as quick and easy mix-and-match meals that are listed in chapter 5.

- **Support:** There are many local celiac support groups throughout the world. Join one of these and check out their gluten-free events and local functions. Join the listservs or follow blogs to help you network, and read about new products. To find local celiac support groups, go to the websites of the Celiac Sprue Association, at www.csaceliacs.info or the Gluten Intolerance Group of North America at www.gluten.net.

- In the resource section at the end of chapter 17, you'll find many more options, including my own site, www.glutenfreeeasy.com, and my blog, www.glutenfreeez.com, listings of many gluten-free events and dining-out cards in 14 languages are provided in chapter 12.

- **Family and Friends:** Educate your family and friends about your dietary needs in order for them to understand how careful you need to be. The tips and suggestions in chapter 14 will help make this easy for you.

Why Can't I Cheat Sometimes?

Most people ask why they can't have gluten just on rare occasions. This is the most common question I get asked, and it seems like a reasonable request; after all, many who are on other types of special diets do "cheat" on occasion. Unfortunately, for those who have celiac disease, this is not an option. Each time gluten is consumed, celiac disease triggers an autoimmune reaction that compromises the body and contributes to damage to the intestinal wall. The future may provide some relief, as there is ongoing research exploring the possibility of taking a pill when gluten is accidently consumed, but at present all the kinks are not worked out. It looks as if these pills may provide more protection from cross-contamination than they would provide for free consumption of gluten. So for now, *gluten should never be consumed.* This is, without question, the most difficult part of caring for your condition. But the rewards of a healthier life, having more energy, and really feeling good outweigh the hardships of 100% compliance.

> **TIP** If you have celiac disease you can never eat gluten without affecting your health.

It may be hard to believe, but even the smallest amount of gluten can cause a reaction. Those with celiac disease must be vigilant when it comes to the risk of cross-contamination. Consider this: someone with celiac disease or non-celiac gluten sensitivity cannot even safely use a toaster that has previously been used to toast wheat-containing bread, or a spatula that has just been used to turn wheat-containing pancakes. Even a spread such as mayonnaise, mustard, peanut butter, or jelly that has previously been spread on wheat-containing bread is no longer safe; just a knife being put back into the jar is enough to cause a reaction! A pinhead's worth of gluten is enough to make someone sick, even if they do not experience any notable symptoms. Left untreated, celiac disease can lead to serious consequences, so it is important for others in your life to understand that you are not being difficult: you really must avoid any trace of gluten, or you will get ill. No exceptions. Again, chapter 14 provides a list of what others need to know about gluten-free living and chapter 7 will give you some suggestions for how to handle the emotional consequences as you adjust to what is most likely a dramatic difference in your diet and lifestyle.

> **TIP** There are many foods that are naturally gluten free; you just need to know where to look.

Simple Gluten-Free Eating

Prior to delving into the vast variety of gluten-free foods available from other sources, such as specialty shops, health food stores, and the Internet, it's good to become familiar with what may be available to you in your local grocery. To minimize any sense of being overwhelmed you may be experiencing when newly diagnosed with celiac disease, we'll keep it simple at this stage. Later in this book, more extensive lists of gluten-free choices will be discussed.

Some supermarkets have elaborate gluten-free sections, but others have only a few items located in the refrigerator or health food aisles. This "starter" meal plan is designed around common, familiar, readily available foods—easy to find, easy to prepare, and gluten free. In chapter 3, there are more extensive lists of gluten-free choices for those of you who are ready to dive in. "Safe Supermarket Shopping" will give you the tools needed to put meals together from your average supermarket.

> **Every effort was made to check the gluten-free status of the brands listed. Manufacturers may change ingredients from time to time. When in doubt, choose an alternate product or contact the manufacturer.**

In the beginning, reading every label of every item you pick up at your local supermarket can seem overwhelming. The following includes some brand name suggestions so you can pick up products more easily. Also, any product that you see with "gluten free" noted on the label can also be used in your meal planning. Since companies often change their formulas, it is important to call companies and to read labels to double-check products' gluten-free status. The brands listed below will give you possible choices to include in your starter meal plan. Many other brands contain gluten-free choices as well and can be substituted in this meal plan. There are many gluten-free brands listed in chapter 10.

Picking Off the Shelf

There are many foods that are safe for those following a gluten-free diet; some are naturally gluten free, and others require a gluten-free alternative. See chapter 3 for more detailed listings of gluten-free foods.

Alcohol: All distilled alcohols (such as vodka, gin, and scotch) are considered gluten free. (The distillation process removes the gluten, but these products most likely will not be labeled gluten free. Note, however, that some of the flavored distilled alcohol products sometimes have flavoring agents added after distillation that could contain gluten). Beer is not distilled, and is made from barley so it is not gluten free. However, many gluten-free beers are now being produced, although some brands may be safer than others and you should do some research before making your selections. Chapter 10 includes a listing of some gluten-free beers. Wine is considered gluten free although some red wines have used wheat flour to seal the barrels, to date wines tested have shown gluten content to be within the safe range of less than 20 parts per million. Hopefully, as they improve regulations in the future, it will make it easier for all to safely select alcoholic beverages.

Beans, Tofu, and Soy: Beans are gluten free, and high in fiber, but on rare occasions gluten may be added to flavored beans. To be safe, buy canned or dried plain, unseasoned beans, or check the packaging to make sure no gluten-containing ingredient has been added. Tofu is also gluten free unless it is baked or marinated in a gluten-containing ingredient, such as soy sauce. Although most soy products are gluten free, except those marinated in a wheat flavoring or those with added barley malt or fillers, soy sauce is usually made from wheat, and cannot be used. However, there are some gluten-free varieties of soy sauce available, such as Eden Tamarai, Jade Dragon, La Choy, Panda (carry-out packets), Wal-Mart's Great Value, and San-J (Organic Tamari Wheat-Free Soy Sauce). Most restaurants' soy sauce and teriyaki sauce usually contain gluten unless the restaurant has a gluten-free menu that specifies otherwise.

Chips (Potato and Corn): Most brands are made from just corn or potato with only oil and salt added and are gluten free. When unsure, pick unflavored chips, which are much less likely to contain gluten. Some brands that are mostly gluten free include Cape Cod, Fritos, Lay's, Ruffles, Tostitos, UTZ, and Wise. Take care with homemade potato and corn chips that may have been fried in a shared fryer that also fried a gluten-containing product (heat in the fryer will not kill the gluten).

Cheese: Real cheeses are gluten free (unless there are gluten-containing ingredients folded into the cheese, as is sometimes the case with blends and cheese spreads). So in the beginning, it is best to pick 100 percent pure cheese products.

Cold Cuts: Many brands have gluten-free choices such as Boar's Head, Hillshire Farms, Hormel, and Wellshire Farms. When you are uncertain, it is safest to pick pure meats that are 100 percent meat, like real roasted turkey or roast beef, with no added fillers. Always ask if it is possible for the slicing machine to be wiped down prior to having your cold cuts sliced, since you cannot be sure if gluten-containing products have been sliced previously on that equipment.

Cereal: Most store brand cereals contain gluten—even some cereals that may appear safe, such as regular Rice Krispies, which have barley gluten included (unless you buy their gluten-free brown rice alternative). When in doubt, always read labels. Now you can find some cereals in the supermarket that are safe to eat, such as Rice Chex, Corn Chex, Honey Nut Chex, Chocolate Chex, Cinnamon Chex, grits, cream of rice, Nature's Path Mesa Sunrise cereal, and Bakery on Main Street products, but in general, most gluten-free cereals will be found in specialty and health food stores.

Corn Tortillas: Most brands are gluten free, but, again, read the labels to make sure there are no added ingredients. If the label says corn, salt, and oil and there is no warning about possible wheat contamination, it is usually safe to use. Some gluten-free brands of corn tortillas include Don Pancho, Food for Life, La Tortilla Factory (Dark & Ivory Teff Gluten-Free Wraps), Manny's (Corn Tortillas), Mission, Que Pasa, Snyder's of Hanover (Corn Tortillas [White, Yellow]), and Trader Joe's (Corn Tortillas, Handmade, Original).

Dairy Products: Milk, half-and-half, cream, cream cheese, cottage cheese (in rare instances gluten is added; so check the label), butter, and ricotta cheese are naturally gluten free. Processed cheese blends, some light sour creams, and on occasion flavored yogurts and other flavored dairy products may contain gluten. Laughing Cow cheese blends and Friendship's light sour cream are gluten free.

Desserts: Most whipped toppings and egg custards are gluten free, except those with cookie dough or toppings mixed in (check labels for added fillers). Many gluten-free desserts are now available; see the recipe selections found in chapters 4 and 11, and the product listings in chapter 10.

Some examples of gluten-free dessert mixes include those sold by Pamela's Products, 1-2-3 Gluten-Free, and Bob's Red Mill.

Eggs: All eggs and egg whites, as well as most egg substitutes, are gluten free.

Fish: All fresh fish is gluten free, unless it is breaded or in a gluten-containing marinade. Though fresh fish in the same case as breaded fish could become cross contaminated. Frozen fish needs to be checked for gluten, because it is often marinated or breaded. Fake crabmeat often contains gluten. So, for now, stick with fresh fish, or buy canned gluten-free choices such as plain Bumble Bee, StarKist, or other gluten-free varieties. (Please note, don't choose the flavored or herb choices, those in pouches, or those that come with crackers; they usually contain gluten.)

Gluten-Free Flours, Grains, and Starches: There are many grains and flours that are naturally gluten free, such as almond, amaranth, bean, buckwheat, coconut, cornmeal, grits, millet, gluten-free oats, potato, quinoa, rice, sorghum, and teff flours please be careful if flavoring agents or fillers are added, because they may contain gluten; also, be on your guard against grain manufacturing processes contaminated with gluten. When in doubt, look for a gluten-free label on the packaging to be sure it is safe. Note that gluten-free grains can be contaminated in transport, especially those weighed and bagged in health food stores.

There are also many gluten-free cereals, bars, breads, rolls, pastas, muffins, and mixes available. Chapter 10 contains listings of where to find gluten-free grains; today, you can find many gluten-free choices available in supermarkets and health food and specialty stores. Fresh potatoes are always gluten free, and 100 percent pure potato starch or flakes are safe. A gluten-free grain found in supermarkets is rice, which is available in a number of varieties: brown, jasmine, instant, long grain, and so forth. However, avoid supermarket rice blends—Rice-a-Roni, and other rice blends are often seasoned with gluten-containing ingredients, so you must always check with manufacturers in these cases.

Ices: Almost all ices and sorbets are gluten free, but don't buy ices that have crunchies, sprinkles, or cookie dough folded in. When in doubt, look for gluten free on the label or check the ingredients to make sure there is no added wheat or barley malt.

Ice Cream: Most ice cream and gelato is gluten free, but it is important to check the labels to make sure that no cookies, wafers, chips, sprinkles, wheat, or barley malt have been added. Most ice creams at ice cream parlors are also gluten free. However, they are often contaminated with gluten because the same scoop is used for all flavors. Most Edy's and Haagen-Dazs flavors are gluten free, except those with cookies or crumbs added.

Meats and Poultry: Most pure meats are gluten free except those that are breaded or marinated in a gluten-containing mixture. Poultry that has a self-basting agent or broth added usually also contains gluten. Make sure you use 100 percent pure poultry, beef, and pork to be safe. Look for those that have no additives listed in the ingredients. If you want to marinate foods, do so yourself by using gluten-free marinades and dressings.

Nuts and Oils: Almost all nuts and vegetable oils are gluten free unless the nuts are coated with a flavoring agent or processed on equipment that has also processed wheat. Butter, margarine, and shortening are also gluten free as long as they have not been cross-contaminated.

Oats: In the past, it was thought that those following a gluten-free diet could not consume oats, even though pure oats do not contain gluten. Recent evidence has shown that if oats are grown and processed so that they do not get contaminated with gluten, they should be safe for many who are following a gluten-free diet. When using oats, make sure they are from a gluten-free source, stating that they are certified gluten free (many sources of gluten-free oats are listed in chapter 10). Before adding oats to your diet, make sure you have been successfully following a gluten-free diet and are symptom-free. Only introduce oats in limited quantities—about 50 grams per day for adults (1/2 cup dry) and 20 to 25 grams per day for children (1/4 cup dry)—to see if it is tolerated. However, some individuals with celiac disease may not be able to include oats in their diets. Although oats do not contain gluten, they do contain the protein avenin, which may activate the immune system in certain individuals. It is thus important to introduce oats carefully, with the support of a health care team. Supermarkets have just started carrying gluten-free oats; but most supermarket brands such as Quaker oats are not gluten-free.

Popcorn: Air-popped fresh popcorn using fresh kernels is gluten free. Flavored popcorn can contain gluten, so it is important to double-check each brand for safety. The following brands are usually gluten free: Newman's Own, Pop Secret, and Jolly Time Popcorn.

Produce: Fresh fruits and vegetables are all gluten free, and frozen and canned fruits and vegetables are usually gluten free unless additives, coatings, sauces, or fillers that contain gluten are used. Dried fruits and fruit juices are also usually gluten free. On occasion, dried flavored fruits or dates may have been dusted with flour (to prevent sticking), so look for 100 percent pure dried fruit.

Pudding: Most puddings are gluten free and flavors in the following powdered and prepared puddings are gluten free: Hunt's (except tapioca), Jell-O, Kozy Shack, Meijer brand, Trader Joe's, and Wegman's store brand.

Rice Cakes: Most flavors of Lundberg and Stop and Shop rice cakes are gluten free. (Some Quaker rice cakes, like the plain large, are gluten free, but other flavors and minis are not, so you will need to double-check.)

Salad Dressings: Many salad dressings are gluten free, but some brands may add fillers or barley malt, so care should be taken. When in doubt, ask for oil and vinegar. In general, many flavors of the following salad dressings are currently gluten free: Kraft, Ken's, Newman's Own, Laura Lynn, Maple Grove, and Walden Farms dressings.

Sauces, Dressings, and Marinades: Many gluten-free choices are available; look for brands that are labeled gluten free or those that have been checked for gluten-free status. Some marinades that claim to be gluten free include Annie's Naturals (Organic Smokey Tomato), Emeril's (BAM!-B-Q Barbecue Sauce, Roasted Red Pepper Pasta Sauce), Jack Daniel's EZ Marinader (Slow Roasted Garlic & Herb), Ken's (Buffalo Wing Sauce, Herb & Garlic, Lemon Pepper), Lawry's (Baja Chipotle, Caribbean Jerk, Havana Garlic & Lime, Mesquite, Tequila Lime), McCormick (Grill Mates, Baja Citrus Marinade, Chipotle Pepper Marinade, Hickory BBQ Marinade, Mesquite Marinade), Wegman's brand (Chicken BBQ, Citrus Dill, Fajita, Greek, Honey Mustard, Lemon & Garlic, Rosemary Balsamic, Santa Fe, Spiedie, Steakhouse Peppercorn, and Tangy), and Zesty (Savory, Thai). See chapter 11 for homemade marinades that can be easily prepared.

Seasonings: Fresh and dried herbs, all whole spices, and garlic and onion powder are gluten free and are safe. Seasoning blends can contain a gluten-containing filler, so do not use these unless they are labeled gluten free or you have checked with the manufacturer first.

Soy Milk: If you are lactose intolerant, you may be using lactaid milk or soy milk. Some gluten-free brands of soy milk include Silk, Trader Joe's, and Westsoy. Double-check other brands of soy milk for gluten—sometimes gluten is added as barley malt.

Sweeteners: Almost all sweeteners are gluten free, including sugar, Sweet 'n' Low, Equal, Splenda, Stevia, agave, honey, molasses, and many more. Barley malt is not gluten free.

Vinegars: All distilled vinegars are gluten free. Vinegars that may contain gluten include malt vinegars and those made with barley, such as rice vinegar (rice vinegar is not distilled and sometimes includes barley).

Yogurts: Almost all flavors in the following brands are gluten free: Albertson's, Brown Cow, Chobani, Colombo (Classic, Light), Horizon, Lowes Food brand, Meijer brand, Publix, Stonyfield, Tillamook, Trader Joe's, Wegman's, Weight Watchers, and Yoplait. Take care not to select yogurt with sprinkles or candy toppings. (Although most Dannon yogurts are probably gluten free, only a few flavors state it on the packaging, so you will need to double-check.)

TIP   Most fresh foods are gluten free.

Easy-Start Gluten-Free Meal Plan

Week 1: All you want to know is what you can eat. This is not the time to learn everything there is to know about gluten-free eating and shopping. This quick-and-easy meal plan makes it a snap to get started.

You can overcome feeling overwhelmed by keeping things simple. The meal plans found in this book make it easy for you to put together quick gluten-free meals with limited meal preparation. Whether you pick up your food from the supermarket, a specialty store, or online, a large variety of gluten-free products are now available. Later, if you are someone who likes to cook, try some of the terrific gluten-free recipes found in chapters 4 and 11.

Breakfast Choices

- Rice Chex or Corn Chex or other gluten-free cereal with milk and blueberries or other fresh fruit

- Corn tortillas, warmed, with scrambled eggs, chopped tomato, and melted cheese

- Gluten-free cream of rice with chopped almonds and milk

- Gluten-free waffles (such as Van's gluten-free waffles) with butter and syrup

- Omelet with onions, peppers, and tomatoes, with two soft corn tortillas and ketchup

- Grits with butter and salt

- Cottage cheese and fruit

- Gluten-free pancakes (some brands that have gluten-free pancakes include Arrowhead Mills, Bob's Red Mill, Gluten-Free Essentials, Gluten Free Pantry, Kinnikinnick, Sylvan, and Van's) with butter and syrup

- Gluten-free yogurt (such as Stonyfield) layered with berries and flax

- Ricotta cheese mixed with sugar and layered with berries

- Hard-boiled eggs mixed with mayonnaise, served on toasted corn tortillas

Lunch Choices

- Sliced turkey with lettuce, tomato, and mayonnaise on warmed corn tortillas or on gluten-free bread with baby carrots

- Grilled sliced chicken over mixed greens, with red peppers, sliced tomato, broccoli florets, and chickpeas, served with oil and vinegar or gluten-free salad dressing

- Toasted gluten-free bread (in dedicated toaster) or warmed corn tortillas, with tuna fish made with mayonnaise, chopped onion, sliced tomato, shredded lettuce, and chopped cucumber

- Grilled salmon or tuna served over mixed greens with shredded carrots, chopped tomatoes, and cucumbers. Serve with oil and vinegar, or favorite gluten-free salad dressing, gluten-free rice crackers, and lemon wedges

- Grilled chicken, salmon, or tuna, with shredded lettuce, sliced tomatoes, baby carrots, and gluten-free rice cakes

- Gluten-free ham on gluten-free toast or warmed corn tortillas with mustard and coleslaw

- Cottage cheese with mixed fruit

- Grilled chicken cutlet marinated in garlic, oil, and lemon, served over chopped romaine lettuce, with gluten-free Caesar dressing, parmesan cheese, and gluten-free rice crackers

- Grilled or broiled sirloin burger with lettuce, tomato, sliced onion, ketchup, and a gluten-free roll if available—if not available, serve over a mixed salad with oil and gluten-free vinegar

- Grilled chicken marinated in garlic, oregano, oil, salt, and pepper, with a sweet potato, butter, and mixed veggies

- Chicken salad made with cooked chicken, mayo, onions, walnuts, and grapes, over a mixed green salad

- Grilled portabella mushroom marinated in garlic and oil, served with mixed green salad

- Peanut butter and jelly on gluten-free rice cakes (such as Lundberg)

Dinner Choices

- Salmon baked with mustard and honey, served with brown rice and steamed green beans

- Hardboiled egg, sliced, with steamed green beans, baby spinach, sliced cucumber, sliced tomato, and chickpeas with oil and vinegar or gluten-free salad dressing

- Grilled chicken cutlet marinated in garlic, oil, and onion powder, served with cooked brown rice, steamed broccoli, and mixed greens served with oil and vinegar or gluten-free salad dressing

- Cooked kidney beans and brown rice added to chopped onions sautéed in olive oil with garlic, and with chopped tomato, chopped red pepper, and hot pepper added to taste, served with a green salad and gluten-free dressing

- Broiled skirt steak with garlic, onion powder, and a dash of salt, served with steamed cauliflower and a medium baked potato with butter or margarine

- Baked flounder cooked with chopped onions, tomatoes, cilantro, garlic, and onion powder, served with steamed spinach, rice, and a mixed green salad with sliced tomato, cucumber, and oil and vinegar or gluten-free salad dressing

- Pork loin cut into two-inch cubes, placed on a skewer with chunks of pineapple, cherry tomatoes marinated in gluten-free Italian dressing, grilled, and served with steamed broccoli and corn with butter or margarine and a dash of sea salt.

- Roasted chicken with carrots, potatoes, and onions, seasoned with garlic, onion powder, salt, pepper, and Italian herbs

- Grilled or baked chicken, shrimp, or veal, placed in a casserole dish and topped with tomato sauce, mozzarella, and parmesan cheese, served with gluten-free pasta

- Gluten-free rice, corn, or quinoa pasta with tomato sauce and a mixed green salad with a favorite gluten-free dressing

- Grilled shrimp over a mixed salad with baby potatoes and a favorite gluten-free salad dressing

- Hand-pressed hamburger or turkey burger with onion and sliced tomato, baked homemade sweet potato fries (note frozen fries sometimes can have gluten coating), and green beans

- Frozen gluten-free pizza baked and served with mixed green salad and gluten-free salad dressing

Snack Choices

- Pear or other fresh fruit

- Canned fruit in its own juice

- Gluten-free yogurt

- Applesauce with cinnamon

- Baby carrots and snow peas with hummus

- String cheese with dried fruit

- Gluten-free pudding

- Gluten-free rice cakes

- Gluten-free nuts with dried fruit (nuts are naturally gluten free unless flavored or processed on gluten-containing equipment; check dried fruit labels to make sure no gluten-containing ingredient has been added)

- A cup of strawberries with Cool Whip

- Plain peanuts or almonds

- Gluten-free rice cakes with cream cheese and jam

- Gluten-free frozen ices

- Gluten-free ice cream

- Gluten-free chips

- Gluten-free snack bar

Foods and Additives That Contain Gluten

The following items all contain gluten; see chapters 3 and 5 for lists of gluten-free alternatives.

Gluten-Containing Foods and Ingredients to Avoid

Wheat

Atta*	Kamut**
Bulgur	Matzoh, matzoh meal
Couscous	Modified wheat starch
Dinkel (also known as spelt)**	Seitan****
Durum**	Semolina
Einkorn**	Spelt (also known as farro
Emmer**	or faro; dinkel)**
Farina	Triticale
Farro or Faro (also known as spelt)**	Wheat bran
Fu***	Wheat flour
Graham flour	Wheat germ
Hydrolyzed wheat protein	Wheat starch

*A fine whole-meal flour made from low-gluten, soft textured wheat used to make Indian flatbread (also known as chapatti flour)

**Types of wheat

***A dried gluten product derived from wheat that is sold as thin sheets or thick round cakes. Used as a protein supplement in Asian dishes such as soups and vegetables.

****A meat-like food derived from wheat gluten used in many vegetarian dishes. Sometimes called "wheat meat."

Barley

Ale*	Malt**
Barley (flakes, flour, pearl)	Malt extract/malt syrup
Beer*	Malt flavoring***
Brewer's yeast	Malt vinegar
Lager*	Malted milk

*Most regular ale, beer, and lager are derived from barley, which is not gluten free. However, there are several new varieties of gluten-free beer derived from buckwheat, sorghum, and/or rice that are gluten free.

**Malt is an enzyme preparation usually derived from sprouted barley that is not gluten free. Other cereal grains can also be malted and may or may not be gluten free depending on the additional ingredients used in the malting process.

***These terms are used interchangeably to denote a concentrated liquid solution of barley malt that is used as a flavoring agent.

	Rye
Rye bread	Rye flour

	Oats*
Oatmeal	Oat flour
Oat bran	Oats

*Celiac organizations in Canada and the United States do not recommend consumption of commercially available oat products as they are often cross contaminated with wheat and/or barley. However, pure, uncontaminated specialty gluten-free oat products from North America are now available, and many organizations allow consumption of moderate amounts of these oats for persons with celiac disease. From: Shelley Case, RD, 2014. *Gluten-Free Diet: A Comprehensive Resource Guide*, 5th edition, Case Nutrition Consulting, Inc., www.glutenfreediet.ca

Gluten-Free Shopping List

When you are first setting up your gluten-free pantry, all you need are enough gluten-free options to get you through a few weeks until you are ready to do more exploring. As you go on, you will begin to establish new staples in place of old ones so you do not need to feel as if you are missing something. Since others in your home may have been spreading their bread with mayo, mustard, peanut butter, and so on, they have contaminated those choices already in your house, so make sure to buy new spreads, and mark them with your name or "GF" so others know not to double-dip in your choices.

TIP Many gluten-free choices can be found in health and natural food stores.

Cereal

Gluten-free cold and hot cereal

Dairy

Butter
Cheese (most cheese is gluten free; cheese spreads and blends some-
  times contain gluten)
Milk
Gluten-free yogurt
Gluten-free pudding

Fats and Oils

Margarine (most brands are gluten free), vegetable oils, and gluten-free
  salad dressings

Grains and Starches

Amaranth
Beans, bean flours, and soy
Gluten-free bread crumbs
Gluten-free bread, bagels. muffins, wraps, and pizza crust
Corn, cornstarch, cornmeal (naturally gluten free)
Corn, rice, or teff tortillas
Gluten-free crackers, rice cakes
Gluten-free pasta, such as rice, corn, quinoa, buckwheat
Mesquite, millet, and montina flour
Potatoes, potato starch
Quinoa
Rice, unflavored, white, brown, instant, jasmine, basmati, and rice flour
Sorghum and sorghum flour
Teff and teff flour
Xanthan gum, guar gum, expandex

Protein

Eggs and egg substitutes
Poultry (is naturally gluten free except when found with marinades or
  when self-basting agents have been added)

Beef and pork (watch out for marinades and fillers)
Fish (watch out for breading and marinades)

Produce

All fresh fruits and vegetables are gluten free
Canned, frozen, and dried fruits and vegetables are gluten free as long
as gluten-containing ingredients have not been added to them

Nuts

Nuts, seeds, and nut butters without added seasonings or coatings are
gluten free

Sauces

Gluten-free ketchup, mustard, relish, barbecue sauce, tomato sauce, salsa
(soy sauce and teriyaki sauce are usually made with wheat, so only buy
those brands that are marked gluten free)

Soup Bases

Gluten-free bouillon cubes and stocks (note that most soup bases contain gluten)

Sweets

Gluten-free cake, cookie, and brownie mixes (check any candy or chocolate that you usually buy for gluten-containing ingredients)

Snacks

Unseasoned nuts
Gluten-free popcorn (e.g., air-popped or gluten-free microwave
popcorn, such as Newman's brand)
Gluten-free pretzels (such as Glutino)
Gluten-free corn and potato chips with gluten-free salsa
Gluten-free yogurt (such as Stonyfield)

Spreads, Dips, and Condiments

Ketchup
Mustard
Mayo
Gluten-free salad dressing
Syrup
Tartar sauce
Tomato sauce
Vegetable oils
Distilled vinegar

Spices and Herbs

Use only 100 percent pure herbs and spices, and check labels for fillers

Your Gluten-Free Shopping List

When shopping for gluten-free choices, make a special effort to choose
foods that are healthier as well including more fruits and vegetables (fresh
and frozen; avoid canned choices whenever possible) and lean proteins.
Try to select choices higher in fiber, as well as lower in fat and sodium.

Remember that gluten can be added or may accidently contaminate many
foods, including those that are naturally gluten free. Make sure you read
labels or contact the manufacturer if a food is in question.

Gluten-Free Shopping List

Produce: (Fresh and frozen fruit and veggies, dried fruits and veggies).

_____

_____

_____

Proteins: (Meats, poultry, fish, eggs, egg whites, milk, yogurt, and cottage cheese. (Check labels for added gluten in marinades, coatings, or flavoring agents.)

_____

_____

_____

Starches: (Gluten-free breads, cereals, pasta, rice, amaranth, beans, buckwheat, corn, millet, quinoa, flour blends, and baking mixes).

_____

_____

_____

Snacks: (Gluten-free crackers, rice cakes, chips, popcorn, nuts, desserts, cheese sticks, hummus, trail mix, bars, cakes, and cookies).

_____

_____

_____

Staples and Condiments: (Gluten-free chicken and beef broth, oils, salad dressings, ketchup, mustard, sauces, and seasonings).

_____

_____

_____

Other: (Gluten-free vitamins, medications confirmed as gluten free, mouthwash, toothpaste, etc.). To confirm your medication is gluten free, visit www.glutenfreedrugs.com.

_____

_____

_____

Discovering What You Can and Can't Eat

Safe Supermarket Shopping

Now that you have the basic tools for living gluten free, you are ready to take the next step. Since safe food choices are a must, knowing what is safe at the supermarket will make it easier to find your favorite gluten-free foods. Let's start by shopping around the perimeter of the store, as this is where most fresh and gluten-free products can be found. Fruits, vegetables, meats, fish, chicken, and dairy are mostly all gluten free. After picking up those items, go to the health food aisle. This is where many gluten-free products, such as gluten-free pasta and gluten-free pancake mixes are located. Then you can go through the rest of the supermarket using the following lists to help make safe choices.

> **TIP** The perimeter of the supermarket is where most gluten-free foods can be found.

What to Eat and What Not to Eat

In the United States, packaged foods regulated by the FDA that contain wheat must state so clearly on the label, but barley and rye do not need to be so listed. Barley is usually listed as barley or malt, and rye is usually only added to wheat-containing foods (which you would be avoiding in any case). New gluten-free labeling laws do spell out what gluten free means (see chapter 6), but indicating gluten free on a label is still only elective and many companies may not provide this information.

Currently, meats and poultry, which are regulated by the USDA, are not required to list wheat on their packaging, because they are not mandated to follow FDA guidelines; doing so is completely voluntary. So even though most meats are gluten free, it is important to watch for marinades, self-basting poultry, modified food starch, and dextrin as possible hidden sources of gluten (if in doubt, call the manufacturer). But since they do not have to write wheat, rye, or barley on their labels, it makes the most sense to buy plain meats and poultry without additives, tenderizers, or self-basting agents, and add seasonings and such on your own.

Reading labels can sometimes be difficult. For example what about seeing a gluten-free product that has wheat listed in the ingredients? This means that although a product was made with wheat, the gluten-containing proteins in it have been removed, and the product is now gluten free, so wheat free and gluten free will not mean the same thing. This is especially important to understand for those who may have a wheat allergy.

Keep in mind that even naturally gluten-free food may contain gluten if it is contaminated during the processing, shipping, or weighing process. If a food product has not been tested to be gluten free there is always a possibility of contamination, and this should always be considered, especially if your symptoms are not improving on a gluten-free diet.

 TIP: READ LABELS CAREFULLY AND SAVE MONEY

Currently, even with the new gluten-free labeling laws, the gluten-free status of foods is not required to be listed on a label, so there are many gluten-free items on the shelves that may not specify their gluten-free status. You might pay three times as much for a comparable product that is marked gluten free (e.g., gluten-free vanilla extract) when one on the shelf right next to it may be just as gluten free but simply not be labeled as such. Read carefully, contact manufacturers, and save money!

Safe, Not Safe, and Questionable Foods Chart

The following charted foods are listed as Safe (S), Not Safe (NS), and Questionable (Q). For specific gluten-free mixes or brands, see the resource section at the end of this book. GF is an abbreviation for gluten free. Note that companies often change their ingredients, so it is important to always read labels to double-check gluten-free status.

	Safe (S)	Not Safe (NS)	Questionable (Q)
BAKING			
Baking chocolate (pure)	(S)		
Baking powder, baking soda	(S) most GF, but double-check		
Brewer's yeast		(NS)	
Carob chips			(Q) most are GF, but some contain barley malt
Carob and cocoa powder	(S)		
Chocolate chips			(Q) usually GF, but some contain barley malt
Coco mix			(Q)
Coconut	(S)		
Coconut (flavored or sweetened)	(S) usually GF		

(continued)

	Safe (S)	Not Safe (NS)	Questionable (Q)
BAKING (continued)			
Cream of tartar	(S)		
Flour (wheat, rye, barley, or gluten-containing flour)		(NS)	
Frosting			(Q) many are GF, but some contain gluten as a filler
Guar gum	(S)		
MSG	(S)		
Vanilla extract	(S)		
Xanthan gum	(S)		
Yeast	(S)		
CANDIES			
Candy, hard			(Q) varies with flavors and brands
Chocolate			(Q) can contain wheat or barley malt
GF Licorice Marshmallows			(Q) some contain gluten
Licorice		(NS)	

	Safe (S)	Not Safe (NS)	Questionable (Q)

CEREALS

Cold cereal			(Q) there are not too many cold GF cereals available; carefully check labels

Note: GF cold cereals are sometimes available and may include grains such as amaranth, puffed amaranth, puffed buckwheat, puffed corn, puffed millet, rice, rice flakes, soy, and teff.

Hot cereal	(S)		

Note: GF hot cereals may be available, but check labels to make sure they come from GF facilities and fields; GF hot cereals may include amaranth, cornmeal [grits], cream of buckwheat, cream of rice, GF oats, quinoa, soy grits, and teff.

Hot cereal such as cream of wheat, barley, regular oats, rye, triticale, or cereals made with malt		(NS)	

CONDIMENTS

Barbecue sauce			(Q) varies by brand
Bouillon cubes (most contain gluten)		(NS) although some GF	
Distilled vinegar (apple cider, rice, balsamic, white, grape, wine)	(S)		
Flavored tomato products			(Q) most are GF

(continued)

	Safe (S)	Not Safe (NS)	Questionable (Q)
CONDIMENTS (*continued*)			
Gravy		(NS) usually contains wheat	
Honey	(S)		
Ketchup	(S) most brand GF		
Malt		(NS)	
Malted vinegar		(NS)	
Marinades			(Q) many questionable ingredients
Miso			(Q) often made with barley
Mustard			(Q) most GF, but some brands may have gluten-containing ingredients
Mustard (yellow)	(S)		
Pickles made with wheat flour		(NS)	
Plain relish, olives, pickles	(S)		
Rice vinegar			(Q) may contain barley malt

(continued)

	Safe (S)	Not Safe (NS)	Questionable (Q)
CONDIMENTS (continued)			
Salad dressing			(Q) many GF but check for malt or wheat
Salsa	(S) most brands GF		
Sauces			(Q) some brands contain wheat
Soy sauce (made with wheat)		(NS) unless labeled GF	
GF soy sauce or GF tamari (must be labeled GF)	(S) if labeled GF		
Stocks and broths (when not homemade)			(Q) may contain wheat
Stuffed olives, pickles	(S) most GF, check labels for brines and flavorings		
Tamari			(Q) some GF, but check labels
Teriyaki sauce		(NS) unless labeled GF	
Tomato sauce and paste	(S)		
Worcestershire sauce			(Q) varies by brand, some contain wheat

	Safe (S)	Not Safe (NS)	Questionable (Q)
DAIRY			
Butter	(S)		
Buttermilk (regular and low-fat)			(Q) check labels
Cheese (hard and soft cheese)	(S)		
Cheese sauces and spreads			(Q) some have gluten-containing fillers
Cottage cheese	(S) most safe, check labels		
Egg substitutes	(S) most safe, check labels		
Eggs	(S)		
Fat-free half-and-half	(S)		
Flavored and lower-fat cottage cheese			(Q) most safe
Flavored cheese			(Q) some have gluten-containing ingredients
Heavy cream	(S)		
Ice cream			(Q) most GF, but check brands, watching out for added ingredients and for cross-contamination

(continued)

	Safe (S)	Not Safe (NS)	Questionable (Q)
DAIRY (*continued*)			
Low-fat sour cream			(Q) most GF
Lower-fat and flavored cream cheese			(Q) most safe but check flavoring agents
Malted milk		(NS) barley	
Milk	(S)		
Milk shakes; flavored milk, coffee creamers, and drinks			(Q) many safe but check flavorings
Regular cream cheese	(S)		
Sour cream	(S)		
Veined cheese (blue cheese, gorgonzola cheese, and stilton)	(S)		
YOGURT			
Flavored yogurt			(Q) some brands contain gluten, but most safe
Frozen yogurt	(S)		(Q) most GF, but check flavors and brands
Plain yogurt	(S)		

	Safe (S)	Not Safe (NS)	Questionable (Q)
DESSERTS			
Cakes, cookies, cupcakes, pies made with gluten-containing ingredients		(NS)	
Flavored gelatin	(S)		
Frostings/icing			(Q) some brands do contain gluten, but most are GF
GF cakes, cookies, pies, waffle cones	(S)		
Ice cream and ices without added gluten-containing ingredients	(S)		
Ice cream with added cakes, cookies, muffins, fillers, or other gluten-containing ingredients		(NS)	
Milk puddings, custard powder, pudding mixes			(Q) most GF
Plain gelatin	(S)		

(continued)

	Safe (S)	Not Safe (NS)	Questionable (Q)

DESSERTS (*continued*)

	Safe (S)	Not Safe (NS)	Questionable (Q)
Sherbet, gelato, nondairy whipped toppings, egg custards			(Q) many GF, but double-check labels
100 percent dairy whipped topping	(S)		

DRINKS

	Safe (S)	Not Safe (NS)	Questionable (Q)
Beer, ale, lager, malted beverages		(NS)	
Cordials (most types, such as Amaretto and Sambuca, are GF unless a flavoring agent is added after distillation)			(Q) most types, such as Amaretto and Sambuca, are GF unless a flavoring agent is added after distillation
GF beers	(S)		
Instant and flavored teas and coffees, fruit-flavored drinks, chocolate drinks, soy milk, wine coolers			(Q) some brands have gluten-containing ingredients
Unflavored tea, coffee, soft drinks, juice, cider, wine, GF beers, pure liquors, distilled alcohol (such as rum, gin, vodka)	(S)		

	Safe (S)	Not Safe (NS)	Questionable (Q)
FATS			
Baking sprays		(NS) contain flour	
Butter, margarine, lard, vegetable oils, cream, shortening	(S)		
Cooking sprays			(Q) most safe but check labels
Lard	(S)		
Mayonnaise			(Q) most GF, but check labels on flavored varieties
Salad dressings			(Q) many GF, but check labels
Shortening	(S)		
Suet			(Q)
FISH			
Canned fish			(Q) most GF, but check labels
Canned fish in vegetable, broth containing HVP (hydrolyzed wheat protein)		(NS)	
Fish patties or cakes or croquettes		(NS) usually not safe	

(continued)

	Safe (S)	Not Safe (NS)	Questionable (Q)
FISH (*continued*)			
Flavored fish in pouches			(Q) gluten-containing flavoring agents may be used
Fresh and frozen unseasoned fish, all varieties	(S)		
Imitation fish products			(Q) often contain wheat
Stuffed, breaded, and marinated fish		(NS)	
FRUITS			
Canned and frozen fruit			(Q) most are GF, but double-check labels
Dates			(Q) most are GF, but some brands are dusted with flour
Fresh, frozen, unflavored dried, canned, and juiced fruits	(S)		
Fruit jams and jellies	(S)		
Fruit pie fillings, dried fruits that have been seasoned			(Q) check the label for type of thickening agent
Fruit with starches added			(Q)

	Safe (S)	Not Safe (NS)	Questionable (Q)

GRAINS AND STARCHES

Note: The grains marked safe below are naturally gluten free, but they can be contaminated with gluten in the fields or during the manufacturing process. To be doubly safe, check the grains you buy to make sure they are marked gluten free. One grain that is often contaminated with gluten is oats—make sure all oats you use are marked and certified gluten free.

	Safe (S)	Not Safe (NS)	Questionable (Q)
Amaranth	(S)		
Arrowroot	(S)		
Artichoke flour			(Q) often mixed with other flours; make sure all ingredients are GF
Barley and barley malt, barley grass		(NS)	

Grains and Starches
BEANS

	Safe (S)	Not Safe (NS)	Questionable (Q)
Baked beans			(Q) some contain gluten, so check labels
Beans (all plain beans, including dai, black beans, chickpeas, fava, lentil, and lima)	(S)		

GRAINS AND STARCHES (continued)

	Safe (S)	Not Safe (NS)	Questionable (Q)
Besan (chickpea flour)	(S)		
Bran			(Q) can be wheat, rye, oat, corn or rice—be sure to check GF status

	Safe (S)	Not Safe (NS)	Questionable (Q)

Grains and Starches
BREAD (continued)

Bread, bagels, biscuits, bread crumbs, cornbread, crackers, doughnuts, English muffins, phyllo, pizza crust, stuffing, wraps containing wheat, rye, barley, spelt, or other gluten-containing grains		(NS)	
GF breads, bagels, biscuits, bread crumbs, cornbread, crackers, doughnuts, English muffins, pizza crust, stuffing, wraps	(S)		

Note: GF choices usually will contain grains such as amaranth, arrowroot, bean (legume flours), buckwheat, corn, flax, millet, potato, quinoa, rice sago, sorghum, soy, tapioca, teff, xanthan gum (some brands may be manufactured in plants that may contain gluten, so double-check labels).

Matzo and Communion wafers		(NS) unless marked GF	

GRAINS AND STARCHES (continued)

Brewer's yeast		(NS)	

(continued)

	Safe (S)	Not Safe (NS)	Questionable (Q)
GRAINS AND STARCHES (continued)			
Buckwheat (100 percent pure)	(S)		
Bulgur		(NS)	
Cassava	(S)		
Channa	(S)		
Chestnut	(S)		
chia Seeds	(S)		
Coconut flour	(S)		

**Grains and Starches
CORN**

	Safe (S)	Not Safe (NS)	Questionable (Q)
Corn canned or frozen			(Q)
Corn arepas, corn malt, corn-starch, corn tortillas (if 100 percent corn)	(S)		
Corn taco shells or corn cakes			(Q)
Flavored corn chips, grits, tortillas, cereal			(Q)
Fresh, corn-starch, plain corn chips, corn syrup	(S)		
Corn noodles			(Q)

	Safe (S)	Not Safe (NS)	Questionable (Q)
GRAINS AND STARCHES (continued)			
Cottonseed	(S)		
Couscous		(NS)	
Dasheen flour			(Q) only safe if gluten-free processing
Dinkle or spelt		(NS)	
Durum or durum wheat		(NS)	
Egg roll and dumpling wrappers		(NS)	
Einkorn		(NS)	
Emmer		(NS)	
Farina		(NS)	
Farro		(NS)	
Flavoring			(Q)
Flax	(S)		
Flour, wheat		(NS)	
Fu		(NS)	
Gliadin		(NS)	
Glutenin		(NS)	
Grits, hominy			(Q) double-check for cross-contamination

(continued)

	Safe (S)	Not Safe (NS)	Questionable (Q)
GRAINS AND STARCHES (continued)			
Hemp			(Q)
Hydrolyzed wheat protein		(NS)	
Job's tears	(S)		
Kamut		(NS)	
Kasha			(Q) double-check for cross-contamination at plant
Kudzu	(S)		
Malt extract, malt		(NS)	
Matzo, matzo meal		(NS)	
Mesquite	(S)		
Millet	(S)		
Milo	(S)		
MIR		(NS)	
Modified food starch			(Q) could be wheat, corn, potato, or tapioca
Montina noodles	(S)		

(continued)

	Safe (S)	Not Safe (NS)	Questionable (Q)
GRAINS AND STARCHES (continued)			
Oats			(Q) only oats, oat bran, and oats from GF sources can be used (see chapter 10)
Ramen noodles made from wheat, wheat starch, spelt, or other gluten-containing ingredients		(NS)	
Soba noodles			(Q) some brands contain wheat
Wheat noodles		(NS)	

Grains and Starches
PANCAKES

	Safe (S)	Not Safe (NS)	Questionable (Q)
Pancakes and waffles and waffle mixes, when made with gluten-containing ingredients		(NS)	
Pancakes, GF, or waffles (frozen, homemade, or mix, or as GF restaurant selection)	(S)		

	Safe (S)	Not Safe (NS)	Questionable (Q)

Grains and Starches
POTATOES

	Safe (S)	Not Safe (NS)	Questionable (Q)
Potato and potato products			(Q) check ingredients of coated products
Potatoes that have been flavored or have added sauces, or fried potatoes (not safe if fried in oil that cooked gluten-containing foods)			(Q)

Grains and Starches
PASTA AND PIZZA

	Safe (S)	Not Safe (NS)	Questionable (Q)
Buckwheat pasta			(Q) check to make sure it is either marked GF or 100 percent buckwheat
GF pasta or pizza crust (usually made from buckwheat, beans, corn, rice, sorghum, quinoa)	(S)		
Pasta, orzo, or pizza made from wheat, wheat starch, spelt, or other gluten-containing ingredients		(NS)	
Quinoa or quinoa pasta	(S)		

	Safe (S)	Not Safe (NS)	Questionable (Q)
GRAINS AND STARCHES (continued)			
Psyllium	(S)		
Grains and Starches **RICE**			
Flavored rice, rice pilaf, risotto			(Q)
Rice noodles that are 100 percent rice	(S)		
Rice, plain, Arborio, rice bran, black, brewer's, brown, calrose, Carolina gold, glutinous, japonica, jasmine, paddy/ rough, pearl, polished, popcorn, red, rosematta, white, wild	(S)		
Risotto mixes			(Q) Flavoring agents could contain gluten
GRAINS AND STARCHES (continued)			
Rye		(NS)	
Sago	(S)		
Semolina		(NS)	

(continued)

	Safe (S)	Not Safe (NS)	Questionable (Q)
GRAINS AND STARCHES (continued)			
Sorghum	(S)		
Soy and soybean flour	(S)		
Spelt		(NS)	
Spring roll wrappers			(Q) some are not 100 percent rice or they may have been fried in oil with gluten-containing foods
Sweet potato flour	(S)		
Tabbouleh		(NS)	
Taco shells			(Q) most are corn and are GF
Tapioca	(S)		
Taro	(S)		
Teff	(S)		
Tortillas, corn, rice	(S)		
Tortillas, wheat		(NS)	
Triticale		(NS)	
Water chestnut flour	(S)		

(continued)

	Safe (S)	Not Safe (NS)	Questionable (Q)
GRAINS AND STARCHES (continued)			
Wheat berries		(NS)	
Wheat nuts		(NS)	
Wheat wonton, eggroll, and dumpling wrappers		(NS)	
Wheat, wheat bran, wheat flour, wheat germ, wheat grass, wheat starch		(NS)	
MEAT AND MEAT SUBSTITUTES			
All meats that do not have marinades, additives, or seasonings added	(S)		
Beef jerky, dried meats, and imitation bacon bits			(Q)
Breaded or flour-coated meats		(NS)	
Deli meats, including bacon, sausages, and pates			(Q) most GF, but some do have added fillers, or barley flavoring agents.
Ham			(Q) some have gluten-containing flavorings

(continued)

	Safe (S)	Not Safe (NS)	Questionable (Q)
MEAT AND MEAT SUBSTITUTES (continued)			
Meat extenders			(Q)
Meat patties			(Q)
Meat substitutes such as seitan		(NS)	
Meatloaf			(Q) bread crumbs often used
Tempeh			(Q) check ingredients
Tofu, flavored			(Q) many seasoned with wheat-containing soy sauce
Tofu, plain	(S)		
TVP (texturized vegetable protein)			(Q) can be made from wheat or soy
Vegetable burgers			(Q) most contain gluten
Veggie crumbles, hot dogs, and sausage			(Q) most contain gluten
NUTS			
Chestnuts	(S)		
Seasoned or dried roasted nuts			(Q)

(continued)

	Safe (S)	Not Safe (NS)	Questionable (Q)
NUTS (*continued*)			
Unseasoned nuts, all varieties	(S)		
OTHER			
Anything breaded		(NS)	
HVP/HPP (hydrolyzed vegetable or plant protein)			(Q) often the source is wheat
Sauces and gravies made from GF ingredients	(S)		
Sauces and gravies made with wheat or other gluten-containing ingredients		(NS)	
POULTRY			
Breaded or floured chicken		(NS)	
Fried chicken			(Q) check the coating, and whether the oil is dedicated for GF frying

(*continued*)

	Safe (S)	Not Safe (NS)	Questionable (Q)
POULTRY *(continued)*			
Plain turkey, chicken, or other poultry that does not have gluten-containing ingredients added	(S)		
Poultry cooked in broth		(NS)	
Poultry patties			(Q)
Stuffed poultry		(NS)	
Turkey, chicken, or other poultry that has had a self-basting product added to it (such as hydrolyzed wheat protein)		(NS)	
SAUCES			
Cocktail sauce			(Q) most safe but some may contain wheat
GF soy sauce or tamari	(S)		
Soy sauce		(NS)	
Tartar sauce	(S)		
Tomato sauce	(S)		

	Safe (S)	Not Safe (NS)	Questionable (Q)
SNACKS			
Air-popped popcorn	(S)		
Chips that contain wheat, rye, or barley		(NS)	
GF pretzels	(S)		
Graham crackers		(NS) unless marked GF	
Most snack and cereal bars contain gluten unless they are labeled GF		(NS)	
Multigrain chips		(NS)	
Plain 100 percent corn, potato, or rice chips	(S)		
Note: Restaurants that make homemade chips in a shared fryer with gluten containing ingredients are not safe, even if they are 100% potato or corn.			
Rice cakes		(NS)	(Q) some brands contain gluten
Rice crackers that are 100 percent rice	(S)		
Seasoned potato, taco, corn, or rice chips			(Q)

	Safe (S)	Not Safe (NS)	Questionable (Q)
SOUPS			
Canned and frozen soups			(Q) most contain gluten; only okay when labeled GF
Homemade broths that do not have bouillon cubes or gluten-containing ingredients added	(S)		
Packaged broths, soup mixes, and bouillon cubes (these often contain gluten)		(NS)	
Restaurant soups			(Q) unless homemade base, most will contain broths or bouillon cubes with gluten
SPICES			
Dried pure herbs and spices	(S)		
Extracts			(Q) most GF, but check labels
Fresh herbs and spices	(S)		
Monosodium glutamate (MSG)	(S)		
Seasoning mixes and blends			(Q)

	Safe (S)	Not Safe (NS)	Questionable (Q)
VEGETABLES			
Flavored canned vegetables			(Q)
Fresh, frozen, and canned vegetables and juices	(S)		
Salad kits			(Q) watch out for dressings and croutons
Scalloped potatoes, batter-dipped vegetables		(NS)	
Sprouted wheat and barley		(NS)	
Squashes	(S)		
Vegetables fried in oil in which other foods have also been fried, or vegetables coated in batter or flour		(NS)	
Vegetables, seasoned or in sauce			(Q)
Wheat grass and wheat grass juice			(Q) although the grass does not contain gluten, it can easily be cross-contaminated if the wheat seed gets into the juice.

> "The most difficult issue is learning what to eat. It is easy to learn what not to eat."
>
> —Peter H. R. Green, MD, Professor of Clinical Medicine, Columbia University

Basic Gluten-Free Foods and Where to Find Them

Most supermarkets have dedicated sections or aisles where they stock their health or specialty foods, but some stores have larger sections than others. It is these dedicated sections that often carry gluten-free choices such as pastas, cereals, flour blends, and crackers. Throughout the rest of the store there may be products that are gluten free as well, some of which are labeled as such, and some of which are not.

Now that you have a list of safe gluten-free foods and have started checking your local stores and some websites, you will be able to put together a more extensive gluten-free meal plan. In the following meal plan, gluten free is abbreviated as GF.

30-Day Meal Plan

Day 1

Breakfast: Mesa Sunrise cereal or other GF cereal with 1% milk and a small banana
Snack: 1 medium pear
Lunch: GF sliced turkey with lettuce, tomato on GF flat bread or corn tortilla with mayonnaise with 1 cup of baby carrots
Snack: GF yogurt
Dinner: Grilled sliced chicken over mixed greens with 1 cup sliced red peppers, 1 medium sliced tomato, 1 cup broccoli florets, ½ cup chickpeas, oil and vinegar or GF salad dressing, and a sprinkle of parmesan cheese
Snack: ½ cup applesauce with cinnamon

Day 2

Breakfast: Two 6 in. corn tortillas, warmed, with scrambled eggs and a slice of low-fat cheese
Snack: GF yogurt

Lunch: GF corn tortillas, with tuna with mayonnaise, sliced tomato, onion, shredded lettuce, and chopped cucumbers

Snack: ½ cup baby carrots, ½ cup hummus

Dinner: Steak kabob with onions, tomatoes, mushrooms, marinated in favorite GF dressing, served over brown rice

Snack: string cheese and a medium sliced pear

Day 3

Breakfast: GF cream of rice with cinnamon, sweetened to taste, and chopped almonds with 1% milk

Snack: 6 oz. fruit in its own juice

Lunch: Roast beef on GF bread with ketchup, shredded lettuce, 1 cup baby carrots, and chopped tomato

Snack: An apple

Dinner: Roasted chicken cooked with butter, garlic, and onion powder over brown rice with steamed broccoli

Snack: GF fat-free pudding

Day 4

Breakfast: GF oats with 1 Tb chopped almonds, 2 Tb raisins, cinnamon, and brown sugar

Snack: GF yogurt

Lunch: Cooked salmon, mixed with mayonnaise, mustard, and dill, served with shredded lettuce and sliced tomato in a gluten-free teff wrap, with baby carrots and sliced cucumber on the side

Snack: String cheese with a medium apple

Dinner: Quick beans and rice: sauté chopped onions in olive oil with garlic, add chopped tomato, chopped red pepper, cayenne pepper, and kidney beans; serve with brown rice and a salad with GF salad dressing

Snack: 10 almonds and a medium apple

Day 5

Breakfast: GF Rice Chex or Corn Chex with 1% milk and strawberries

Snack: GF yogurt

Lunch: GF sliced turkey on GF toast with mustard; also, coleslaw

Snack: Mixed green salad with mandarin orange wedges and GF salad dressing

Dinner: Baked chicken cutlet with garlic and onion powder with steamed cauliflower and a medium sweet potato with butter, brown sugar, and cinnamon
Snack: Strawberries with whipped cream

Day 6

Breakfast: Egg whites sautéed in olive oil with chopped green onions and chopped red pepper, served with two toasted soft corn tortillas
Snack: GF yogurt
Lunch: American cheese melted on GF toast with sliced tomato and roasted red pepper
Snack: Grapes
Dinner: Broiled flounder cooked with GF salsa, steamed green beans, and brown rice
Snack: A medium pear and 5 almonds

Day 7

Breakfast: Certified gluten-free oats with 2 Tb raisins, 1 tsp cinnamon with brown sugar, and 1% milk
Snack: GF fruit yogurt
Lunch: Cottage cheese with melon
Snack: GF rice cakes
Dinner: Baked skinless chicken cutlet, topped with GF honey mustard with steamed asparagus, a baked potato, and sour cream
Snack: GF vanilla ice cream with mini M&Ms

Day 8

Breakfast: GF waffles with butter and syrup and 1% milk
Snack: Small banana with peanut butter
Lunch: Greek salad with lettuce, tomatoes, cucumbers, feta, olives, onions, and chickpeas, served with GF salad dressing
Snack: GF yogurt
Dinner: Grilled hamburger with sautéed onions, lettuce, tomato, and onion, and baked GF sweet potato fries
Snack: GF pudding

Day 9

Breakfast: Poached eggs over toasted GF English muffin with cheddar cheese
Snack: Jell-O
Lunch: GF ham and Swiss with mustard on corn tortilla
Snack: GF snack bar
Dinner: 2 hardboiled eggs, sliced, with ½ cup green beans, steamed and then chilled, 2 cups chopped spinach, half a cucumber, sliced, a small boiled potato, peeled and sliced, and a medium sliced tomato, served with oil and vinegar or GF salad dressing
Snack: GF chocolate pudding

Day 10

Breakfast: GF cereal with 1% milk and blueberries
Snack: Hummus with baby carrots
Lunch: Tuna melt: GF tuna with mayonnaise over GF toast with sliced tomatoes and melted mozzarella
Snack: Fruit salad
Dinner: Grilled salmon with dill, and cooked millet with steamed green beans
Snack: GF chocolate chip cookies and 1% milk

Day 11

Breakfast: GF pancakes with sliced banana, whipped butter, and syrup
Snack: GF rice cakes
Lunch: Large mixed salad with grilled chicken, chickpeas, roasted peppers, parmesan cheese, and GF dressing
Snack : GF rice pudding
Dinner: Roasted pork loin, baked with GF honey mustard, corn, and steamed broccoli
Snack: GF whipped cream with blueberries

Day 12

Breakfast: GF oatmeal with raisins, cinnamon, brown sugar, and 1% milk
Snack: GF ice pop

Lunch: Broiled or grilled hamburger with cheddar over mixed greens with sliced onion and tomato
Snack: GF snack bar
Dinner: Flounder with garlic, onion, oregano, and lemon over cooked brown rice with mixed vegetables
Snack: Baked apple with cinnamon and brown sugar

Day 13

Breakfast: Scrambled eggs with Canadian bacon and toasted GF multi-grain bread
Snack: Grapes
Lunch: Stuffed tomato with tuna fish and GF brown rice crackers
Snack: GF yogurt
Dinner: Chicken, red pepper, and onion kabob, marinated in GF Italian dressing and grilled over cooked millet
Snack: GF ice cream

Day 14

Breakfast: GF cereal with 1% milk and mixed berries
Snack: GF rice cakes
Lunch: GF turkey and cheddar on GF wrap with mustard
Dinner: Roasted chicken with garlic and rosemary with new potatoes and green beans
Snack: GF ices

Day 15

Breakfast: GF grits with shredded cheese and butter
Snack: GF yogurt
Lunch: Turkey burger over a salad with GF salsa and GF corn chips
Snack: GF three-bean salad
Dinner: Grilled pork and pineapple with GF barbeque sauce, corn, and green salad
Snack: GF cookies and milk

Day 16

Breakfast: GF cereal with 1% milk and sliced peaches
Snack: GF rice cakes

Lunch: Deviled eggs with a mixed green salad and GF dressing
Snack: GF yogurt
Dinner: Stuffed peppers with beef, rice, onion, garlic, and tomatoes
Snack: Mixed fruit salad

Day 17

Breakfast: Frittata with sliced potatoes, egg, cheese, tomatoes, onions, and mushrooms
Snack: GF ice pop
Lunch: GF potato pancakes with sour cream and applesauce, with a mixed salad and GF dressing
Snack: GF yogurt
Dinner: GF chicken enchiladas with rice and beans
Snack: GF cookies and milk

Day 18

Breakfast: GF French toast with butter, syrup, and sliced banana
Snack: Half a grapefruit with brown sugar
Lunch: Fresh cold shrimp platter over salad with lemon and GF cocktail sauce
Snack: Sliced apple with peanuts
Dinner: Roasted turkey with cranberry sauce, sweet potato with butter, and green beans
Snack: GF pudding

Day 19

Breakfast: Cooked hot teff cereal with dried berries, flax seeds, and maple syrup
Snack: Peaches in their own juice
Lunch: Chicken salad served with toasted corn tortillas
Snack: GF snack bar
Dinner: Cornmeal-crusted catfish with mixed vegetables, and baked potato with butter
Snack: GF ice cream

Day 20

Breakfast: Ricotta cheese, layered with berries and GF cereal
Snack: String cheese

Lunch: GF roast beef and GF horseradish sauce with GF lentil crackers
Snack: 1 oz. plain mixed nuts
Dinner: Chicken fajitas with GF salsa, sour cream, and warmed corn tortillas
Snack: Cappuccino (no flavoring agents)

Day 21

Breakfast: GF waffles with peanut butter, raisins, and 1% milk
Snack: Fruit smoothie
Lunch: GF turkey rolled with Swiss cheese in lettuce leaves with mustard
Snack: GF snack bar
Dinner: GF pizza with salad and GF dressing
Snack: GF ice pops

Day 22

Breakfast: GF polenta with melted mozzarella cheese and sliced tomato
Snack: GF yogurt
Lunch: Cornmeal-crusted chicken fingers with apricot preserves
Snack: Baked apple with cinnamon, walnuts, and brown sugar
Dinner: Chicken breast stuffed with spinach and blue cheese, with a sweet potato topped with melted butter
Snack: Fruit kabob

Day 23

Breakfast: GF oats with sunflower seeds, raisins, and brown sugar
Snack: GF pudding
Lunch: Grilled cheese on GF bread with baby carrots
Snack: GF rice cakes
Dinner: Grilled chicken cutlet with tomato sauce and melted mozzarella with GF pasta
Snack: GF cookies and milk

Day 24

Breakfast: GF toasted bagel with cream cheese, onion, tomato, and lox
Snack: Jell-O
Lunch: GF tuna salad over roasted red peppers and sliced cucumbers with brown rice crackers

Snack: GF three-bean salad
Dinner: Grilled tuna with GF soy sauce, ginger, and garlic over cooked millet with mixed vegetables
Snack: GF ice cream

Day 25

Breakfast: GF blueberry muffin with 1% milk
Snack: Sliced peaches and cottage cheese
Lunch: GF chili in a baked potato with a mixed green salad and GF dressing
Snack: GF snack bar
Dinner: Beef, onion, tomato, and mushroom kabobs marinated in GF Italian dressing with minced garlic, broiled or grilled and served over brown rice
Snack: GF coffee cake and milk

Day 26

Breakfast: GF pumpkin pancakes with butter, syrup, and 1% milk
Snack: GF rice cakes
Lunch: GF cheese enchiladas with rice and beans
Snack: Pea pods and hummus
Dinner: Grilled chicken with GF honey mustard, on a GF roll with lettuce and tomato
Snack: GF chocolate cake with 1% milk

Day 27

Breakfast: GF cornbread with 1% milk
Snack: Mixed dried 100 percent fruit and GF nuts
Lunch: Grilled eggplant with melted mozzarella and a mixed green salad with GF dressing
Snack: GF yogurt
Dinner: Roasted chicken with brown rice and mixed vegetables
Snack: GF pudding

Day 28

Breakfast: GF cereal and 1% milk with sliced strawberries
Snack: GF fruit rollups

Lunch: Baked potato stuffed with broccoli florets and melted cheddar
Snack: GF snack bar
Dinner: Grilled steak with sautéed mushrooms and onions, with oven baked fries
Snack: GF pudding

Day 29

Breakfast: Hot teff cereal with dried berries, maple syrup, and cinnamon
Snack: GF yogurt
Lunch: GF pasta with mixed vegetables, black olives, baby shrimp, and GF Italian salad dressing
Snack: GF rice pudding
Dinner: GF hot dogs with sauerkraut and GF baked beans
Snack: GF ice cream

Day 30

Breakfast: Cantaloupe stuffed with 1% cottage cheese
Snack: GF snack bar
Lunch: GF turkey rolled with coleslaw, Swiss cheese, and mustard, served with GF crackers
Snack: Dried apricots
Dinner: GF pasta with tomato sauce, ricotta cheese, and grilled zucchini
Snack: GF chocolate chip cookies and 1% milk

Essential Do's and Don'ts

Do	Don't
Find restaurants with gluten-free menus	Stop going out because it is more difficult to find gluten-free choices
Find delicious gluten-free combos to replace gluten-containing choices	Start eating plain, boring, repetitive meals because you are confused about what to eat
Be excited about all the new interesting food choices you are making	Start feeling depressed because you can't do things exactly as you are used to
Bring gluten-free dining out cards to your favorite restaurants	Try to just pick things off a menu without letting the restaurant know of your special needs
Stock up on gluten-free choices at home	Let gluten-free supplies run low at home
Bring gluten-free snacks, crackers, and choices with you on the go	Go on trips and to events without packing some gluten-free choices
Have a dedicated toaster and dedicated spreads and dips for your gluten-free eating	Use the same toaster or spreads as other family members
Have a special shelf to store your gluten-free staples at home	Mix your gluten-free choices in with all other family foods, making them difficult to find (or fair game to be eaten by someone else)
Choose more whole grains and higher-fiber gluten-free choices like legumes	Use only prepackaged gluten-free blends (typically low in fiber and high in fat)
Pay attention to labels for serving size, fat, calories, carbohydrates, and fiber	Stop reading labels because you feel overwhelmed
Pick foods higher in calcium, such as milk and gluten-free yogurt; take gluten-free supplements if you don't get adequate dairy	Continue using products you have before without checking to make sure they are gluten free

Planning and Cooking Simple Gluten-Free Meals

Tips for Gluten-Free Cooking

Eating gluten free doesn't have to mean complicated, boring, or tasteless. But in the beginning, getting familiar with an array of completely new or modified favorite recipes may present a bit of a learning curve. Having a plan can make a huge difference.

Delicious gluten-free meals are easy when you use these tips to get started:

- Start with recipes that don't usually contain gluten; this way, you won't have to make any modifications.

- Or begin with those recipes that only need a small amount of changes so you will have a better chance of success. For example, substitute a gluten-free broth for regular broth, or use rice flour or potato starch as a thickener in place of wheat flour—these are easy modifications that are sure to work.

- Use fresh, flavorful ingredients.

- Keep a tabbed notebook or a folder on your computer with information on gluten-free ingredients and sources for quick access to information.

- Check sauces, dressings, and seasoning agents to ensure that they are gluten free.

- Make sure you mark spreads such as peanut butter, butter, margarine, mayonnaise, and jam so that others don't accidently double-dip and cross-contaminate your food.

- Use a designated gluten-free toaster or gluten-safe Toast-It toaster bags, and cover cooking surfaces such as baking sheets with aluminum foil to help prevent cross-contamination.

- Store gluten-free products on top shelves so gluten-containing foods don't accidently get mixed into safe foods.

- Have dedicated colanders and measuring utensils for your gluten-free cooking.

- Use labeled containers with scoops to keep your gluten-free ingredients easier to access.

- Premix your own gluten-free flour blends for easy use, or buy already-mixed gluten-free blends and keep them on hand for quick recipe development.

- Sign up for gluten-free cooking classes. You'll save a lot of time and money by learning the right way to work with gluten-free grains right from the start.

- Get involved with local celiac support groups and trade recipes with others.

Stocking a Gluten-Free Kitchen

- Keep gluten-free ingredients on hand for easy-to-prepare meals.

- Stock up on gluten-free grains, as well as staples such as gluten-free pasta, polenta, and rice.

- Keep a supply of favorite gluten-free broths, sauces, and dressings.

- Make sure packaged rice, corn, quinoa, buckwheat, teff, amaranth, millet, oats, and potato products are from gluten-free sources.

- Have gluten-free crackers, breads, pasta, and chips available.

- Stock gluten-free cereals and bread crumbs for quick coatings for fish and chicken and as an easy-to-use base for pie crusts.

- Have gluten-free flours available, such as amaranth, bean flour, brown rice flour, corn flour, cornmeal, buckwheat flour, millet, nut flours, sorghum, and teff (make sure you keep them refrigerated or in the freezer to help them stay fresh longer).

- Keep gluten-free starches on hand, such as arrowroot, cornstarch, potato starch, and tapioca flour to be used as thickening agents.

- Keep your freezer stocked with gluten-free breads, bagels, bread crumbs, waffles, and pizza crusts.

- Purchase premade gluten-free frozen meals (for quick meals when you don't have the time to cook).

- Have premixed gluten-free mixes, such as cake, cookie, and flour blends.

 TIP: GLUTEN-FREE CHICKEN CUTLETS

"My family likes chicken cutlets. I make them like regular cutlets by dipping them in egg first but then coat them in a mixture of almond flour, coconut flour, rice flour, and Romano cheese. Next, I fry them in a pan with olive or coconut oil. I don't really measure anything, but I do use more almond flour than anything else."—Janice Ciacco

Janice, her daughter Samantha, and mom Chris have celiac disease, and her son Joey has additional food intolerances.

Budgeting Tips

Many people say that gluten-free foods can be expensive, and yes that can be true. Gluten-free flours, breads, cakes, cookies, and pastas cost more then their gluten-containing versions.

This is for several reasons: When farmers grow gluten-free grains, special precautions are needed to prevent them from getting contaminated with any gluten. Farmers can't rotate gluten-free crops with gluten-containing crops. They also can't harvest with the same equipment, or transport crops in the same containers, which will end up costing more money. For manufacturers, it means separate production lines, more cleaning of equipment, separate work stations, and sometimes testing of foods for any possible contamination. All this drives up the prices.

There are things you can do to save money:

- Make and freeze some gluten-free baked goods until you need them, instead of buying everything premade.

- Buy less expensive gluten-free flours and products, such as beans and bean flours, corn and corn flour, rice flour, potatoes, and potato starch.

- Keep gluten-free flours in the freezer or refrigerated to prevent them from going bad.

- Buy foods that are naturally gluten-free such as fresh fruits and vegetables, dairy products, eggs, fresh meat, chicken, and fish. If you limit most of your more expensive gluten-free choices to pasta, breads, and desserts you can really limit your expenses.

- Keep track of the difference in cost between using gluten-free choices and regular products as there are some tax deductions that can be taken for those who have been diagnosed with celiac disease. This is not something that can just be automatically taken off your taxes, talk to your accountant about the best way to do this.

Quick-and-Easy Gluten-Free Recipes

Use these recipes to prepare quick, easy, delicious, gluten-free meals.

ALLERGY INFORMATION: Since people often have multiple allergies, I have included an allergy guide next to the tips for each recipe using the following codes: GF = gluten free, MF = milk free, SF = soy free, EF = egg free, NF = nut free, PF = peanut free, FF = fish free, SFF = shellfish free, V = vegetarian, VG = vegan.

If a recipe can be modified to remove an allergen, this information is also included. Some common substitutions include:

1 cup of milk	1 cup almond, coconut, rice, or soy milk
Cooking spray	Vegetable oil, coconut oil, butter, or margarine **Note: Some cooking sprays have soy oil. For soy free, use soy free oil spray or vegetable oil.
Whipped cream	Dairy-free gluten-free whipped toppings such as Cool Whip or whipped coconut milk
1 egg	Egg Beaters (contains eggs) or gluten-free egg-free egg substitute, ¼ cup mashed tofu, or 1 Tb ground flax or ground chia seeds mixed with 2 Tb hot water

Mayonnaise	Veganaise (vegan, egg-free mayonnaise, sour cream, or plain yogurt)
Peanut butter or nut spreads	Nut-free spreads, SunButter, or soynut butter
Margarine (with soy)	Butter or soy-free margarine such as Earth Balance buttery spread
Chocolate chips (with soy and dairy)	Soy-free, dairy-free chocolate chips such as from Enjoy Life Foods, nut-free chocolate chips
Wine	Broth, water, or juice

TIP: MORE GREAT SUBSTITUTIONS

Check out great allergen substitutions at Cybele Pascal's Ingredient Smarts, http://cybelepascal.com/ingredient-smarts

Every care has been made to try to accurately list allergens and provide allergy recommendations but since products and ingredients often change, please always double-check the label and call manufacturers on any questionable products.

Breakfast Recipes:

- Banana Pancakes

- Quick-and-Easy Coconut Pancakes

- Cornmeal Breakfast Cakes

- Toasty Cinnamon Sticks

- Eggs & Salsa Omelet in a Corn Tortilla

- Ricotta Surprise

- Yogurt Parfait

Banana Pancakes   Serves 4

A yummy, delicious pancake, perfect for Sunday brunches.

1 cup brown rice flour
¼ cup tapioca flour
2 tsp gluten-free baking powder

½ tsp gluten-free baking soda
2 Tb sugar
1 tsp cinnamon powder
¼ tsp nutmeg
2 eggs
¼ cup 1% buttermilk
2 bananas, sliced
Gluten-free cooking spray or vegetable oil

1. Sift all dry ingredients together in a large mixing bowl.

2. Beat eggs and buttermilk together in a small bowl.

3. Add wet ingredients to dry ingredients and stir until well combined.

4. Coat a hot griddle with cooking spray or vegetable oil.

5. Drop batter by ¼-cupfuls onto hot griddle. Place banana slices carefully onto pancakes.

6. When bubbles begin to form, flip pancakes and continue cooking until browned on the bottom.

Nutritional information per serving: 205 calories, 6 grams protein, 40 grams carbohydrates, 3 grams fat, 72 milligrams cholesterol, 263 milligrams sodium, 2 grams fiber, 104 milligrams calcium, less than 1 milligram iron

Tip: Sprinkle with pecans and serve with warm maple syrup.

**Allergy Tip: This recipe is GF, SF, NF, PF, FF, SFF, V. To keep this recipe soy free, use soy-free vegetable oil in place of the cooking spray. To make milk free, use any milk substitute for the buttermilk and add 1 teaspoon of vinegar. To make egg free, use any gluten-free egg-free egg substitute. To make vegan, use gluten-free alternatives for both the milk and the eggs.

Quick-and-Easy Coconut Pancakes   Serves 4

¾ cup skim milk
2 Tb melted butter
1 egg
¾ cup all-purpose gluten-free baking blend (or homemade flour blend; see chapter 5)
¼ cup coconut flour

2 tsp baking powder

2 Tb sugar

½ tsp salt

Gluten-free cooking spray (or vegetable oil)

1. In a large bowl, mix together milk, butter, and egg.

2. In a small bowl, mix together all dry ingredients.

3. Blend dry ingredients into wet ingredients.

4. Spray a skillet with cooking spray and heat over a low heat.

5. Ladle pancake mix onto griddle.

6. Cook until brown on one side and bubbling. Turn pancakes.

7. Serve with butter and syrup.

Nutritional information per serving: 261 calories, 6.1 grams protein, 39.3 grams carbohydrates, 9 grams fat, 69 milligrams cholesterol, 492 milligrams sodium, 2 grams fiber, 110 milligrams calcium, 1 milligram iron

Tip: Coconut flour adds a nice flavor to pancakes; another great gluten-free flour that can be used in place of coconut flour is mesquite flour (it has a sweet, nutty flavor).

**Allergy Tip: This recipe is GF, SF, NF. (Note that some people consider coconut a nut. Check with your allergist to see if you can consume coconut safely. Also, always check gluten-free flour blends for any possible nuts.), PF, FF, SFF, V. To keep this recipe soy free, use soy-free vegetable oil in place of the cooking spray. To make milk free, use any milk-free substitute. To make egg free, use any gluten-free egg-free egg substitute for the whole eggs. To make vegan, use gluten-free alternatives for the milk, butter, and egg.

> **TIP** Reduce the amount of fat in your diet by replacing whole eggs with egg whites or a low-fat egg substitute.

Cornmeal Breakfast Cakes   Serves 4

A simple-to-prepare rustic breakfast cake that you are sure to love.

1 cup gluten-free yellow cornmeal
½ tsp salt
¾ cup 1% milk
1 Tb honey or maple syrup
1 Tb butter
2 egg whites
Gluten-free cooking spray (or vegetable oil)

1. Mix cornmeal and salt in a large bowl.

2. In a small saucepan, heat milk, honey, and butter to a low simmer.

3. Pour mixture over cornmeal; stir to combine. Let sit for 5 minutes.

4. In an electric mixer, beat egg whites in a small bowl until stiff white peaks form. Gently fold egg whites into the cornmeal mixture.

5. Coat a hot griddle with cooking spray or vegetable oil. Pour batter by ¼-cupfuls and spread to ¼ inch thick.

6. Cook for 2–3 minutes on each side until golden brown.

Nutritional information per serving: 203 calories, 6 grams protein, 44 grams carbohydrates, 3.5 grams fat, 10 milligrams cholesterol, 336 milligrams sodium, less than 1 gram fiber, 57 milligrams calcium, 1 milligram iron.

Tip: Serve with butter and syrup or honey or agave, or make a maple butter whip: take 2 parts butter or margarine, softened, and blend with 1 part honey or syrup. (Also great with cinnamon.)

**Allergy Tip: This recipe is GF, SF, NF, PF, FF, SFF, V. To keep this recipe soy free, use soy-free vegetable oil in place of the cooking spray. To make milk free, use any milk-free substitute and replace the butter with vegetable oil. To make egg free, use any gluten-free egg-free egg substitute for the egg whites. To make vegan, use gluten-free alternatives for the milk, butter, and egg whites.

Toasty Cinnamon Sticks   **Serves 3**

Kids will love these—or make them as a treat for the kid inside you!

6 pieces of gluten-free bread, with crust removed
2 eggs

¼ cup skim milk
1 tsp vanilla extract
2 tsp cinnamon
2 tsp butter melted
Gluten-free cooking spray (or vegetable oil)
2 tsp powdered sugar
¼ tsp cinnamon
Optional toppings (maple syrup or jam)

1. Cut each piece of bread into 3 strips each.

2. Mix together eggs, skim milk, vanilla, cinnamon, and butter.

3. Soak breadsticks in egg mixture until egg mixture is well absorbed.

4. Spray a large skillet with cooking spray or coat with vegetable oil.

5. When skillet is hot, place cinnamon sticks on pan and brown on both sides.

6. Sprinkle with sugar and cinnamon and serve with a little maple syrup or jam.

Nutritional information: 251 calories, 6.6 grams protein, 29 grams carbohydrates, 11.7 grams fat, 48 milligrams cholesterol, 107 milligrams sodium, 1.6 grams fiber, 93 milligrams calcium, 2.5 milligrams iron

Tip: Delicious served with fresh berries or sliced bananas.

**Allergy Tip: This recipe is GF, SF, NF, PF, FF, SFF, V. To keep soy free, use soy-free vegetable oil and double-check the bread. To keep nut free, check that the bread does not contain nuts. To make milk free, use any milk-free substitute and replace the butter with vegetable oil or margarine. To make egg free, use a gluten-free egg-free egg substitute for the egg, and make sure your gluten-free bread is egg free. To make vegan, use gluten-free alternatives for the milk, butter, and egg, and use gluten-free vegan bread.

Eggs and Salsa Omelet in a Corn Tortilla   Serves 2

This simple dish is ready in just minutes.

Gluten-free cooking spray or olive oil
4 eggs
⅛ tsp onion powder

¼ cup chunky gluten-free salsa
4 corn tortillas

1. Beat eggs and onion powder together.

2. Spray a large skillet with cooking spray and heat until hot, then lower temperature to medium heat.

3. Pour eggs into the hot skillet and cook until eggs are set, then pour the salsa in the middle of the eggs and fold eggs over the salsa like an omelet. Remove eggs from the pan and set aside.

4. Continue to heat skillet and warm each corn tortilla on both sides and serve half of the omelet with 2 of the warm corn tortillas.

Nutritional Information: 253 calories, 15.5 grams protein, 23.3 grams carbohydrate, 10.9 grams fat, 472 milligrams cholesterol, 272 milligrams sodium, 3.3 grams fiber, 98 milligrams calcium, 2.4 milligrams iron

Tip: Eggs are a quick and easy gluten-free breakfast choice. Try filling with any veggie and cheese for a terrific omelet.

**Allergy Tip: This recipe is GF, MF, SF, NF, PF, FF, SFF, V. To keep this recipe soy free use olive oil in place of the cooking spray.

Ricotta Surprise   Serves 2

If you like dessert fillings like those found in Italian pastries, you will love these. What a great way to start the morning!

1 cup skim ricotta cheese
2 Tb light cream cheese
2 Tb sugar
½ cup favorite gluten-free cereal
1 cup mixed berries
½ tsp cinnamon

1. Mix together ricotta cheese, cream cheese, and sugar until smooth.

2. Layer cheese mixture, cereal, and berries in two parfait glasses.

3. Sprinkle with cinnamon.

4. Chill until ready to serve.

Nutritional information: 309 calories, 16.5 grams protein, 32.8 grams carbohydrates, 12.5 grams fat, 46.5 milligrams cholesterol, 252 milligrams sodium, 1.3 grams fiber, 382 milligrams calcium, 3.4 milligrams iron.

Tip: This is quick, easy, and delicious. It can be prepared in to-go cups or containers ahead of time for a quick grab-and-go breakfast.

**Allergy Tip: This recipe is GF, EF, SF, NF, PF, FF, SFF, V. To keep this recipe soy free, check cereal for soy. To keep this recipe nut free, make sure cereal does not contain nuts or peanuts.

Yogurt Parfait   Serves 2

Light, quick, and delicious. Perfect for those mornings when you don't have a lot of time but want a special start for the day.

2 (6-oz) containers gluten-free lite vanilla yogurt (such as Stonyfield)
1 small banana, sliced
½ cup blueberries (or other favorite berry)
2 Tb whipped cream or gluten-free, dairy-free whipped topping (such as Cool Whip)
2 gluten-free cookies such as gluten-free animal crackers or gluten-free graham crackers crumbled (optional)

1. Place a piece of cheesecloth over a medium cup and hold in place with a rubber band.

2. Pour yogurt in cheesecloth and leave in refrigerator for a few hours, or overnight, if possible. Save creamy part of yogurt and discard liquid in the cup.

3. Layer yogurt with gluten-free cookies, blueberries, and banana, top with whipped cream or whipped topping, and serve.

Nutritional information: 225.6 calories, 8 grams protein, 44.7 grams carbohydrates, 2.5 grams fat, 5 milligrams cholesterol, 101 milligrams sodium, 4.4 grams fiber, 305.1 milligrams calcium, less than 1 milligram iron.

Tip: Any kind of fruit and gluten-free cookie or cereal can be used to make a delicious parfait. The creamy part of the yogurt, also known as yogurt cheese, makes a great spread.

**Allergy Tip: This recipe is GF, EF, SF, NF (To make sure you are allergy safe always check gluten-free cookies for eggs, soy, and nuts), PF, FF, SFF, V.

Breads:

- Popovers
- Socca
- Stuffed Arepas
- Gluten-Free, Dairy-Free Biscuits

Popovers   **Serves 6**

These are light, crispy, and custardy in the middle. Delicious with fruit-flavored butter or fresh preserves.

3 eggs
¾ cup nonfat milk
¾ cup gluten-free flour blend (see basic flour blends, formula 1 in chapter 5, or use a store-bought blend)
1 tsp salt
1 tsp xanthan gum
3 Tb butter (or reduce the amount of fat by using light butter or light trans fat-free margarine)

1. Preheat oven to 375 degrees F.

2. Separate butter equally in each popover tin, and place popover pan in the oven to heat.

3. Beat eggs, and blend into milk.

4. Mix flour with salt and xanthan gum.

5. Blend flour mixture into egg mixture.

6. Fill each popover tin about ⅔ full (do this quickly, taking care not to let the pan cool too much during the process).

7. Bake for about 30–35 minutes, until puffed.

8. To keep the popovers from falling, don't open the oven while baking.

9. Remove from the oven and poke popovers with a fork to keep from them from falling.

Nutritional information: 171 calories, 5.5 grams protein, 18.8 grams carbohydrates, 8.6 grams fat, 121.6 milligrams cholesterol, 489 milligrams sodium, less than 1 gram fiber, 73 milligrams calcium, less than 1 milligram iron.

Tips: Make sure you use a popover pan—it is much deeper than a typical muffin pan. Although you can make a popover in a different pan, you won't get that extra puff or height. These are also delicious with honey butter: softened butter or margarine creamed with honey.

**Allergy Tip: This recipe is GF, SF (to be safe always check gluten-free flour blends for soy), NF (to be safe always check gluten-free flour blends for nuts), PF, FF, SFF, V. To make milk free, use any milk substitute and replace the butter with margarine or vegetable oil (Note that most margarines contain soy). To make this recipe vegan, use gluten-free alternatives for the milk, butter, and eggs (note that it won't puff as much).

Socca   Serves 4

Often found in France and Northern Italy, socca are a real treat. Not only are they quick and easy to make, but they have fabulous taste and texture and can be used in many ways.

1 cup chickpea flour
1 cup water
2 Tb olive oil
½ Tb rosemary, freshly chopped (or favorite herbs)
½ tsp sea salt
¼ tsp pepper
¼ cup onion or shallots, sliced thin (optional) (or 2 Tb minced dried onions)
Gluten-free cooking spray (or olive oil)

1. Mix together chickpea flour, water, 1 Tb olive oil, rosemary, salt, pepper, and shallots, and let mixture sit for about 30 minutes covered, at room temperature. (Mixture will resemble a thick cream.)

2. Preheat oven to broil.

3. Spray a 9½-in. round nonstick skillet with cooking spray (or coat with vegetable oil) and heat on low until hot.

4. Pour about ½ cup batter into pan and swirl around to coat pan like a crêpe in a nice round shape (use a heat-safe rubber spatula to loosen up the sides).

5. Cook socca until brown on both sides. If you like them crispy, slide each socca onto a cookie sheet or a pizza pan, drizzle top with ¼ Tb olive oil, and brown under the broiler.

Nutritional information: 153 calories, 5.2 grams protein, 14.3 grams carbohydrates, 8.3 grams fat, 0 milligrams cholesterol, 306 milligrams sodium, 2.7 grams fiber, 14.3 milligrams calcium, 1.2 milligrams iron.

Tips: Although socca is traditionally made on a different type of pan and in a much hotter oven, cooking it this way cuts the fat in half and works easily for home cooks. Socca can be used as a flatbread with dips or can be topped with any of your favorite toppings. If you wish to add toppings, broil until it just starts to crisp, lightly sprinkle with cheese or tomato or other favorites, and put back under the broiler to finish. Keep toppings light so you don't drown out the flavor of the socca. An Indian version of socca can be made using lentil flour.

**Allergy Tip: This recipe is GF, MF, EF, SF, NF, PF, FF, SFF, V, VG. To keep this recipe soy free, use olive oil in place of the cooking spray.

Stuffed Arepas   Serves 4

A delicious Hispanic flatbread, often served as a sandwich for eggs or cheese. It can be made from precooked corn or masa harina, as below—a great find!

1 cup instant gluten-free masa harina (precooked cornmeal)
1½ cups boiling water
½ tsp salt
Gluten-free cooking spray (or vegetable oil)
2 Tb parmesan cheese
2 oz hard provolone cheese
4 pieces roasted red pepper

1. In a medium bowl, mix together masa harina, boiling water, and salt until well combined. Let mixture sit for about 5 minutes.

2. Preheat oven to 350 degrees F.

3. Wet your hands with cold water and separate mixture into four balls; flatten these with your hands into patties.

4. Spray a large skillet with cooking spray (or coat with vegetable oil) and heat it over medium heat until hot.

5. Place each patty in the skillet and cook for 5–7 minutes on each side until it browns and puffs up a little and the center is mostly set (the middle will be a little soft, like polenta).

6. Slice each arepa open and fill it with provolone, red pepper, and parmesan cheese. Place on a baking sheet and bake at 350 degrees F until the cheese melts.

Nutritional information: 176 calories, 7.6 grams protein, 24.4 grams carbohydrates, 5.7 grams fat, 12 milligrams cholesterol, 456 milligrams sodium, 3.5 grams fiber, 178 milligrams calcium, 2.3 milligrams iron.

Tip: Arepas are easy to prepare and make a quick sandwich bread. Can be filled with eggs for breakfast, pulled chicken or pork for a savory dish, or even grilled chicken with pickled onions—the sky is the limit.

**Allergy Tip: This recipe is GF, EF, SF, NF, PF, FF, SFF, V. To keep this recipe soy free, use a soy-free vegetable oil in place of the cooking spray. To make milk free, omit the cheese or use a milk-free cheese (note that some contain soy). To make vegan, omit the cheese or use a vegan-friendly gluten-free substitute.

Gluten-Free, Dairy-Free Biscuits   Serves 10

Chris Howard from Long Island makes these for her grandchildren who have celiac disease and other food intolerances.

Gluten-free cooking spray or olive oil
1½ cups of hazelnut flour
⅓ cup or arrowroot flour
⅙ cup of tapioca starch
¾ cup of almond meal
¼ cup coconut oil
2½ Tb olive oil
1 tsp xanthum gum

2½ tsp baking powder
1 egg
1 tsp salt
⅔ cup plain almond milk

1. Preheat oven to 400 degrees F.

2. Mix together all dry ingredients.

3. In a separate bowl blend together liquid ingredients.

4. With a fork, work all ingredients together, then work dough until it sticks together. If too wet add additional almond meal, if too dry a bit of additional oil.

5. Spray a cookie sheet with cooking spray.

6. Use ¼ cup cookie scoop to place dough balls on a cookie sheet.

7. Bake for about 12 minutes until they spring back to touch.

Nutritional information: 255 calories, 5 grams protein, 7.8 grams carbohydrates, 24 grams fat, 19 milligrams cholesterol, 577 milligrams sodium, 3.2 gram fiber, 75 milligrams calcium, 1.4 milligram iron.

Tip: When working with nut flours, the fat content will be much higher. Even though it is a healthier type of fat, use nut flours in moderation.

**Allergy Tip: This recipe is GF, MF, SF, PF, FF, SFF, V. To keep this recipe soy free, use a soy-free vegetable oil in place of the cooking spray. Double-check the nut flours to make sure they are not contaminated with peanuts. To make egg-free or vegan, use a gluten-free alternative for the egg.

Appetizers:

- Apple Cranberry Quinoa Salad

- Artichoke Cheese Dip

- Baked Vidalia Onion Dip

- Black Bean and Mango Salsa

- Black Bean Dip with Corn Chips

- Sesame Noodles

- Cornmeal Crusted Chicken Tenders
- Hot Crabmeat Dip
- Layered Taco Dip
- Parsnip and Carrot Fries

Apple Cranberry Quinoa Salad   Serves 6

Quinoa is a high-protein grain that is easy to cook and used in many gluten-free recipes. The dried fruit provides a boost of antioxidants. Catherine Brittan, a registered dietitian, put together this delicious recipe.

2 tsp butter or margarine or oil
1 shallot, minced
¼ cup dried cranberries
¼ cup diced dried apples
½ tsp salt
2½ cups gluten-free vegetable or chicken broth
3 cinnamon sticks
1 cup quinoa
3 green onions, finely chopped

1. Melt butter in a large saucepan over medium heat. Add shallot and sauté for 5 minutes. Stir in cranberries, apples, salt, broth and cinnamon sticks; bring to a boil.

2. Add quinoa and return to a boil. Cover, reduce heat and simmer for 15–20 minutes until quinoa is tender. Remove from heat and discard cinnamon sticks.

3. Stir in green onion.

Nutritional information: 192 calories, 6.9 grams protein, 32.4 grams carbohydrates, 3.8 grams fat, 4.4 milligrams cholesterol, 472 milligrams sodium, 3.6 gram fiber, 10.3 milligrams calcium, 1.2 milligram iron.

Tip: Change it up. Try any combination of dried fruit. This salad can be a side dish for 8 or a main dish for 4 served over salad greens.

**Allergy Tip: This recipe is GF, EF, SF, NF, PF, FF, SFF, V. If you are vegetarian, make sure you use the gluten-free vegetable broth; if you are soy free as well, double-check to make sure the broth doesn't contain soy. To make milk free and vegan, use vegetable oil or margarine in place of the butter.

Artichoke Cheese Dip   Serves 20

This is a terrific lower-fat version of a classic party favorite.

1 cup grated parmesan
12 oz part-skim shredded Mozzarella cheese
1 cup low-fat mayonnaise
1 can (14 oz) artichoke hearts, drained
1 tsp garlic powder
Gluten-free crackers or veggie sticks

1. Preheat oven to 400 degrees F.

2. Blend all ingredients together in a food processor.

3. Pour into a 1-quart casserole dish.

4. Bake for about 25 minutes, until bubbly.

5. Serve with veggie sticks or gluten-free crackers.

Nutritional information: 110 calories, 6 grams protein, 3.5 grams carbohydrates, 7.8 grams fat, 17 milligrams cholesterol, 284 milligrams sodium, less than 1 gram fiber, 169 milligrams calcium, less than 1 milligram iron.

Tip: Add some gluten-free bread crumbs to this mixture, and stuff the uncooked mixture into mushroom caps and bake until the mushrooms are cooked for a yummy stuffed mushroom appetizer.

**Allergy Tip: This recipe is GF, NF, PF, FF, SFF, V. Note sometimes shredded cheese has gluten added so make sure you check labels. To make soy free, make sure the mayonnaise is soy free and double-check the the crackers. To make milk free, use milk-free cheeses (note that some may contain soy). To make vegan, use a gluten-free vegan substitute for the cheeses and mayonnaise (note that many vegan choices will contain soy).

Baked Vidalia Onion Dip   Serves 12

So simple to prepare and it will disappear as quickly as you can make it—a cheesy treat!

2 large finely minced Vidalia onions

2 cups shredded Swiss cheese
2 cups low-fat mayonnaise
1 cup parmesan cheese
Veggie sticks or gluten-free crackers

1. Preheat oven to 400 degrees F.

2. Mix first four ingredients together.

3. Place all mixed ingredients in a casserole dish.

4. Bake for about 20–25 minutes, until bubbling.

5. Serve with gluten-free crackers and veggie sticks.

Nutritional information: 240 calories, 8 grams protein, 6 grams carbohydrates, 19 grams fat, 29 milligrams cholesterol, 466 milligrams sodium, less than 1 gram fiber, 285 milligrams calcium, less than 1 milligram iron.

Tip: Any kind of cheese can be used in this recipe—it's a sure party hit!

**Allergy Tip: This recipe is GF, NF, PF, FF, SFF, V. To make milk free, use milk-free cheese (may contain soy). To make soy free, use soy-free mayonnaise and check the crackers. To make vegan, use gluten-free cheese substitute and vegan mayonnaise.

Black Bean and Mango Salsa   Serves 12

This salsa gives a fresh, colorful, finished touch to any meal. A real crowd pleaser.

2 (10½-oz) cans black beans, drained and rinsed
1 ear of corn, kernels only (about 1 cup frozen corn, if fresh is unavailable)
1 mango, peeled chopped
Juice of 2 limes
1 jalapeno pepper, chopped
1 red pepper, chopped
1 red onion, chopped
¼ cup cilantro, chopped

1. Mix all ingredients together.

2. Refrigerate mixture until ready to use.

3. Add a dash of sea salt if so desired.

Nutritional information: 63 calories, 3 grams protein, 13.2 grams carbohydrates, less than 1 gram fat, 0 milligrams cholesterol, 99 milligrams sodium, 2.9 grams fiber, 20 milligrams calcium, less than 1 milligram iron.

Tips: Great served over chicken or fish! To remove the kernels from an ear of corn, remove husk from the outside of the corn and run a knife down each side of the corn over a small bowl, removing and saving all kernels.

**Allergy Tip: This recipe is GF, MF, EF, SF, NF, PF, FF, SFF, V, VG.

Black Bean Dip with Corn Chips   Serves 6

A great party dip that is loaded with flavor and fiber—leftovers work great as a sandwich spread.

2 Tb olive oil
1 large onion, chopped
1 Tb minced garlic
1 tsp dried oregano
1 tomato, chopped
10.5-oz can black beans, drained and rinsed
2 Tb lime juice
1 Tb gluten-free hot sauce (to taste)
1 tsp ground cumin
1 tsp chili pepper
¼ cup cilantro, chopped
¼ cup (2 oz) gluten-free vegetable broth (such as Pacific brand)
1 tsp salt
1 tsp pepper
6 oz 100% corn chips

1. Heat oil and sauté onion, garlic, and oregano together until onion starts to brown.

2. Add tomato, black beans, lime juice, hot sauce, cumin, chili pepper, cilantro, and vegetable broth. Cook for about 5–10 minutes; if too dry, add a little water. Then add salt and pepper.

3. Put all ingredients through a food processor until very smooth.

4. Refrigerate overnight before serving.

5. Serve with corn chips; taste and add extra hot sauce if so desired.

Nutritional information: 236 calories, 4.4 grams protein, 29 grams carbohydrates, 12.7 grams fat, 0 milligrams cholesterol, 741 milligrams sodium, 5 grams fiber, 91.7 milligrams calcium, 1.5 milligrams iron.

Tip: Beans are a great way to increase the fiber in your diet. Bean dips can keep well refrigerated for about a week. Extra gluten-free broth can be saved by freezing in ice cube trays, and later transferring to a ziplock freezer bag.

**Allergy Tip: This recipe is GF, MF, EF, SF, NF, PF, FF, SFF, V, VG. For soy free, make sure the broth and corn chips that you use do not contain soy.

Sesame Noodles   Serves 6

This is a rich, delicious side dish that can stand alone as a meal or work great as part of an appetizer buffet selection.

1 pound of brown rice linguini
2 Tb gluten-free light soy sauce (such as LaChoy or San-J gluten free)
1 tsp gluten-free hot sauce
1 Tb sesame oil
1 Tb cider vinegar
1 tsp sugar
1 clove minced garlic (about 1 tsp)
1 Tb peanut or vegetable oil
4 Tb toasted sesame seeds
6 scallions, chopped

1. Boil linguini until just cooked; rinse thoroughly under cold water. Make sure pasta is dry before mixing with other ingredients.

2. Combine all remaining ingredients and toss with pasta.

3. Chill until ready to use. Heat slightly in a microwave to soften noodles prior to serving. Top with additional chopped scallions if desired.

Nutritional information: 368 calories, 7.2 grams protein, 61 grams carbohydrates, 7.5 grams fat, 10 milligrams cholesterol, 200 milligrams sodium, 1.7 grams fiber, 71.3 milligrams calcium, 3 milligrams iron.

Tip: These are great served warm with a chopped cucumber salad and grilled chicken breasts.

**Allergy Tip: This recipe is GF, MF, EF, NF, PF, FF, SFF, V, VG. To make soy free, omit soy sauce, check the hot sauce for soy, and use soy-free vegetable oil, and soy-free gluten-free vegetable broth with some extra salt added.

Cornmeal-Crusted Chicken Tenders   Serves 4

Chicken fingers are always a hit. Make them ahead of time and freeze them so you can always have a batch ready to go.

1 pound uncooked plain chicken tenders
2 Tb potato starch
¼ tsp salt
¼ tsp pepper
2 eggs
¼ cup instant mashed potato flakes (most are gluten free, but double-check the label)
¼ cup cornmeal
2 tsp grill seasoning blend (see tip)
2 Tb vegetable oil

1. Place chicken, potato starch, salt, and pepper in a gallon-size zipper bag. Shake to coat chicken.

2. Beat eggs in a shallow dish.

3. In a separate shallow dish, mix potato flakes, cornmeal, and grill seasoning.

4. Remove chicken from bag, dip it in the egg mixture, and roll it in the cornmeal mixture until it is well coated.

5. Heat oil in a large nonstick skillet over medium high heat. Place chicken in skillet and cook for 3–4 minutes on each side until cooked through. (Turn chicken often to prevent burning.)

6. Remove from skillet and place on paper towel–lined plate to drain.

Nutritional information per serving: 286 calories, 30 grams protein, 17 grams carbohydrates, 11 grams fat, 171 milligrams cholesterol, 205 milligrams sodium, less than 1 gram fiber, 29 milligrams calcium, 2 milligrams iron.

Tips: Chicken tenders make the perfect-sized chicken fingers. You can also buy premade gluten-free chicken tenders; Bell and Evans is one brand (check to make sure gluten free is marked on the packaging). Serve with gluten-free honey mustard dressing (see sauce recipes in this book, or buy premade gluten-free choices). Also, if you are unsure about the gluten-free status of your grill seasoning blend, make your own by combining dehydrated garlic and onion, salt, black pepper, sage, thyme, rosemary, red pepper, dehydrated parsley, dehydrated orange peel, paprika, and dehydrated green bell peppers. (When making your own seasoning blend, it is handy to make extra and keep it in a jar in your spice cabinet. It makes a great holiday gift.)

**Allergy Tip: This recipe is GF, MF, SF, NF, PF, FF, SFF. To keep milk free and soy free, make sure the mashed potato flakes do not contain milk or soy. Also to keep this recipe soy free, use soy-free vegetable oil in place of the cooking spray. To make egg free, substitute an egg-free substitute for the eggs.

Hot Crabmeat Dip   Serves 4

This crabmeat dip makes the perfect start for a great evening of entertaining. It can be made with baby shrimp or lobster in place of the crab if so desired.

2 cans (6 oz each) lump crabmeat (*see tip)
4 oz gluten-free low-fat cream cheese
¼ cup light mayonnaise
1 Tb minced dried onions
1 tsp gluten-free red curry paste (such as Taste of Thai)
1 tsp dried parsley flakes

1. Preheat oven to 375 degrees F.

2. Drain and rinse crabmeat.

3. Mix drained crabmeat with remaining ingredients and place in a 1-quart oven-safe baking dish.

4. Sprinkle with parsley.

5. Bake for 20 minutes, until bubbly.

6. Serve with favorite gluten-free crackers or gluten-free chips.

Nutritional information per serving: 167 calories, 16 grams protein, 5 grams carbohydrates, 9 grams fat, 96 milligrams cholesterol, 467 milligrams sodium, 0 grams fiber, 68 milligrams calcium, 1.2 milligrams iron.

Tips: For added crunch, top with any kind of chopped nuts before baking. *Make sure you use real crabmeat—imitation crabmeat often contains gluten.

**Allergy Tip: This recipe is GF, NF, PF, FF. To make soy free, use a soy-free mayonnaise and a soy-free vegetable oil. To make milk free, use a dairy-free cream cheese. To make egg free, use eggless mayonnaise.

Layered Taco Dip   Serves 12

This dip includes many favorite Mexican toppings, is easy to make, and is very inexpensive. Put it together, refrigerate it, and pull it out when your guests arrive. Leftovers work great as part of a homemade taco salad.

16-oz jar gluten-free salsa
1 cup shredded low-fat cheddar cheese
1 cup shredded lettuce
2 green onions, chopped
8 oz gluten-free fat-free sour cream
16 oz can gluten-free refried beans
15.5-oz can black beans (drained)
7 oz can corn kernels drained
2 tomatoes, chopped
2 avocados, peeled and chopped
2-oz can black olives, sliced (drained)

1. In a glass bowl no more than 6 inches high, layer ingredients as desired.

2. Serve with veggie sticks, or gluten-free corn chips.

Nutritional information: 187 calories, 8.7 grams protein, 22 grams carbohydrates, 8.5 grams fat, 11.5 milligrams cholesterol, 604 milligrams sodium, 6 grams fiber, 228 milligrams calcium, 1.7 milligrams iron.

Tip: This is yummy if just warmed in the microwave for about a minute. If you like things spicy, add some chopped jalapeno peppers or hot sauce while layering.

**Allergy Tip: This recipe is GF, EF, SF, NF, PF, FF, SFF, V. Double-check that the refried beans to make sure they are soy free. To make milk free, use a milk-free sour cream or milk-free plain yogurt and milk-free cheese (note that these products sometimes contain soy). To make vegan, omit the cheese and sour cream or use gluten-free, dairy-free substitutes.

Parsnip and Carrot Fries   Serves 4

Registered dietitian Catherine Brittan shares a healthier option to French fried potatoes.

4 carrots
4 parsnips
1 Tb olive oil
¼ tsp black pepper
½ tsp kosher salt
¼ tsp paprika
¼ cup grated parmesan cheese
Gluten-free nonstick cooking spray or vegetable oil

1. Preheat oven to 425 degrees F.

2. Peel carrots and parsnips and cut into approximately 2½" × ½" strips.

3. In a large resealable plastic bag, mix olive oil, pepper, salt, paprika, and cheese. Add carrot and parsnip strips a few at a time and shake to coat.

4. Place on a baking sheet coated with cooking spray. Bake for 20–25 minutes until tender.

Nutritional information: 140 calories, 3.5 grams protein, 21.3 grams carbohydrates, 5.2 grams fat, 4 milligrams cholesterol, 512 milligrams sodium, 4.6 grams fiber, 106 milligrams calcium, less than 1 milligram iron.

Tip: These "fries" can be spiced any way you like. Try Italian seasoning or a Mexican flavor combination of cumin and chili powder.

**Allergy Tip: This recipe is GF, EF, SF, NF, PF, FF, SFF, V. To keep this recipe soy free, use soy-free vegetable oil in place of the cooking spray. To make milk free or vegan, omit the parmesan cheese or use a dairy-free, gluten-free alternative.

Soups, Salads, and Sandwiches:

- Italian Tuna Salad

- Portabella Mushroom Burgers

- Shrimp Salad–Stuffed Tomatoes

- Easy Chicken and Rice Soup

- Cheddar Quesadillas

- Turkey Avocado Melt

- Roasted Peppers and Tomato Salad

Italian Tuna Salad   **Serves 2**

Most people think of tuna as something that you find at the local deli. But this tuna fish salad is so different and so delicious that you won't want to leave a bite.

6 oz canned gluten-free solid white tuna in water, drained (fresh grilled
     tuna can be used as well)
½ cup pitted green olives, chopped
¼ cup red onions, chopped
2 Tb good-quality olive oil
1 Tb capers
2 Tb lemon juice
2 gluten-free teff wraps (such as La Tortilla gluten-free wraps or 4
     toasted corn tortillas)
Optional:
     1 tomato, chopped
     1 cup lettuce, shredded
     1 cucumber, chopped

1. Drain tuna and place in a bowl; break into small pieces with a fork.

2. Add olives, onions, oil, capers, and lemon juice to the tuna and
   blend well.

3. Serve in teff wraps or corn tortillas with tomato, lettuce, and
   cucumber. Or serve as part of a salad platter.

Nutritional information: 474 calories, 25 grams protein, 42 grams
carbohydrates, 2.3 grams fat, 36 milligrams cholesterol, 910 milligrams
sodium, 6.5 grams fiber, 69 milligrams calcium, 2.3 milligrams iron.

Tip: This recipe works great with salmon as well.

**Allergy Tip: This recipe is GF, EF, MF, SF, NF, PF, SFF. Double-check tuna
for soy and the wraps for any added allergens such as soy, dairy, or nuts.

Portabella Mushroom Burgers   **Serves 4**

If you have never had portabella mushrooms before, you will be surprised and thrilled about how wonderful they truly are. Leftovers work great in salads and wraps and mixed into spreads.

4 portabella mushroom caps
½ tsp salt
½ tsp pepper
2 crushed garlic cloves
2 Tb olive oil
1 Tb balsamic vinegar
1 tomato, sliced
4 slices roasted red peppers
4 thin slices red onion
4 lettuce leaves

1. Rinse and dry mushroom caps.

2. Mix mushrooms with salt, pepper, garlic, olive oil, and balsamic vinegar, and marinate in a zipper bag for about 30 minutes.

3. Preheat oven to 350 degrees F.

4. Place mushrooms gill-side down on a baking sheet and bake for about 10–15 minutes, until cooked through.

5. Serve each mushroom with sliced tomato, roasted red pepper, red onion, and lettuce leaves.

Nutritional information: 121 calories, 5 grams protein, 10.7 grams carbohydrates, 10.7 grams fat, 0 milligrams cholesterol, 305 milligrams sodium, 3.4 grams fiber, 79 milligrams calcium, less than 1 milligram iron.

Tip: Portabella mushrooms have a meaty, satisfying texture that makes a nice sandwich. Try one on your favorite toasted gluten-free roll.

**Allergy Tip: This recipe is GF, EF, MF, SF, NF, PF, FF, SFF, V, VG.

Shrimp Salad–Stuffed Tomatoes   **Serves 4**

Tomatoes are perfect for stuffing, especially fresh-picked summer tomatoes, and there is no better filling than shrimp salad. You can also use cherry tomatoes, cut in half, as a perfect appetizer size.

4 medium tomatoes

8 oz precooked shrimp, shells and tails removed and cut into ½-inch pieces

1 celery stalk, chopped

4 Tb green onion, chopped

4 Tb reduced-fat gluten-free mayonnaise

1 Tb ketchup

2 Tb parsley, chopped

¼ tsp salt

¼ tsp pepper

1 Tb lemon juice or hot sauce

Parsley to garnish

1. Cut tops off tomatoes and hollow out, reserving pulp and discarding liquid.

2. Mix tomato pulp thoroughly with all remaining ingredients except parsley garnish.

3. Refrigerate all ingredients overnight to allow the flavors to blend.

4. Stuff filling into tomatoes; garnish with parsley and serve.

Nutritional information: 127 calories, 13 grams protein, 6 grams carbohydrates, 5.4 grams fat, 113 milligrams cholesterol, 407.6 milligrams sodium, 1.7 grams fiber, 42 milligrams calcium, 2.2 milligrams iron.

Tip: Use lemon juice or hot sauce to taste.

** Allergy Tip: This recipe is GF, MF, NF, PF, FF. To make soy-free use soy-free mayonnaise, plain yogurt, or sour cream. To make egg free, use a gluten-free vegan mayonnaise (check the label as it may contain soy).

Easy Chicken and Rice Soup   Serves 10

Quick chicken soup like mom used to make is always something that warms you from the inside out. This soup is so good that no one will believe that you were able to just throw it together.

Gluten-free cooking spray (or vegetable oil)

1 large onion, chopped

4 celery stalks, sliced thin

1 cup baby carrots, sliced

1 potato, cut into ¼-inch pieces

96 oz (3 32-oz containers) low-sodium gluten-free chicken broth (such as Pacific brand)

2 (6-oz) boneless skinless chicken breasts

1 cup cooked brown rice

1. Spray a large pot with cooking spray (or coat with vegetable oil), and sauté veggies.

2. Add chicken stock and simmer for about 1 hour.

3. Cut chicken cutlets into 2-inch pieces and add to simmering broth, along with cooked rice, until chicken is just cooked about 5–10 minutes.

4. Serve hot.

Nutritional information: 94 calories, 9.8 grams protein, 11 grams carbohydrates, 1 gram fat, 16 milligrams cholesterol, 194 milligrams sodium, 1.3 grams fiber, 14.5 milligrams calcium, less than 1 milligram iron.

Tip: Leftover gluten-free pasta or cooked beans work great in place of the brown rice in this soup as well.

**Allergy Tip: This recipe is GF, MF, EF, NF, PF, FF, SFF. To keep soy free, use a soy-free broth and a soy-free cooking spray or vegetable oil. To make vegetarian or vegan, use vegetable broth, omit the chicken, and add tofu (note that tofu is made from soy) or beans with additional vegetables.

Cheddar Quesadillas   Serves 2

These are the best quesadillas I've ever had. You won't miss the typical flour tortillas at all.

2 (6-inch) corn tortillas

2 Tb shredded light gluten-free cheddar cheese

¼ avocado, sliced

½ jalapeno pepper, chopped (optional)

2 Tb black olives, chopped

½ cup drained gluten-free salsa (a mini strainer works great)

2 Tb fat-free sour cream

1. In a sauté pan on low heat, warm both sides of the tortillas.

2. While each tortilla is still in the sauté pan, place ½ the cheese, avocado, jalapeno, and olives on one half of each tortilla.

3. When cheese starts to melt, place salsa and sour cream on same side and fold tortilla in half.

4. Heat several minutes more and serve.

Nutritional information: 139.5 calories, 5.1 grams protein, 20 grams carbohydrates, 5.4 grams fat, 6.4 milligrams cholesterol, 516 milligrams sodium, 4 grams fiber, 164.5 milligrams calcium, less than 1 milligram iron.

Tip: Wrap in aluminum foil for a quick grab-and-go meal.

**Allergy Tip: This recipe is GF, EF, SF, NF, PF, FF, SFF, V. To keep soy free, make sure the tortillas, sour cream, and cheese do not contain soy. To make milk free, use a milk-free cheese and omit the sour cream (if you are soy free as well check the cheese and the cheese alternative for soy). To make vegan, use gluten-free vegan cheese and sour cream substitutes.

Turkey Avocado Melt   **Serves 2**

Avocado and cheddar give a nice, creamy texture and a burst of flavor to this terrific sandwich. Pickles, roasted peppers, and bacon are also great additions.

4 slices of your favorite whole-grain gluten-free bread
2 Tb gluten-free brown mustard
4 oz gluten-free honey turkey (such as Boar's Head), sliced paper thin
⅛ avocado, peeled and sliced
1.5 oz shredded reduced-fat gluten-free cheddar cheese
2 slices red onion
2 slices tomato
Gluten-free cooking spray or vegetable oil

1. Toast bread in a gluten-safe toaster or in the oven

2. Spread mustard on bread.

3. Make up each sandwich with turkey, avocado, cheddar, red onion, and tomato.

4. Spray a skillet with cooking spray and brown each sandwich on each side until cheese melts, then serve. Can be sprayed with cooking spray and browned under the broiler as well.

Nutritional information: 362 calories, 19.8 grams protein, 39.7 grams carbohydrates, 14.1 grams fat, 35 milligrams cholesterol, 1094 milligrams sodium, 2.3 grams fiber, 366 milligrams calcium, 3.3 milligrams iron.

Tip: Many people don't realize that they can be as careful as possible with their gluten-free foods and then turn around and contaminate them with gluten in a toaster that has previously toasted regular wheat bread. To protect your food, have a dedicated gluten-free toaster, use toaster-safe bags, or use your oven with aluminum foil on the rack.

**Allergy Tip: This recipe is GF, NF, PF, FF, SFF. Always check breads for any nuts or eggs. To make soy free, use soy-free cooking spray or vegetable oil, and check the bread, cheese, and turkey as well. To make milk free, use a milk-free cheese, omit the sour cream or use a gluten-free vegan alternative, and double-check the bread (if you are soy free as well, check the cheese and sour cream substitutes). To make vegetarian, omit the turkey. To make vegan, omit the turkey and use gluten-free vegan substitutes for the cheese and sour cream (check these for soy if you are soy free as well).

Roasted Peppers and Tomato Salad   Serves 4

This summer salad makes the perfect side dish for a barbecue.

2 cucumbers, sliced
2 cups cherry tomatoes, cut in half
¼ cup red onion, chopped
½ cup roasted peppers, chopped (if jarred, rinse and drain)
2 Tb basil, freshly chopped

Dressing:
1½ Tb olive oil
2 tsp wine vinegar
1 tsp gluten-free Dijon mustard
1 tsp oregano, freshly chopped (or ¼ tsp dried)
2 tsp brown sugar

1. Whisk together all dressing ingredients.

2. Toss all ingredients together with dressing, and refrigerate until ready to serve.

Nutritional information: 100 calories, 2 grams protein, 12.3 grams carbohydrates, 5.4 grams fat, 0 milligrams cholesterol, 39 milligrams sodium, 2.3 grams, fiber, 38 milligrams calcium, less than 1 milligram iron.

Tip: For a sensational taste, make your own roasted peppers. To roast peppers, put them on a baking sheet that has been covered with aluminum foil, and put them into a 450-degree F oven and cook until the peppers start to turn black on the outside. Cool and then peel and discard seeds and skin. Roasted peppers can be refrigerated for several days and stored in a glass jar in the refrigerator.

**Allergy Tip: This recipe is GF, MF, EF, SF, NF, PF, FF, SFF, V, VG.

Entrees:

- Chicken in Vodka Sauce with Mushrooms

- Blackened Mahi Mahi

- Asian Rubbed Flank Steak

- Eggplant Rollatini

Chicken in Vodka Sauce with Mushrooms   Serves 4

This Italian favorite is perfect served with gluten-free pasta. See tips for making extra vodka sauce.

2 Tb light margarine
2 Tb garlic, chopped
1 pound of chicken tenders
¼ cup brown rice flour
½ tsp salt
⅓ cup vodka
14 oz can diced tomatoes
8 oz mushrooms, sliced
4 Tb fat-free half-and-half
2 Tb parmesan cheese

1. Combine rice flour and salt in a medium bowl.

2. Melt margarine in a large skillet over medium heat.

3. Sauté garlic in margarine for 2–3 minutes.

4. Meanwhile, toss chicken in rice flour and salt.

5. Brown chicken in skillet on both sides until just cooked, and remove from pan.

6. Remove pan from heat, add vodka, and then return to heat.

7. Add diced tomatoes with liquid and simmer.

8. Add mushrooms and simmer until mushrooms are cooked. Add chicken back to pan, and add half-and-half with Parmesan cheese. Simmer for a few minutes until sauce starts to thicken, and serve.

Nutritional information: 457.7 calories, 21 grams protein, 34 grams carbohydrates, 21.2 grams fat, 49.4 milligrams cholesterol, 1,064 milligrams sodium, 3 grams fiber, 118 milligrams calcium, 2.4 milligrams iron.

Tip: To make vodka sauce separately, (1) melt margarine in a large skillet and sauté garlic for 2–3 minutes; (2) add about 1 Tb of rice flour and salt and stir until thickened; (3) add vodka and diced tomatoes, with their juice, and stir until all ingredients are combined; (4) add half-and-half and Parmesan cheese and continue stirring; (5) simmer for a few minutes, until the sauce starts to thicken; (6) serve immediately. You can use vodka sauce with any pasta dish, or over grilled shrimp or other fish—delicious!

**Allergy Tip: This recipe is GF, EF, NF, PF, FF, SFF. To make milk free, use a milk-free cheese and rice milk in place of the half-and-half. To make soy free, use soy-free margarine or butter and check any dairy substitutes for soy. To make vegetarian, omit the chicken. To make vegan, omit the chicken and use gluten-free, dairy-free vegan cheese and half-and-half.

Blackened Mahi Mahi   Serves 4

This spicy favorite will take you right back to the islands.

1 Tb lemon pepper
½ tsp cayenne pepper
1 tsp oregano
1 tsp thyme
1 tsp white pepper
3 Tb butter (or trans-fat free margarine), melted
16 oz (4 [4-oz each]) mahi mahi fish fillets
Gluten-free cooking spray (or vegetable oil)

1. In a small bowl, mix together lemon pepper, cayenne pepper, oregano, thyme, and white pepper.

2. Spray a heavy cast iron skillet with cooking spray (or coat with vegetable oil) and heat over medium-high heat until very hot.

3. Brush each fillet with melted butter and sprinkle with pepper spice mix on both sides. Press mixture into fish with hands.

4. Place fish in skillet. Cook until fish has a charred appearance—about 2–3 minutes. Turn fish over and continue to cook until fish is blackened and easily flakes with fork.

Nutritional information: 181 calories, 21 grams protein, less than 1 gram carbohydrate, 9 grams fat, 106 milligrams cholesterol, 401 milligrams sodium, less than 1 gram fiber, 27.4 milligrams calcium, 1.5 milligrams iron.

Tips: Make sure you have good ventilation and the fan on when cooking this fish—it will smoke!

**Allergy Tip: This recipe is GF, EF, SF, NF, PF, SFF. To keep this recipe soy free, use soy-free vegetable oil in place of the cooking spray. To make milk free, use margarine instead of butter.

Asian Rubbed Flank Steak   **Serves 4**

This recipe is a barbecue favorite, easy to make and loaded with flavor.

1 lb flank steak

Marinade:

¼ cup gluten-free soy sauce (such as La Choy or San-J gluten free)
3 Tb pineapple juice
¼ tsp black pepper
1 clove garlic, minced
½ tsp ginger, freshly chopped

Dry Spice Rub:

½ tsp cinnamon
¼ tsp ground cloves
¼ tsp dry ginger
¼ tsp allspice

½ tsp garlic salt
1 Tb black peppercorns, crushed
1 tsp anise seeds, crushed

1. Mix all marinade ingredients in a gallon size zipper bag. Add flank steak and turn to coat. Seal bag and place in refrigerator for 1–2 hours.

2. Mix dry rub ingredients in a small bowl.

3. Preheat broiler.

4. Remove steak from marinade. Discard marinade.

5. Press dry rub onto both sides of steak and place on broiler pan.

6. Place under broiler and cook for 3–4 minutes on each side, or to desired doneness.

Nutritional information: 204 calories, 25 grams protein, 2 grams carbohydrates, 10 grams fat, 48 milligrams cholesterol, 503 milligrams sodium, less than 1 gram fiber, 18.7 milligrams calcium, 2.4 milligrams iron.

Tip: This recipe works great with any steak.

**Allergy Tip: This recipe is GF, MF, EF, NF, PF, FF, SFF.

Eggplant Rollatini   Serves 4

Grilling the eggplant cuts down the amount of fat used in the traditional recipe and saves time, since you skip the breading step.

1 medium eggplant
1 Tb olive oil
½ cup water
1 tsp garlic powder
¾ cup skim ricotta cheese
3 Tb basil, freshly chopped
4 oz skim mozzarella (shredded)
2 cups tomato sauce
2 Tb grated Parmesan cheese

1. Preheat oven to 350 degrees F.

2. Peel eggplant and slice lengthwise into 8 pieces.

3. Mix together olive oil, water, and garlic powder.

4. Dip eggplant slices in liquid mixture.

5. Grill eggplant until just cooked on both sides.

6. Mix chopped basil with ricotta.

7. Roll eggplant with 1½ Tb ricotta mixture in each piece of eggplant.

8. In a casserole dish, pour ½ cup tomato sauce, and place each eggplant roll in a single layer on top of the sauce.

9. Top with the rest of the sauce, cover with sliced or shredded mozzarella cheese, and sprinkle with Parmesan cheese.

10. Bake for about 15–20 minutes, until cheese is melted and hot.

Nutritional information: 251 calories, 16.2 grams protein, 18 grams carbohydrates, 12.7 grams fat, 34.6 milligrams cholesterol, 914 milligrams sodium, 6.5 grams fiber, 407 milligrams calcium, 1.9 milligrams iron.

Tip: Can be made as either an appetizer or a main dish.

**Allergy Tip: This recipe is GF, EF, SF, NF, PF, SFF, FF, V. Always check the label when buying shredded cheese to make sure gluten or soy has not been added. To make milk free, use dairy-free cheese substitutes (many of these contain soy). To make vegan, use gluten-free, dairy-free dairy substitutes for the cheese (if you are soy free, check for soy as well).

Desserts:

- Yogurt Pie
- Quick-and-Easy Cheesecake
- Chocolate Dream Treats
- Bananas Foster
- Frozen Banana Cream
- Quick-and-Easy Gluten-Free Cookie Truffles
- Chocolate-Covered Peanut Butter Balls
- Gluten-Free Brownies

- Blancmange
- Gelatin Chews

Yogurt Pie   Serves 8

What a wonderful way to get some extra calcium into your diet; a dessert that is easy and inexpensive to make.

18-oz package gluten-free ginger snaps, crushed
2 Tb butter, melted
1 small banana, sliced
2 (6-oz) 90-calorie gluten-free fruit yogurts (such as Stonyfield)
1 (3-oz) packet gluten-free cherry Jell-O
8 oz fat-free Cool Whip

1. Mix cookie crumbs with butter and press into a 9-inch pie plate.

2. Arrange banana slices over pie crust.

3. Blend together yogurt, Jell-O, and Cool Whip and pour into pie crust.

4. Freeze pie until set, then serve.

Nutritional information: 289 calories, 2 grams protein, 42 grams carbo-hydrates, 11.8 grams fat, 8 milligrams cholesterol, 66 milligrams sodium, less than 1 gram fiber, 106.5 milligrams calcium, less than 1 milligram iron.

Tip: Any fruit-flavored yogurt works well in this pie.

**Allergy Tip: This recipe is GF, EF, NF, PF, SFF, FF, V. When buying gluten-free gingersnaps make sure eggs or nuts have not been added.

Quick-and-Easy Cheesecake   Serves 10

Any cheesecake recipe can easily be made gluten free. Using a gluten-free cereal makes the crust a snap.

1 cup Rice Chex (finely ground) (or use Honey Nut or Cinnamon Chex and you can eliminate the brown sugar and slivered almonds in this recipe)
2 Tb slivered almonds
2 Tb dark brown sugar
½ tsp cinnamon

¼ tsp nutmeg

3 Tb melted butter

2 (8-oz) packages reduced-fat cream cheese

¾ cup sugar

2 eggs

½ cup reduced-fat sour cream

1 tsp almond extract

Crust:

1. In a food processor, blend Rice Chex, almonds, brown sugar, cinnamon, and nutmeg until finely ground.

2. Add butter and blend until mixed.

3. Press into a 9-inch pie pan to form crust.

Filling:

1. In a large bowl, beat cream cheese, sugar, eggs, sour cream, and almond extract until smooth and well mixed.

2. Pour into prepared shell.

3. Bake at 350 degrees F for 45–55 minutes or until set.

4. Allow to cool completely before serving.

Nutritional information: 250 calories, 6.9 grams protein, 24 grams carbohydrates, 14.2 grams fat, 80 milligrams cholesterol, 212 milligrams sodium, less than 1 gram fiber, 89 milligrams calcium, 2.1 milligrams iron.

Tip: This is a delicious, easy-to-prepare cheesecake recipe. Why not top it with your favorite fruit preserves or fold in some jam or gluten-free chocolate chips for a nice addition?

**Allergy Tip: This recipe is GF, PF, SFF, FF, V. To make milk free, use milk-free alternatives for the cream cheese and sour cream and use margarine. To make egg free, use an egg-free egg substitute. To make nut free, omit the almonds.

Chocolate Dream Treats   Serves 30

Everyone loves candy, and these creamy, decadent treats will make you savor every bite.

1 (4.4-oz) bar gluten-free milk chocolate (such as Hershey's)
1 (4.25-oz) bar gluten-free dark chocolate (such as Hershey's)
1 (8-oz) container gluten-free mascarpone cheese
1 tsp gluten-free vanilla extract
1 oz shot gluten-free liquor (cordial, such as Amaretto)

1. Melt chocolate in top of a double boiler (or in the microwave).

2. Remove from heat and stir in cheese, vanilla, and liquor.

3. Pour chocolate into molds or pour about 1 Tb each into mini-muffin paper cups dusted with cocoa or powdered sugar.

4. Refrigerate to set and serve.

Nutritional information per serving (serving size 1 treat): 56 calories, 1 gram protein, 4.6 grams carbohydrates, 3.5 grams fat, 5.6 milligrams cholesterol, 32.5 milligrams sodium, less than 1 gram fiber, 11.1 milligrams calcium, less than 1 milligram iron.

Tip: If desired, top with shredded coconut and dried fruit.

**Allergy Tip: This recipe is GF, EF, NF, PF, SFF, FF, V. Double-check the labels as some mascarpone cheese can have wheat added and some chocolate contains gluten (often listed as flavorings or barley malt) or nuts.

Bananas Foster   Serves 4

This simple-to-prepare bananas Foster is a lightened-up version of that traditional New Orleans favorite.

2 Tb lite butter or margarine
2 bananas, sliced
1 tsp cinnamon
2 Tb brown sugar
2 Tb dark rum
2 cups low-fat gluten-free vanilla ice cream

1. Melt butter or margarine in a skillet over medium heat.

2. Add bananas, cinnamon, brown sugar, and rum to the skillet, and heat until the bananas start to caramelize—about 5 minutes; add a tiny bit of water if pan gets too dry.

3. You can keep the banana mixture refrigerated until ready to use; just microwave it before serving.

4. Serve ice cream topped with caramelized bananas.

Nutritional information: 221 calories, 3.7 grams protein, 37.4 grams carbohydrates, 5.2 grams fat, 17.5 milligrams cholesterol, 109 milligrams sodium, 2 grams fiber, 107 milligrams calcium, less than 1 milligram iron.

Tip: Traditionally, this recipe is made with a lot of butter and brown sugar, set on fire when the rum is added, and then ladled over ice cream. It is naturally gluten free and is a decadent way to have your ice cream.

** Allergy Tip: This recipe is GF, SF, NF, PF, SFF, FF, V. To keep soy free, use butter instead of margarine. Make sure you check the ice cream to make sure it is soy free and nut free.

Frozen Banana Cream   **Serves 4**

Cool, light, delicious, and easy to prepare.

4 small bananas (peeled, cut into 2-inch pieces, and frozen)
2 cups strawberries (frozen)
2 Tb strawberry jam
⅛–¼ cup water
4 mint sprigs (optional)

1. Puree bananas, strawberries, and jam in a food processor.

2. Gradually add water until desired texture is achieved, but be careful not to add too much water.

3. Garnish with mint or some berries and serve immediately.

Nutritional information: 170 calories, 1.8 grams protein, 39.4 grams carbohydrates, .6 grams fat, 0 milligrams cholesterol, 4.6 grams fiber, 19.4 milligrams calcium, less than 1 gram iron.

Tip: Any berry or jam works well in this recipe. To make it easier to use the bananas, peel them before freezing, and then package them in a freezer bag. Bananas are hard to peel after they are already frozen!

**Allergy Tip: This recipe is GF, MF, EF, SF, NF, PF, SFF, FF, V, VG.

Quick-and-Easy Gluten-Free Cookie Truffles   **36 Servings**

This recipe was adapted from a traditional popular recipe to a gluten-free version by Barbara Barbona from the Gluten Intolerance Group of Long Island.

2 boxes of Gluten Free K-Too's Chocolate Sandwich Creme Cookies (or 1½ boxes of gluten-free Glutino Chocolate Vanilla Creme Cookies)
8 oz low-fat cream cheese (softened)
16 oz gluten-free semi-sweet or milk chocolate chips (Nestles or Hershey's work well)
2 teaspoons vegetable oil

1. In a food processor, grind cookies until they resemble bread crumbs.

2. Combine cookie crumbs and cream cheese.

3. Roll mixture into truffle-sized balls.

4. Microwave chips with oil for about 1 minute and stir; if still whole, microwave for 10–15 seconds more until melted.

5. Dip truffles in melted chocolate and place on wax paper or aluminum foil until chocolate is hard.

Nutritional information: 127 calories, 1 grams protein, 16.6 grams carbohydrates, 7 grams fat, 3.6 milligrams cholesterol, 1.6 grams fiber, 14 milligrams calcium, less than 1 gram iron.

Tip: Before the chocolate is firm you can roll truffles into coconut, chopped nuts, or gluten-free sprinkles.

**Allergy Tip: This recipe is GF, SFF, FF, V. To make soy free, use soy-free chocolate chips, vegetable oil, and double-check the cookies.

Chocolate-Covered Peanut Butter Balls   **Serves 24**

1 cup creamy peanut butter
1 cup powdered sugar
1 tablespoon salted butter melted
3 teaspoons vegetable oil
¼ cup powdered sugar
¼ cup crushed gluten-free cereal such as Corn Chex
2 cups gluten-free milk chocolate chips

1. Combine peanut butter, ¾ cup powdered sugar, and melted butter.

2. Cover a baking sheet with parchment paper.

3. Rub 1 teaspoon of vegetable oil in the palms of your hands, and roll peanut butter into 1½-teaspoon-sized balls. If the mixture is too gooey to roll, add a little extra powdered sugar to it.

4. Combine the ¼ cup of crushed cereal with ¼ cup powdered sugar and roll peanut butter balls in it, then flatten them a little. Refrigerate for about 10 minutes.

5. Meanwhile put chocolate chips in a microwave safe bowl with 2 teaspoons vegetable oil and heat for 1 minute, and stir until all chips are melted. If needed, microwave for an additional 10 seconds.

6. Put fresh parchment paper on a baking sheet, and dip each peanut butter ball in chocolate, using 2 teaspoons to help coat both sides. Place on clean parchment paper and refrigerate until set.

7. When hard, store in a container in a single layer and refrigerate until ready to serve.

Nutritional Information: 161 calories, 2.6 grams protein, 18.5 grams carbohydrate, 10 grams fat, 1.3 milligrams cholesterol, 46 milligrams sodium, 1.5 milligrams fiber, 4.8 milligrams calcium, .7 milligrams iron

Tip: Stick a lollipop stick in each peanut butter ball before they are cooled and make them peanut butter balls on a stick. Generally peanut balls are made with paraffin wax to keep them from melting, I prefer to keep them refrigerated until ready to serve.

**Allergy Tip: This recipe is GF, EF, SFF, FF, V. To make milk free, use margarine and milk-free chocolate. To make soy free, use soy-free vegetable oil, and check the chocolate chips, cereal, and peanut butter for soy.

Gluten-Free Brownies   36 Servings

Who could be happy without a brownie recipe as part of their collection? Barbara Bonavoglia, who shared this recipe, is wonderful at adapting classic favorites into delicious gluten-free options.

Gluten-free cooking spray or vegetable oil
1 cup (2 sticks) of butter or margarine

2 cups sugar

2 tsp. vanilla extract

4 eggs

1 cup gluten-free flour blend (see below)

1 tsp. xanthan gum

¾ cup gluten-free cocoa powder (such as Hershey's)

½ tsp. baking powder

¼ tsp. salt

1 cup chopped nuts (optional)

Gluten-Free Flour Blend:

2 cups white rice or brown rice flour

⅔ cup potato starch (not flour)

⅓ cup tapioca starch/flour

1. Heat oven to 350 degrees F.

2. Spray a 13 × 9 × 2" baking pan with cooking spray.

3. Microwave butter or margarine in large bowl until melted. Stir in sugar and vanilla. Add eggs, one at a time, beating well after each addition.

4. Add gluten-free flour, cocoa powder, baking powder, salt and xanthan gum. Beat until well blended.

5. Stir in nuts. Pour into pan.

6. Bake brownies 30–35 minutes or until brownies begin to pull away from sides of pan.

7. Cool completely before serving.

Nutritional information per serving: 138 calories, 1.8 grams protein, 16 grams carbohydrates, 7.9 grams fat, .5 grams fiber, 34 milligrams cholesterol, 79 milligrams sodium, 18 milligrams calcium, less than 1 milligrams iron.

Tip: Add some gluten-free chocolate chips for extra gooey brownies.

**Allergy Tip: This recipe is GF, SF, SFF, FF, V. To keep soy free, use a soy-free vegetable oil in place of the cooking spray, butter instead of margarine (or a soy-free margarine) and make sure your flour blend does not contain soy. To make milk free, use margarine (if you are also soy free use a soy-free margarine). To make egg free, use an egg-free alternative. To make nut free, omit the nuts (make sure the chocolate and flour blend are nut free). To make vegan, use margarine and an egg substitute such as flax and water.

Blancmange   Serves 4

French for "white food." This recipe for an economical, light pudding is from Rosemary Kass.

⅓ cup sugar
3 Tbs. cornstarch
¼ tsp salt
½ tsp cinnamon
2¼ cups 2% milk
1½ teaspoons of vanilla extract

1. Dissolve cornstarch in ¼ cup milk.

2. In a small saucepan, combine sugar, salt, and corn starch mixture.

3. Over low heat, slowly add milk, stirring constantly, until mixture boils. Boil one minute. Remove from heat and blend in vanilla extract.

4. Pour into dessert cups and top with cinnamon. Refrigerate until ready to serve.

Nutritional information per serving: 156 calories, 4.5 grams protein, 28.7 grams carbohydrates, 2.7 grams fat, 0 grams fiber, 11 milligrams cholesterol, 210 milligrams sodium, 165 milligrams calcium, less than 1 milligram iron.

Tip: Serve with a gluten-free cookie and berries with whipped cream to really wow your guests.

**Allergy Tip: This recipe is GF, EG, SF, NF, PF, SFF, FF, V. To make milk free and vegan, use rice, almond, coconut, or soy milk.

Gelatin Chews   Serves 6

This is a fun, easy recipe that works great when cut into shapes for kids' parties. Adults can add some vodka for a treat with a punch.

2-½ cups boiling water
2 pkg. gluten-free gelatin dessert mix (8-serving size each), any flavor

1. Mix boiling water into gelatin dessert mix, stir until completely dissolved.

2. Pour into a 13" × 9" pan and refrigerate until set.

3. Cut into desired shapes and serve.

Nutritional information per serving: 203 calories, 6 grams protein, 23.8 grams carbohydrates, 0 grams fat, 0 milligrams cholesterol, 100 milligrams sodium, 0 grams fiber, 0 milligrams calcium, 0 milligrams iron.

Tip: Most gelatin dessert mixes, like Jell-O brand, are gluten free. You can make a variety of inexpensive, quick, and easy treats with them.

**Allergy Tip: This recipe is GF, MF, EG, SF, NF, PF, SFF, FF.

TIP: A BETTER BANANA CAKE

"I turned a yellow cake mix into a delicious gluten-free banana cake by replacing the butter with two very ripe mashed bananas, adding a little canola oil (about a ¼ cup), sprinkling in some ground flax seed, and adding chocolate chips. I baked it in a square pan sprayed with cooking spray, and followed the instructions on the box for cooking times."

—Dahlia Alese, Farmingville, NY

Quick-and-Easy Gluten-Free Meal Tips

Breakfast

Morning can be a hurried time of the day, but that is no reason not to have a great breakfast.

- Premake gluten-free pancakes and freeze them; when ready, microwave and serve.

- Frozen gluten-free waffles are available at many stores. Make sure you use a dedicated gluten-free toaster to cook them.

- Use boxed egg substitute or egg whites to make a quick omelet.

- Use a whole grain gluten-free roll with cream cheese and jelly for a grab-and-go breakfast.

- Make a homemade smoothie or buy yogurt smoothies.

Lunch

There is no reason to have the same old, same old everyday. Planning ahead can make lunch something to look forward to.

- Almond butter and sliced bananas on gluten-free bread makes a great make-ahead lunch

- Grilled cheese on gluten-free bread can be done with many different cheeses, and can go a bit gourmet by adding extras such as roasted peppers, sliced tomatoes, sliced pears, or apples.

- Early in the week prep chopped lettuce, red cabbage, peppers, onions, carrots, and celery. Have assorted other ingredients on hand (dried, fruit, fresh fruit, peas, beans, corn, shredded cheese, chopped nuts, and other veggies such as cucumbers, mushrooms, zucchini, or sprouts). Every day throw together a different combination, and top with your favorite gluten-free salad dressing.

- Make chicken or tuna salad and serve in lettuce leaves or with gluten-free crackers instead of bread. Do the same with gluten-free cold cuts and cheese.

Dinner

The trick to making gluten-free cooking quick and easy is to find ways to prep some items that can be used throughout the week.

- Grill several chicken cutlets to use during the week. Day one, serve with tomato sauce and melted mozzarella cheese and gluten-free pasta. Day two, serve sliced chicken over a mixed salad with dried cranberries and goat cheese. Day three, serve with gluten-free barbecue sauce, corn niblets, and a mixed a salad. Day four, serve chicken with salsa and corn chips.

- Microwave a potato and fill with some cheese and veggies.

- Boil gluten-free pasta in the same pot with frozen mixed veggies for a one-pot meal.

- Make use of your grill by mixing chicken or fish or beef with veggies and seasonings in an aluminum foil packet, and grill or roast for a delicious meal with easy clean-up.

Snacks and Treats

- Mix together gluten-free cereal, nuts, and dried fruit for a yummy trail mix.

- Melt gluten-free chocolate chips in the microwave and dip strawberries and apples in it.

- Blend gluten-free flavored yogurt with some vanilla almond milk for a delicious shake.

- Layer gluten-free yogurt and gluten-free cereal or berries in a parfait glass.

- Try hummus with baby carrots or celery.

Quick-and-Easy Substitutions

Finding Quick Substitutes for Your Favorite Foods

We are all creatures of habit, and we like to keep things exactly the way we are used to them. Our habits follow us everywhere—especially the ways we like our food. Many people will say that their mom's lasagna is the best, yet everyone's mom can't have the best lasagna. But it is the lasagna, or pot roast, or chicken soup that you have always eaten, that is at the heart of your soul, that is the one you are looking for.

Thus, the hardest part of changing your diet will always be finding ways to have your favorite foods the way you like them, and if you can't do this you will always feel like you are missing something. So whether you cook, grab-and-go, or dine out, you need to stay gluten free while finding wonderful substitutes for the foods you love.

Consider the foods that you normally eat that contain gluten: breads, pastas, and desserts. For some of these, you can find good substitutes, and for others the key will be tweaking the ingredients in favorite recipes so that they still work while eliminating the gluten that makes you sick. Learning how to work with gluten-free grains will help you achieve better textures and flavors in your recipes. You'll want to stock up on dried and frozen gluten-free pasta or try some homemade pasta recipes like those in chapter 11. Pick up gluten-free breads, bread crumbs, flat breads, bagels, cereal, crackers, pancakes, muffins, and waffles—both frozen and mixes—and keep them stocked at home.

Make sure your spices, seasonings, condiments, and packaged foods are all gluten free. Carry gluten-free bars, chips, fruits, nuts, and snacks with you when you are out and need something quick to eat. The trick is being prepared, so that you won't ever feel deprived by whatever choices (or lack of choices) may be available wherever it is that you are.

Using Gluten-Free Grains and Flour Blends

Create substitutes for your favorite traditionally gluten-filled foods and add new flavors to your meals by learning how to work with gluten-free grains in place of wheat, rye, and barley. In chapter 3, you learned which grains are gluten free, but now you need to know how to use them.

Some gluten-free grains, especially the flours, have a shorter shelf life than wheat flours, so it is best to keep them in a cool, dry place, in an airtight container, to help extend their freshness. Storing them in a freezer may help to extend the shelf life even longer.

> **TIP**   Keeping gluten-free grains in the refrigerator or freezer helps keep them fresh longer.

Gluten-Free Grains

Some of the most commonly used gluten-free grains are

Amaranth: This is one of the ancient grains. Its tiny seeds are high in fiber, iron, and protein. They are easy to use and are found as seeds, puffed, or ground into flour.

Arrowroot Flour: This is a starch that can be used in equal amounts to replace cornstarch in recipes. It is a great alternative for those who cannot have corn.

Bean Flours: High-protein flours such as bean flours help provide a better texture to baking blends. Try them in desserts, bread, and homemade pasta blends. Since some people are allergic to beans, it is always important to let others know when you include them in your recipes. Note that some people lack the enzyme to digest fava beans (a condition called favism); they will get anemia when they consume fava beans. These individuals, mostly men of Mediterranean descent, must avoid fava beans.

Buckwheat: Buckwheat, contrary to its name, is not from the wheat family but from the rhubarb family, and it is gluten free. It is found as whole groats, such as kasha, and as a flour, and is great for making pancakes, breads, and crêpes. Buckwheat is full of flavor and nutrients.

Corn: Corn is naturally gluten free, is widely available in many forms, and is used in many Spanish dishes. It is a versatile and inexpensive grain.

Corn Flour: Corn flour is often used in cornbread, tortillas, and muffins.

Cornmeal: Ground dried corn, found in many Mexican dishes. Precooked cornmeal is also available, such as masa harina, which is great for dishes such as arepas and corn empanadas (breads and patties often served stuffed with cheese and meat).

Cornstarch: A starch made from corn, often used in Asian cooking and in puddings, sauces, and baking.

Expandex: A modified food starch made from tapioca starch that can be used in breads and baked products for a texture similar to gluten-containing baked foods.

Guar Gum: A powder made from a plant that works well to provide texture to baked products. It has a high fiber content, so you need to take care not to use too much in recipes because it can cause stomach problems for those who have sensitive stomachs. A bit of a laxative.

Mesquite: Not to be confused with mesquite cooking, ground mesquite pods make a delicious gluten-free flour addition with a mocha coffee aroma and a taste of cinnamon and chocolate.

Millet: A delicious small grain with a sweet taste that is quick and easy to prepare. It comes whole, puffed, and as flour.

Nut Flours: Nut flours are made from ground nuts and work great in baked recipes and, when added to the flour blends, are especially flavorful in desserts. Some nice gluten-free flour blends will include almond, hazelnuts, and chestnuts. Since nuts are usually a common allergen, it is important to alert others about the ingredients when serving nut-based flour products.

Potato: All potatoes are gluten free, and potato flours and starches are often used in gluten-free cooking.

Potato Flour: This is a heavier product than potato starch and has a strong potato taste. When buying premade potato products, double-check to make sure the manufacturer hasn't added gluten to the product.

Potato Starch: When added to gluten-free flour blends, it helps lighten up baked products.

Quinoa: Quinoa is a high-protein grain loaded with nutrients. It needs to be rinsed three times before cooking to remove its outer sapone coating, unless it is purchased prerinsed. Quinoa is delicious and works well as a pilaf, in stews, casseroles, and pasta flour blends. When cooking it whole, wait until the small tail-looking end pops out—then you'll know it's done.

Rice: All rice is generally gluten free unless it has become contaminated by other foods. It is important to double-check any flavored rice products, or rice that has been produced in a plant that handles gluten-containing grains. Rice flours are great when added to almost all flour blends, because they don't overpower the flavors in the recipe, and they have nice texture. Rice flours come in both fine and medium grinds; heavier grinds will require more liquid in recipes. One hundred percent rice paper is also a great choice for dumplings and stuffing.

Sorghum: A small, round grain about the size of barley. Sorghum takes on the flavor of other ingredients found in recipes and is ideal for putting together gluten-free flour blends. It is available whole and as a flour. When whole sorghum is toasted it will puff like tiny popcorn kernels, with a sweet, nutty taste.

Soy Flour: This flour has a nutty taste and is higher in fat and protein. Soy flour works great with other grains, especially when combined with stronger-flavored ingredients such as chocolate, dried fruit, and nuts, and it is often found in gluten-free cookies and mixes. Soy has a short shelf life, so only buy it when you are going to use it. Its higher protein content gives a nice texture to baked goods. Some people with celiac disease are often sensitive to soy proteins. Often the soy found in baked goods is soy lecithin, or the fat component of the soy, which does not usually include the soy protein.

Sweet Rice Flour: Sweet or sticky, or glutinous, rice does not contain gluten. It works well in sauces and is sometimes called sweet rice flour. It is soft and fine and doesn't have that gritty texture that other rice flours sometimes have. Make sure you check mixes that include glutinous rice to make sure that other gluten-containing ingredients are not added.

Tapioca Flour or Tapioca Starch: Tapioca is a very light starch and is often added to baked goods in flour blends. It keeps well and gives a nice crispy texture and golden color to breads. It is also used to lighten up otherwise heavy gluten-free baked goods.

Teff: Teff is a tiny grain that is high in iron and that is available as both a light and dark grain. It is great in flour blends and delicious cooked whole as a hot cereal. It has a nice sweet aroma when cooking, and it gives an earthy hearty texture to baked goods.

Xanthan Gum: A product that has been produced by the fermenting of corn sugar. Xanthan gum can be used as a thickener or to produce a texture similar to that which gluten gives to bread recipes.

Cooking with Gluten-Free Grains

Now that you know what some ingredients are, you will need to know how to measure, combine, and cook them. If you have trouble finding any ingredient, see chapter 10 and the resource section at the end of this book for sources of gluten-free grains.

When working with gluten-free grains, difficulties come when you try to work with them the same way you would work with wheat. Wheat has specific properties that are not found in other single grains, so knowing how to combine different flours and enhancers can make the difference between a dense, tasteless product and a delicious treat.

Gluten-Free Thickeners

In order to thicken a sauce or a stew, use gluten-free thickening agents:

- Arrowroot
- Cornstarch
- Gluten-free flours
- Potato starch
- Tapioca flour

Baking Powder

Baking powder sometimes contains gluten. When gluten-free baking powder is unavailable, make your own at home: 1 part baking soda +1 part gluten-free starch +2 parts cream of tartar = homemade baking powder.

Substitutes for Small Amounts of Flour in Recipes

When a recipe calls for just a few tablespoons of flour as a coating or part of the recipe, any of the following flours can be used:

- Almond Meal
- Bean
- Millet

- Rice

- Sorghum

- Tapioca

The next section will give you some ideas about how to make your own flour blends, as well as teaching you what ingredients work well together to obtain better textures.

You can work to achieve your own favorite flour blend or use some of the combinations suggested here. I am indebted to Carol Fenster, whose flour blends have been the inspiration and starting place for many of these flour blends.

Gluten-Free Baking Blends

The following are some all-purpose flour combinations that can be used in many recipes throughout this book. For recipes that require some extra texture, such as breads and pasta, add 1 tsp of xanthan gum, guar gum, or expandex for every 2–3 cups of blend.

Gluten-Free Flour Blend #1   *Makes 4½ cups*

Works well in any basic recipe—if it is a little too wet when blending into a dough, add some rice flour.

1½ cups sorghum flour
1½ cups potato starch or cornstarch
1 cup tapioca flour
½ cup chickpea, corn, almond, or hazelnut flour
[Printed with permission from *Gluten-Free 101* by Carol Fenster (Savory Palate, 2008).]

Gluten-Free Flour Blend #2   *Makes 5½ cups*

Great in gluten-free pasta and bread recipes.

1 cup sorghum or millet flour
¾ cup brown rice flour
2 cups potato starch
1 cup tapioca starch
½ cup garbanzo bean flour, or soy flour

Gluten–Free Flour Blend #3 *Makes 5 cups*

Gives a nice golden crispy texture to baked foods.

1½ cups sorghum flour
½ cup brown rice flour
1½ cups potato starch or cornstarch
1 cup tapioca flour
½ cup chick pea or almond flour or corn flour

Baking Combinations

Combinations of these flours make great baked products.

Base Flours

Combine with modifiers and starches for improved texture.

- Buckwheat

- Chestnut

- Millet

- Rice

- Sorghum

Texture-Enhancing, Flavorful Grains

HP means higher protein (provides stability).

- Amaranth

- (HP) Bean and nut flours

- Buckwheat

- Corn

- Flax

- Job's tears

- Mesquite

- Quinoa

- Teff

Modifiers and Starches

Lightens product and provides crisper crust.

- Arrowroot
- Cornstarch
- Glutinous or sweet rice flour
- Potato starch
- Tapioca flour and starch

High-Protein Additions

HP choices provide better consistency by holding together well.

- (HP) Bean and nut flours
- (HP) Beans (flours, or puréed)
- (HP) Eggs (powder or whole)
- (HP) Cheese
- (HP) Milk
- (HP) Nuts (flours, or butters)

Fruit Blends

These help provide good texture and stability to baked products.

- Fruit butters
- Fruit sauce or purees (such as apple or pear)
- Mashed bananas

Leavening Agents (for baked goods such as bread, pizza, cakes)

Reduces crumbling, helps products rise. Very small amounts of these are added to recipes.

- Xanthan gum (add to dry ingredients), usually 1–2 tsp for every 2–3 cups gluten-free flour blend
- Guar gum (add to dry ingredients), usually 1–2 tsp for every 2–3 cups gluten-free flour blend

- Expandex (add to dry ingredients), usually 1–2 tsp for every 2–3 cups gluten-free flour blend

- Gelatin (soften in water), use twice as much as the gums above, usually 1 Tb for every 2–3 cups of gluten-free flour blend

- Cider vinegar, 1–2 tablespoons helps with leavening in baked goods such as breads and pizza crusts.

TIP: MEASURING AND STORING GLUTEN-FREE FLOURS

(Excerpted from 1,000 *Gluten-Free Recipes* by Carol Fenster)

Measuring

Measure dry ingredients by whisking the flour a few times to aerate or fluff it and then lightly spooning it into a measuring cup before leveling it off with a knife. Don't use the measuring cup as a scoop; you'll get up to 20% more flour that way and don't pack the flour down into the cup. Don't use spouted measuring cups (which are for liquids) to measure dry ingredients such as flour or sugar because you may get more than necessary.

Storing

Use storage containers that fit with your storage needs. Any of the following options will work:

1. Heavy-duty freezer (food-quality) bags
2. Plastic (food quality) storage containers
3. Original containers the flours are sold in

Be sure to refrigerate or freeze flours if you live in a warm climate; otherwise store them in a dark, dry area. Certain flours should be refrigerated at all times (e.g., brown rice flour, amaranth, millet, sorghum, or any flours with amounts of oil because they have a tendency to turn rancid). Don't allow storage containers to sit in direct sunlight or near any heat source that causes condensation to form inside. This will cause the flour to clump and deteriorate quicker. Be sure to clean out storage containers periodically to assure that old flours are used up or thrown away before you add new flour to the container.

Cooking Beans and Gluten-Free Grains

Except for lentils, soak beans overnight prior to cooking for best results.

Grain or Bean	Amount of Grain	Amount of Water	Cooking Time	Yield
Amaranth (whole)	1 cup	3 cups	20–25 minutes	3 cups
Black beans*	1 cup	4 cups	1½ hours	2¼ cups
Brown rice	1 cup	2½ cups	35–45 minutes	3½ cups
Buckwheat groats	1 cup	2 cups	15 minutes	2½ cups
Chickpeas*	1 cup	4 cups	2–3 hours	2 cups
Kidney beans*	1 cup	3 cups	1½ hours	2¼ cups
Lentils	1 cup	2¼ cups	20–30 minutes	2¼ cups
Lima beans	1 cup	4 cups	1 hour	2 cups
Millet	1 cup	2¼ cups	25–30 minutes	3½ cups
Navy beans*	1 cup	3 cups	1½ to 2 hours	2⅔ cups
Pinto beans*	1 cup	3 cups	1 hour	2½ cups
Polenta (corn grits)	1 cup	4 cups	25 minutes	2½cups
Quinoa	1 cup	2 cups	10–15 minutes	2¾ cups
Gluten-free rolled oats	1 cup	3 cups	5–8 minutes	3½ cups
Sorghum (whole)	1 cup	3 cups	50–60 minutes	4 cups
Soybeans*	1 cup	4 cups	3+ hours	3 cups
Split peas	1 cup	3 cups	45 minutes	2 cups
Teff	1 cup	3 cups	20 minutes	3½ cups

(continued)

Grain or Bean (continued)	Amount of Grain	Amount of Water	Cooking Time	Yield
White rice	1 cup	2 cups	20–30 minutes	3 cups
Wild rice	1 cup	3 cups	35–50 minutes	4 cups

*Soak prior to cooking (best overnight)

Conversions

When converting recipes it is important to know how to alter measurement amounts. When working with dry ingredients,

3 tsp = 1 Tb
4 Tb = ¼ cup
16 Tb = 1 cup

When working with wet ingredients,

2 Tb = 1 oz.
1 cup = 8 oz.
1 cup of butter = 2 sticks
2 cups = 16 oz. (1 pint)
4 cups (32 oz.) = 1 quart
4 quarts (128 oz.) = 1 gallon

Easy Mix-and-Match Meals: Combining Gluten-Free Dishes and Ingredients

Sometimes all you need to know is how to combine foods and you can have a delicious meal.

Someone said to me once, "I don't have time to cook—I'm lucky if I find the time to boil rice noodles." People who are following a gluten-free diet are doing it because they have to. Some love to cook, some hate to cook, and some have no time to cook. Since the diet needs to be followed at all times, finding easy ways to throw meals together is essential for everybody.

Looking at what food you have on hand and combining it with seasonings or sauces makes meal planning a breeze. The following chart teaches you how to combine foods in three steps for easy mix-and-match meals. Open your refrigerator, and see all the possibilities for a meal.

Mix-and-Match Food Chart

The following combos give you choices from many food groups. The possibilities are endless—add your own!

1. Pick food choices from categories below.

2. Combine your selections with seasonings, sauces, or sweeteners.

3. Heat and serve.

Starches

- Cooked gluten free: Pasta, oats, grits, corn, amaranth, beans, buckwheat, flaxseed, millet, polenta, potatoes, quinoa, rice, teff, sweet potato (baked, grilled, fried), butternut squash, chili, plantains (baked, grilled or fried), pumpkin

- Gluten-free cereals (both hot and cold)

- Gluten-free breads, wraps, pancakes, waffles, crackers, pizza crust, rice cakes, corn tortillas, chips, and arepas

Fruits and Vegetables

- Fresh, frozen, canned, or dried fruit

- Fresh, frozen, canned, or dried vegetables, squash, and mixed greens

- Grilled fruits or vegetables (e.g., eggplant, onions, zucchini, peppers, apples, pears, papaya, pineapple)

- Shredded or cubed vegetables (e.g., carrots, beets, zucchini)

- Fruit and vegetable juices

Proteins (cubed, sliced, strips, or shredded)

- Chicken, turkey, fish, tofu, beans, beef, pork

- Gluten-free deli meats, cheese (hard and soft), eggs, milk, buttermilk

- Nuts, nut butters, and seeds

- Yogurt (plain and gluten-free flavored)

- Hummus or bean dips

Sauces/Seasonings/Fats

- Gluten-free salad dressing, ketchup, mustard, syrup, honey, maple syrup, molasses, agave, relish, sugar, oils, distilled vinegars, soy sauce, barbecue sauce, yogurt sauce, tomato sauce, garlic sauce, cheese sauce, tahini, hot sauce

- Jams and jellies

- Fats and oils (such as olive, soy, peanut, corn, walnut, almond, hazelnut, canola, and vegetable), butter, margarine, avocado, gluten-free broths and stocks, half-and-half

- Wines and distilled liquor

- Herbs (e.g., basil, oregano, thyme, sage, rosemary, mint)

- Gluten-free spices (e.g., garlic and onion powder, pepper, mustard, paprika, salt)

- Gluten-free olives, capers, pickles, salsa

 TIP: QUICK-AND-EASY GLUTEN-FREE COATINGS

Looking to make breaded cutlets or fish but out of gluten-free bread crumbs? No problem! Process gluten-free cereal, corn chips, or potato chips in a food processor and mix together with seasonings such as garlic, onion power, and dried herbs, and you're ready to go.

Easy Mix-and-Match Meals at Home

These combinations are different from the standard meal plans provided earlier because all these suggestions are based on what you have on hand and require little cooking or preparation. The purpose here is to see what you have in your refrigerator or cabinet and then to combine choices in order to have a quick-and-easy gluten-free meal. Use the mix-and-match food chart to find ideas of how to combine foods.

For example, if you looked in your refrigerator and found a baked potato, some grilled onions, a cooked hamburger, shredded cheese, and salsa, you could make salsa-stuffed potato skins. Cut the potato open and scoop out the center then mash the potato with the leftover hamburger and stuff it back into the shell (it will be a little overstuffed). Top the stuffed potato with grilled onions, salsa, and shredded cheese, then microwave until the potato is hot and the cheese is bubbling. There are so many possibilities!

The following combos provide many ideas for breakfast, lunch, and dinner.

Breakfast Combos

- Gluten-free waffles or pancakes with butter and syrup or peanut butter and raisins

- Cottage cheese and mixed fruit

- Corn grits with melted cheese

- Toasted corn tortilla, folded and filled with scrambled eggs and cheddar

- Gluten-free cereal (such as Rice Chex, Corn Chex, or Mesa Sunrise) with skim milk and berries or sliced bananas

- Gluten-free rice cakes spread with peanut or almond butter and raisins

- Gluten-free cooked leftover teff with maple syrup and berries or dried fruit

- Instant quinoa cereal

- Gluten-free oatmeal with cinnamon, honey, and toasted walnuts

- Scrambled eggs served over toasted corn tortillas with gluten-free salsa

- Gluten-free French toast with butter and syrup

- Gluten-free yogurt and gluten-free cereal or flax topping

- Scrambled eggs and cheese with leftover gluten-free fries

Lunch Combos

- Baked potato with broccoli florets and melted cheddar cheese
- Store-bought gluten-free pizza crust with tomato sauce, shredded mozzarella, and sliced mushrooms
- Gluten-free wrap with roasted turkey, lettuce, tomato, and mayonnaise
- Gluten-free bread toasted with peanut butter and jelly
- Gluten-free instant polenta with tomato sauce and goat cheese
- Toasted corn tortilla with guacamole and salsa
- Grilled chicken breast with gluten-free barbecue sauce on a toasted gluten-free roll
- Leftover rice mixed with chopped onions, tomatoes, feta cheese, leftover shrimp or chicken, and gluten-free salad dressing
- Gluten-free ham and Swiss cheese with mustard on a gluten-free roll or tortilla
- Leftover gluten-free pasta with mixed veggies, cheese, olives, and gluten-free Italian salad dressing
- Hummus with corn chips and Greek salad
- Tuna with mayo and pickle relish, with chopped lettuce and tomato and gluten-free crackers
- Large salad, with chickpeas, leftover tuna, or chicken, and gluten-free salad dressing

Dinner Combos

- Use leftovers to create kabobs, such as tuna, chicken, or beef with a combo of tomato, onion, and pepper kabob marinated in gluten-free salad dressing
- Chili stuffed in a baked potato
- Leftover grilled burger or chicken breast with salsa and shredded cheese
- Leftover pork or chicken with gluten-free barbecue sauce on a roll with a salad

- Leftover gluten-free pasta with tomato sauce and ricotta cheese
- Roasted chicken with leftover brown rice or millet and mixed vegetables
- Large salad with veggies—toss with salmon or tuna and gluten-free salad dressing and chickpeas
- Leftover gluten-free breaded chicken breasts, heated with tomato sauce and mozzarella cheese
- Any baked fish with gluten-free salad dressing, served with salad and leftover rice or potatoes
- Grill a steak and serve with salad or veggies and gluten-free baked beans
- Gluten-free premade soup with a salad
- Leftover gluten-free sausage, sautéed with onions and peppers
- Leftover shrimp with gluten-free mayonnaise and chopped onions with corn tortillas

Reading and Translating Labels

What You Need to Know about Reading Labels

Food labels provide us with necessary information about the foods that we eat. Along with the name of the food, ingredients, nutritional information, and serving sizes, food labels also might include a suggested recipe, or maybe something designed to appeal to us, such as "New and Improved Flavor" or "Supports a Healthy Heart." In order to ensure that labels and claims on foods are accurate, the government has stepped in. However, in spite of laws, labels still can be confusing to understand. Luckily, with the new FDA labeling laws, figuring out whether a product contains gluten or not has become easier, but it is still a little tricky, so it is important to understand all the rulings.

Additives and Flavoring Agents

There are many ingredients that can be made from wheat starch, such as caramel color, dextrin, glucose syrup, maltodextrin, and modified food starch. Fortunately, in the United States, in most packaged foods when wheat is the source of starch, food labels must say so. However, when it comes to meat, poultry, and egg products, wheat is not yet required to be listed, so on these types of products, make sure to check the labels for caramel, maltodextrin, glucose syrup, modified food starch, dextrin, marinade, or self-basting poultry agents, because they *could* contain hidden traces of wheat (in these cases it is often important to check with the manufacturer). If a product contains caramel, it is most likely not a concern, because caramel is usually made from corn, and if it is made from wheat it rarely contains close to 20 parts per million, which is considered a safe limit for those who need to follow a gluten-free diet (but to be safe, if not sure, it's better to avoid it).

Natural flavoring agents can be made from rye or barley. When barley is present in foods it usually is listed as malt or barley, and when rye is used, it is mostly found in bakery products.

Pure herbs and spices are always gluten free, provided there is no cross contamination and that no anticaking ingredients have been added to them (even when they are, most do not contain gluten). However, since blended seasoning agents can contain gluten as an added ingredient, it should always be checked.

Understanding the New Gluten-Free Labeling Laws in the United States and Canada

In the United States

FDA Gluten-Free Labeling Laws

On August 2, 2013 the FDA issued its final rule for the labeling of gluten-free foods. The compliance date for manufacturers to abide by this law was set at August 5, 2014. Note that it is not mandatory for manufacturers to provide the gluten-free status of their products (it is still elective), but for those companies that do, there are now rules that must be maintained. Since this rule is voluntary, there may be food products that meet all of the proposed definitions for gluten-free labeling without the manufacturers' listing them as being so. Therefore, you may still find that some foods are gluten free even if they do not claim it on their food labels.

Gluten is defined as the proteins that are naturally occuring in a prohibited grain and that may cause adverse health effects in people with celiac disease.

A prohibited grain is one of the following or related grains:

- Wheat (triticum)

- Rye (secale)

- Barley (hordeum)

- Crossbreeds of wheat, rye, or barley (e.g., triticale, a cross between wheat and rye)

Thus, if something is labeled gluten free, it would mean that a food bearing this claim is inherently gluten-free or it:

- Does not contain an ingredient that is a gluten-containing grain (e.g., spelt, wheat)

- Does not contain an ingredient derived from a gluten-containing grain that has not been processed to remove gluten (e.g., wheat flour)

- Does not contain an ingredient that is derived from a gluten-containing grain that has been processed to remove the gluten (e.g., wheat starch), if the use of that ingredient causes the food to have gluten levels that are 20 parts per million (ppm) or more.

Other terms used that are synonymous with "gluten free" and will fall under this gluten-free ruling include:

- "No gluten"

- "Free of gluten"

- "Without gluten"

Only these claims can be used to indicate gluten-free status, there is no symbol that is recognized by the FDA that would in itself mean gluten free.

Why Did They Select Less than 20 Parts per Million As a Safe Amount of Gluten?

Some people ask why zero ppm wouldn't be the standard for the amount of gluten in a gluten-free product, but zero ppm of gluten would be impossible to achieve—there is so much risk for cross-contamination that to maintain this type of criteria outside of a lab environment is next to impossible. But less than 20 ppm is so small that it is the amount that has been determined by experts to be safe for those with celiac disease (even if many servings are consumed daily)—which is why less than 20 parts per million is the worldwide standard for gluten-free foods.

So how small is less than 20 ppm? Just so you can think about it with a little more clarity . . .

One part per million is equal to:

- One penny in $10,000

- One minute in two years

- One dime in a one-mile-high stack of pennies

There are some companies that may want to note if their product has been tested to 5 or 10 ppm, which is allowed as long as their product does not exceed the amount declared.

What about Oats?

Overall, oats that are not certified gluten free are often contaminated with gluten that has more than 20 ppm; however, for the new gluten-free labeling law, certified gluten-free oats are not required for a final food product to be labeled "gluten free." Though manufacturers would still need to make sure that there was less than 20 ppm in the final product—which would most likely require the use of certified gluten-free oats anyway.

Testing

- Although the term gluten free would mean a product had less than 20 ppm, manufacturers are not required to test their products to make sure they meet this guideline. However, if the FDA decided to check manufactured items and found a product to have 20 ppm or more, the product would be considered misbranded. It would therefore be in a manufacturer's best interest to test their gluten-free products to make sure they fall below 20 ppm.

- If a manufacturer chooses to elect to analyze their foods they can select methods most appropriate for them. They are not obligated to use any specific method. Remember, testing is elective.

- To date, current testing methods have not been established for fermented or hydrolyzed foods products. More research needs to take place in this area to make sure the products are truly gluten free.

- Compliance would be monitored by the FDA through review of food labels, as well as on-site inspections of food manufacturers, and analysis of food samples. Manufacturers of foods that are found to contain gluten at more than the 20 ppm levels would face the charge of misbranding.

- The FDA has identified two sandwich enzyme-linked immuno-sorbent assays (ELISA)–based methods of testing for possible enforcement of food labeling compliance; however, there are possible limitations with using these testing methods. New methods may be utilized in the future.

Certifications

Since testing is elective on gluten-free products, consumers may want to select a certified gluten-free product to ensure minimum testing is done on their gluten-free selections. There are many verifications available, some of the most recognized and respected are listed below. For details on each certification be sure to check each company's website.

Certified Gluten-Free Certification Organization (GFCO Mark)
www.gfco.org
253-218-2956

The Celiac Sprue Association (CSA)
www.csaceliacs.org
877-CSA-4-CSA

The Coeliac Society of Australia
www.coeliacsociety.com.au
(02) 948788 50

Asociacion Celiaca Argentina in Buenos Aires
www.celiaco.org.ar

> **TIP** If a product is not certified gluten free, and is not labeled gluten free even though it is a naturally gluten-free product such as rice, there is no guarantee that it hasn't been contaminated with gluten in the harvesting, transport, and packaging processes.

Exceptions

- Although worldwide less than 20ppm has been accepted as the level that would constitute a gluten-free food, in Europe they also have "very low-gluten foods" that will have from 21 to 100 ppm.

- Other statements manufacturers can use that will not constitute a safe gluten-free product include statements such as: "Not made with gluten containing ingredients," or "made with no gluten containing ingredients". Do not take these statements to mean that these food items are gluten free. Voluntary statements such as "processed in a facility that also processes wheat" are also allowed, but if the product is labeled gluten free it still needs to meet the less than 20 ppm rule.

Cross-Contamination

As discussed in the previous chapter, cross-contamination can happen in the manufacturing or packing of processed foods, just as it can happen in your own home. Manufacturers will sometimes use the same plant to make more than one kind of food, so if a company produces a food that contains gluten—for example, bread—and also produces a gluten-free food (such as gluten-free cookies), there could be a risk of gluten cross-contamination. If a product is labeled gluten free this should not be too much of a concern because gluten-free labeled products are required to have less than 20 ppm of gluten.

The contamination issue is a little more complicated, because it falls under what the FDA calls "advisory labels." This means manufacturers will now give consumers more information about whether their product was in contact with a food that is one of the top eight allergens. For instance, you might see "This food was manufactured in a plant that also processes peanuts," or "may contain wheat," which would be more important for those with food allergies.

Enforcement

- If a food bears the claim "gluten free" in its labeling and does not meet these requirements it will be deemed misbranded.

- If a food bears the term "wheat" in its ingredients and makes a gluten-free claim, it will be deemed misbranded unless the ingredient list or the "contains wheat" statement is immediately followed by an asterisk (or other symbol) that immediately precedes the following: "The wheat has been processed to allow this food to meet the Food and Drug Administration (FDA) requirements for gluten-free foods." (Note that these foods would still not be safe for those with a wheat allergy.)

- If a person sensitive to gluten eats a product labeled gluten free and becomes ill, they can report the incident to the Center for Food Safety and Applied Nutrition's Adverse Event Reporting Systems called "CAERS" at 240-402-2405, or to the an FDA Consumer Complaint Coordinator in the state where the food was purchased.

Restaurants, Cafeterias, & Buffets

The FDA suggests that the use of an FDA defined food labeling claim "gluten free" should be consistent with regulatory definitions established for food manufacturers (requiring less than 20 ppm of gluten). Although enforcement and compliance regulations may not currently be in the works, if a complaint is made that a restaurant is serving foods that are mislabeled as gluten free, the FDA may step in. Some restaurants may choose to use terminology that is not consistent with the current labeling regulations, such as "no added gluten," or "without gluten" which would be sidestepping the laws intention. This would be misleading to consumers and could add another layer of confusion. More regulations may need to be included to better provide safe information from restaurants to consumers.

Medications

Although there is currently no ruling on the use or identification of gluten in medications, on December 21, 2011, FDA's Center for Drug Research and Evaluation (CDER) issued a Federal Register notice (76 FR 79196) to request public comments to help in its evaluation of options that would help individuals with celiac disease in limiting their gluten exposure from drug products. It is hoped that these laws will be passed soon.

Keeping Up To Date on New Regulations

The FDA lists many papers to help answer questions about their labeling laws. Some links that may be helpful include:
www.tinyurl.com/q6zezf7
www.gpo.gov/fdsys/pkg/FR-2013-08-05/pdf/2013-18813.pdf
www.fda.gov/Food/GuidanceRegulation/GuidanceDocumentsRegulatoryInformation/LabelingNutrition/ucm053455.htm
www.fda.gov/Food/GuidanceRegulation/GuidanceDocumentsRegulatoryInformation/LabelingNutrition/ucm053455.htm

United States Department of Agriculture (USDA)

The above information pertains to all foods regulated under the FDA rule, but the FDA doesn't govern all foods. The United States Department of Agriculture (USDA) regulates meats, poultry, and egg products, and at this time it has not yet initiated the same rules for listing food allergens or for stating gluten-free status of foods. Although many USDA-regulated companies have elected to list allergenic ingredients on their labels and to comply with FDA guidelines, additional regulations need to be added in the future. One positive step is that the USDA has stated it will maintain the same definitions as the FDA when a USDA regulated manufacturer chooses to make a gluten-free claim.

Tips when buying USDA regulated products (meat, poultry, and egg products):

- Buy from companies that report they will state any gluten-containing ingredients on their labels.

- Don't get overwhelmed by a list of complicated ingredients. Try to buy meats and poultry where the only ingredients listed are beef or poultry.

- Check a manufacturer's allergy statement for wheat. If there is an allergy statement it is more likely that it would indicate all allergens. If there is no allergen statement and questionable ingredients are listed, there is no way to know if the product contains gluten without contacting the manufacturer.

- If in doubt, and you can't contact the manufacturer, don't buy it.

Alcohol and Tobacco Trade Bureau (TTB)

The TTB has issued an interim policy of gluten-free labeling of alcoholic beverages under its jurisdiction as follows:

1. If a product had originally included any gluten containing grain such as wheat, barley, rye, crossbred varieties, or ingredient derived from these grains, it cannot be labeled gluten free.

2. Alcohol products can be labeled gluten free if no gluten containing ingredient was used in the raw ingredients and finished products are not contaminated with gluten.

3. For products that started with a gluten-containing ingredient and then were processed, treated, or crafted to remove gluten, labeling as gluten free is allowed if one of these two statements is included:

a. "Product fermented from grains containing gluten and {processed or treated or crafted} to remove gluten. The gluten content of this product cannot be verified, and this product may contain gluten." OR

b. "This product was distilled from grains containing gluten, which removed some or all of the gluten. The gluten content of this product cannot be verified and this product may contain gluten."

FDA Labeling Laws for Other Allergens

In 2004, the Food Allergen Labeling and Consumer Protection Act, known as FALCPA, stated that by January 1, 2006, food manufacturers had to identify in plain English any ingredient from a list of eight major food allergens. This means that if the food contains milk, eggs, fish, crustacean shellfish, tree nuts, peanuts, wheat, or soybeans, the label is required to say so. The law allows this to be done in one of two ways—either by listing it in the ingredients or by adding a "contains" statement at the end of the ingredient list. Here's an example of the former:

> **Ingredients:** Enriched flour (wheat flour, malted barley, niacin, reduced iron, thiamin mononitrate, riboflavin, folic acid), sugar, partially hydrogenated soybean oil and/or cottonseed oil, high fructose corn syrup, whey (milk), eggs, vanilla, natural and artificial flavoring, salt, leavening (sodium acid pyrophosphate, monocalcium phosphate), lecithin (soy), mono- and diglycerides (emulsifier).

In this option, if an ingredient contains a food that is an allergen, it says so in parentheses next to the food. "Enriched flour" has a parenthetical list next to it that clearly states wheat; "whey" has a parenthetical list next to it that clearly says milk, and eggs are also clearly listed. (Parentheses are not needed—eggs are eggs!) Using the second option, the list of ingredients would not have these clarifications in parentheses. It would simply conclude the list with the statement:

> Contains Wheat, Milk, Eggs, and Soy

In Canada

The regulatory agencies in Canada are Health Canada (HC) and the Canadian Food Inspection Agency (CFIA). Food companies are responsible for the administration of the Food and Drug Act including the labeling of all foods, poultry, meat, and egg products. Canada does have a gluten-free regulation. Food companies that want to make a gluten-free labeling claim must meet section #B.24.018 which states:

> It is prohibited to label, package, sell or advertise a food in a manner likely to create an impression that it is a gluten-free food if the food contains **any gluten protein** or modified gluten protein, including any gluten protein fraction, referred to in the definition "gluten in subsection B:01.010.1(1)."

The definition of "gluten" can be found in the subsection B.01.010.1 (1) which refers to any gluten protein found in any of the following cereals or grains; barley, oats, rye, triticale, and wheat. Although in this subsection no specific threshold is mentioned, based on current scientific evidence, levels of gluten less than 20 ppm would be protective for the majority of the people with celiac disease. Therefore, Health Canada considers gluten-free foods to be prepared under good manufacturing practices that contain levels of gluten not exceeding 20 ppm as a result of cross-contamination, meeting the health and safety intent of B.24.018 when a gluten-free claim is made.

When There Are No Labels, Part 1: Gluten Free on the Run

It is impossible to plan for every situation where there will be food selections to choose from. In many cases, it will even be hard to find out your how your food was prepared. So what do you do? Going hungry isn't the answer. A solid knowledge base will help make it possible for you to find safe foods wherever you are:

- Review the many food choices that are naturally gluten free in chapter 2.

- Carry a copy of the chart of safe foods found in chapter 3 so you can quickly review your options at any time.

- When in doubt, always opt for fresh choices such as fruits, veggies, plain meats, chicken, eggs, dairy, and fish.

- Carry gluten-free salad dressings, crackers, and seasoning packets with you to help spruce up your meals.

- Carry gluten-free trail mix, dried fruit, nuts, and cheese with you so you can have something quick when you aren't able to easily find something to eat.

- Bring a favorite entree and dessert with you to parties and events so you'll have something both safe and special.

- Carry the dining out sheets in Chapter 12 to make things easier in ethnic restaurants.

- Call ahead to restaurants and catering halls so you do not have to figure out everything in front of a group of people or a busy staff.

The most important thing to do is to be prepared. Even when you are not in an ideal situation, you can always have delicious food choices available to you.

When There Are No Labels, Part 2: Gluten Free at the Deli, Fast-Food, and Chain Restaurants

There are many times you may be on the road or in a hurry when you will want to grab something quick to eat. Although you may not like eating fast food, some circumstances may dictate this as the only choice. Knowing what to buy at the deli or in a fast food restaurant will make these times so much easier.

At the Deli

Although we usually think of a deli as a sandwich stop, there are many choices for the gluten-free diner as well. Why not pick up a fresh salad? Tuna, chicken, and egg salad are good choices, as long as bread is not added to the recipe to extend the salad—and be sure to ask whether the same scoops and spatulas are used when spreading on wraps and bread to avoid cross-contamination. Grilled chicken can be a good choice if the marinade is gluten-free and the grill is covered with aluminum foil to protect your food. Fresh fruit, canned and dried fruits, and packaged gluten-free chips and nuts are available in most delis. Many brands of cold cuts are gluten-free, as are most cheeses, so if you have gluten-free crackers, you can throw together a quick meal.

Gluten-free products typically found at delis:

- Applegate Farms gluten-free organic deli meats and cheese

- Boar's Head deli meats, cheeses, and condiments

- Carl Buddig deli meats

- Foster Farms deli meats

- Hebrew National salami, bologna, and hot dogs

- Hormel Natural choice deli meats

- Hormel Cure 81 ham

- Jennie-O deli meats

- Thumann's gluten-free deli meats, cheese, condiments, and pickles

**Please note that many other brands may also be gluten-free—make sure to check with the manufacturer.

TIP Be careful of cross-contamination from the meat slicer and grill. Ask to have the slicer wiped down and for them to change their gloves before your meat is sliced, and for the grill to be covered with aluminum foil before your food is cooked.

Brands that sometimes contain gluten

- Dietz & Watson

- Organic Valley

This is a partial listing; if in doubt on a particular brand see if you can check the label or contact the manufacturer.

Avoid

- Dietz & Watson scrapple, bockwurst, fat-free beef franks, and gourmet lite franks.

- Any deli meat that contains hydrolyzed vegetable protein, modified food starch, or wheat.

Also question

- All condiments, salads, and soups—they may contain bouillon cubes, soup bases, seasoned mustards, malt vinegars, and salad dressings that are not gluten-free.

- Corned beef is sometimes cooked with rye seed.

**Note that many brands may contain gluten; double-check by contacting the manufacturer whenever you are trying a new brand or product.

> **TIP** Always ask the deli manager if he or she can provide you with a list of ingredients on questionable products. If you use the same deli on a regular basis, go during slow times, when staff may be available to answer your questions.

At Fast Food and Chain Restaurants

Many chains regularly change their menu items, so make sure you look for regular updates by calling their headquarters or checking their websites to make sure your food choices are safe. This list is a partial listing of options; gluten-free restaurants are opening up all over the country. The easiest way to view a restaurant's gluten-free options is to type "gluten free" and the restaurant name in a search engine. Some chains specify wheat free but not gluten free, so their offerings may not be safe to consume.

In general, watch out for French fries or other fried products, which are often fried in the same oil as breaded products. Fries are only safe if made in a dedicated fryer. Also note that some locations may have a gluten-free menu but the staff may not be well trained in preventing cross-contamination. Ask a lot of questions, and use your best judgment when making your choices.

If you are new to an area and trying to find a gluten-free restaurant, there are many apps available to help you, including findmeglutenfree. com or urbanspoon.com. But even if a site states that a restaurant has gluten-free choices, you should still call to confirm that they are conscious of cross-contamination issues.

Arby's

cds.arbys.com/pdfs/nutrition/nutrition-info.pdf

1 (800) 487-2729×4315

Arby's posts allergen information on its site listing gluten-free options. Check regularly for updates.

Baja Fresh

www.bajafresh.com/mexican-food-nutrition

1 (877) 225-2373

Allergen information is not posted on the site, but the company recommends that you e-mail any questions concerning allergens.

Baskin Robbins

www.baskinrobbins.com/content/baskinrobbins/en/nutritioncatalog.html

1 (800) 859-5339

Many Baskin Robbins products are classified as wheat-free but not gluten free. And even if a flavor is gluten free, it can be cross-contaminated by a shared ice cream scoop, so it should be avoided unless a fresh container of gluten-free ice cream is being scooped using a clean scoop. All ice cream with gluten-containing ingredients such as cookies or crumbles should always be avoided.

Bertucci's Italian Restaurant

www.bertuccis.com/menu/gluten-free-menu.html

508-351-2500

A good variety of items on their menu are gluten free, including some pasta options.

Bloom's Deli

www.bloomsnewyorkdeli.com

Full gluten-free menu available, including gluten-free pancakes, French toast, and hamburger buns.

Bonefish Grill

www.bonefishgrill.com/menu

Gluten-free and regular menu. Grill base contains gluten and a shared grill is used, but they will prepare foods in a separate pan if you request it.

Boston Market

www.bostonmarket.com/ourFood/index.jsp?page=nutrition

1 (800) 365-7000

Boston Market has a large listing of gluten-free items on its website, but remind them when ordering not to place a corn muffin on top of your chicken.

Boston Pizza

www.bostonpizza.com

A variety of gluten-free pasta and pizza options.

Buca di Beppo

www.bucadibeppo.com

Gluten-free salads and entrees but make sure to remind server so they will modify your menu option.

Bugaboo Creek Steakhouse

www.Bugaboo.com

Gluten-free steaks, ribs, chicken, trout, and some sides.

Burger King

www.bk.com/cms/en/us/cms_out/digital_assets/files/pages/MenuGlutenFree.pdf

1 (305) 378-3535

Burger King lists wheat-free products on its website. At the top of the list, it is mentioned that these items are not for those with severe gluten intolerance. Therefore the gluten-free status of these choices is in question.

Burtons Grill

www.burtonsgrill.com

Gluten-free and vegetarian menus, gluten-free buns for the burgers and fries. At service they bring out gluten-free choices on different shaped plates, making it easy to identify an error during service.

Café Formagio

www.Cafeformagio.com

They serve a huge selection of delicious Italian cuisine and almost every menu item can be made gluten free.

Canyons Restaurant

www.canyonsrestaurant.com

A variety of gluten-free options.

Carvel

www.carvel.com/nutrition

Carvel's lists many of its ice creams as gluten-free on its website. Make sure to avoid sprinkles, crunchies, and any gluten-containing cookie or crumb toppings.

Carrabba's Italian Grill

www.carrabbas.com/Content/menu-gluten-free

Carrabba's Italian Grill has a gluten-free menu on its website. Make sure to request the gluten-free versions of these items. Note they use a gluten-containing grill base and share the same grill with gluten-free orders. Make sure you ask for a manager and request your food be prepared in a separate sauté pan, not on the grill.

Charlie Brown's Steakhouse

www.charliebrowns.com

Many items on the menu are gluten free, but not the buns and bread.

Chick-Fil-A

www.chick-fil-a.com/Food/Allergen-Gluten-Diabetic

Chick-Fil-A's website states that several items may fit into your gluten-free diet as per their suppliers, but this is not guaranteed and should only be used as a guide when making selections.

Chipotle Mexican Grill

www.chipotle.com/en-us/menu/special_diet_information/special_diet_information.aspx

Chipotle offers many gluten-free items, mostly the salad bowls (not the burrito bowls). As stated on the Chipotle website "If you are highly sensitive and would like us to change our gloves, we would be happy to do that at your request."

Cheeseburger in Paradise

www.cheeseburgerinparadise.com/Our-Menu/Gluten-Free-Menu.aspx

Cheeseburger in Paradise has a gluten-free menu on their website.

Chili's

www.Chilis.com

1 (800) 983-4637

Chili's website provides a listing of "Suggested Menu and Beverage Options for Wheat/Gluten Allergies" bundled in a PDF for those with other types of food allergies as well; there are not many gluten-free options listed. This PDF states that Chili's is not able to guarantee that any menu item is completely free of allergens.

Dairy Queen

www.dairyqueen.com

Has a listing of gluten-free menu items available on their website.

Don Pablo's

www.donpablos.com

Many gluten-free Mexican options with a separate gluten-free menu available.

Dunkin' Donuts

www.dunkindonuts.com/content/dunkindonuts/en/menu.html

1 (800) 859-5339

Gluten-free items are not listed on the website, but a few items are listed as wheat free. There has been recent press about the upcoming release of gluten-free donuts so check the website regularly for any changes.

Eat'n Park

www.eatnpark.com

A variety of gluten-free options including gluten-free buns.

First Watch

www.firstwatch.com

A full listing of gluten-free options, including bread and pancakes.

Five Guys Burgers and Fries

www.fiveguys.com

Their burgers without the buns and fries are gluten free. Allergy information is available on their website.

Fleming's Prime Steakhouse & Wine Bar

www.flemingsprimesteakhouse.com

Many gluten-free options including appetizers, entrees, and some desserts too.

Garlic Jim's

www.garlicjims.com

Delivery gluten-free pizzas and salads. Menu available on-line.

Hardee's

www.hardees.com/menu/nutritional_calculator_landing

1 (877) 799-STAR

Hardee's website provides a list of product ingredients. The company also claims that some food items are "wheat- and wheat gluten-free," although this is not an acceptable method for listing gluten-free foods. Many foods may be wheat free yet contain other forms of gluten, so you need to ask questions in order to be safe.

Joe's Crab Shack

www.joescrabshack.com

A variety of seafood bowls with sausage are gluten free.

Kentucky Fried Chicken

www.kentuckyfriedchicken.com/nutrition/#

1 (800) 225-5532

Kentucky Fried Chicken does have an allergy listing on its website that indicates wheat, gluten, and other common allergens. There are not many gluten-free options.

Legal Sea Foods

www.legalseafood.com

Separate gluten-free seafood menu. Note they don't offer a gluten-free cocktail sauce to go with their raw bar, but they do offer gluten-free rolls.

Longhorn Steakhouse

www.longhornsteakhouse.com/menu/nutritional_information.asp

Longhorn Steakhouse has a list of gluten-sensitive menu items. As stated on the menu: *"To ensure that your meal is prepared properly, please request that all items be prepared in separate containers."*

Long John Silver's

www.ljsilvers.com/nutrition/

Long John Silver's has an allergy listing on its website that lists wheat-free and gluten-free items and items containing other common allergens, as well as an ingredient listing.

Mama's Restaurant

www.mamas-restaurant.com

Full Italian gluten-free menu including homemade ravioli and homemade cannolis.

McDonald's

www.mcdonalds.com

1 (800) 244-6227

McDonalds provides "ingredients statements" on its website. They note some allergens, but instead of stating wheat next to sandwiches and burgers, they just write the word "Bun." So wheat isn't clearly listed, making it difficult to easily identify safe gluten-free choices.

Mitchell's Fish Market

www.mitchellsfishmarket.com

A variety of gluten-free seafood options on their menu.

Nizza Restaurant

www.nizzanyc.com

Full gluten-free menu, including homemade chickpea flatbreads (socca) with a Mediterranean flair.

Olive Garden

www.olivegarden.com/menu/gluten-allergen/

The Olive Garden has a gluten-free/allergen-free menu on their website. The website mentions that customers need to ask their servers for the gluten-free versions of these menu items.

Outback Steakhouse

www.outback.com/menu/pdf/glutenfree.pdf

Outback Steakhouse has a downloadable gluten-free menu that is basically their usual menu with items that should be removed. Since it is the same as the regular menu items, double-check when they serve you that they didn't make any errors (like leaving the croutons on your salad).

Panera Bread

www.panerabread.com

Panera bread does have a list of products that do not have gluten-containing ingredients, but because they bake daily they cannot guarantee the gluten-free status of these choices.

Pica Pica

www.Picapica.com

The menu of authentic Venezuelan cuisine is 100 percent naturally gluten free.

P.F. Chang's

www.pfchangs.com/menu/

P.F. Chang's has a gluten-free menu on their website. As stated on the menu, let your server know that you have a food allergy, ask for the gluten-free soy sauce, and double-check when you are served.

Qdoba Mexican Grill

www.qdoba.com/

Allergen listings of all their menu items are available on their website.

Red Brick Pizza

www.redbrickpizza.com
Almost all their menu items including pizza and wraps can be made gluten free. They keep the gluten-free pizza in a separate area from the regular pizza, and will get toppings from the refrigerator if you don't feel comfortable with the toppings on display.

Red Mango

www.redmangousa.com
A large variety of gluten-free frozen yogurt and toppings.

Red Robin

www.redrobin.com
Has a listing of how to make menu items gluten free, plus it is dated when the information was checked and posted so you can see when last updated. There is a warning notice that they cannot be sure of cross-contamination.

Risotteria

www.risotteria.com
Gluten-free risotto, salads, desserts, and more.

Romano's Macaroni Grill

www.macaronigrill.com
They have a listing of all their menu choices with allergen information so you can see which items can be made gluten free.

Ruby Tuesday

www.rubytuesday.com/faq/nutrition/
Has a downloadable allergen/sensitivity menu guide on its website.

Shanes Rib Shack

www.Shanesribshack.com
Has many gluten-free options including entrees and sides.

Starbucks

www.starbucks.com
Few items at Starbucks are gluten-free, but they do offer fruit, some gluten-free bars, and gluten-free beverage choices.

Subway

www.subway.com/nutrition/nutritionlist.aspx
Subway has an allergy listing on its website that indicates wheat, gluten, and other common allergens.

Swiss Chalet

www.Swisschalet.com

Their ribs and chicken are gluten free, but most other items on the menu contain gluten.

Taco Bell

www.tacobell.com/nutrition/allergens

1 (800) TACOBELL

Taco Bell has its gluten-free menu items listed on its website. There are not a lot of choices considering many products are corn based and could be easily converted to gluten free.

Taco Del Mar

www.tacodelmar.com

A large variety of gluten-free Mexican options.

Ted's Montana Grill

www.tedsmontanagrill.com

All items that can be made gluten free are listed online including burgers without buns and a variety of salad options.

Thaifoon

www.thaifoon.com

A variety of Thai options that can be prepared gluten free.

The Melting Pot

www.meltingpot.com

A variety of fondues are available gluten free but you need to take extra care when ordering. Let your server know you can't have the bread for dipping, and that the beer in the fondue should be gluten free. If you are eating with friends who are not gluten-free, make sure they don't dip their bread in your fondue.

UNO Chicago Grill

www.unos.com/nutrition.php

UNO Chicago Grill does have a gluten-free menu, but states on its website: "... however, we cannot be responsible for individual reactions to any food products or guarantee that the food we serve is free from any allergen."

Wendy's

www.wendys.com/en-us/living-without-gluten

1 (614) 764-3100

Wendy's has a "Living Without Gluten" web page where it lists gluten-free menu items, and items at risk for possible cross-contamination.

White Castle

www.whitecastle.com

At this time allergen information is not readily available on the White Castle website, though ingredients are available for review.

ZPizza

www.Zpizza.com

They offer a large variety of toppings for their gluten-free pizza crust.

Handling Your Feelings—And Knowing You're Not Alone

It's Okay to Get Upset

Never! The word seems to carry its own special punishment. If you're like most people, being told that you can never have something only makes you want it more. If you have ever given up your favorite foods for Lent, or leavened bread for Passover, you know how hard it can be to completely abstain from something you love to eat.

Of course, Lent and Passover eventually come to an end, and then you can start eating the forbidden foods again. But with celiac disease and gluten sensitivity, that's not an option. You can never eat foods containing gluten again—for the rest of your life.

Living gluten free isn't what you would expect. It's not just one food that you can't have, but anything that has even the smallest amount of wheat or rye or barley is totally off-limits.

This is why being gluten intolerant can be emotionally painful, especially at first. It's no fun needing to be careful about every little thing you put in your mouth, especially while everyone around you is happily eating whatever they want.

If you're like most people who can no longer eat gluten, you will particularly miss wheat. Those of us who live in the Western world eat wheat at nearly every meal and use it in almost all recipes. Foods containing wheat are served at parties, at family gatherings, in restaurants and bars, at work, and in classrooms. You literally can't avoid it. You can find entire communities that are children free or pet free, but try to find a single block, anywhere in the world, that is totally gluten free, and you're out of luck.

Now for the good news: there's nothing special or natural about eating wheat. People in many cultures eat little or none of it. Over thousands of years, we have learned how to cultivate it, harvest it, mill it, and cook it so that it is tasty to most people. But because it is not especially well-suited to human digestion, some of us simply can't tolerate it. This brings us to another piece of good news. You are anything but alone. Although you may feel lonely and isolated when you first learn that you are gluten intolerant, remember that more than 1 in 100 have celiac disease, an unspecified percentage of the population have a wheat allergy, and an estimated 5 to 6 percent of the population could be non-celiac gluten sensitive.

This book is dedicated to helping you find foods that you fully enjoy while living a sane and healthy gluten-free life. In this chapter, we'll focus on the feelings that can arise for people who can no longer eat gluten.

These feelings are very common. Who wouldn't react strongly to suddenly learning that for the rest of their life they need to live with so many restrictions?

This chapter offers useful strategies for handling your feelings about your gluten sensitivity when you're angry, bored, depressed, embarrassed, hurt, or overwhelmed.

Dealing with Anger

It's not fair! Everyone else is munching on the bread and splitting appetizers I can't touch, while I just sit here biting my nails. Why do people who are supposed to be my friends always order only one appetizer I can have, like grilled shrimp, and then pass everything around the table, leaving me with only one shrimp? Don't they remember that I can't eat any of those other things? Don't they see that I'm just sitting here, starving?

If I give up and order my own separate appetizer, it's obvious that some of them think I'm being petty or neurotic—and half the time it arrives five minutes after my entrée.

I know it's not their fault that I'm gluten intolerant, but they seem completely blind to my situation, even though I've told them about it a thousand times. It makes it hard to enjoy going out to eat with a group. Sometimes I get really mad at them for not noticing my dilemma or making it easier for me.

Why did this have to happen to me?

It's okay to get mad. It isn't fair that you have to be so careful about everything you eat. You didn't choose to be gluten intolerant, and your condition isn't the result of something you did or any decision you made.

It's also important to express your anger, but in a healthy and nonthreatening way—and at an appropriate time and place (not during dinner, perhaps!). Maybe afterward, on your way home, you can say, "I know this is nobody's fault, but sometimes I get angry when people seem to completely forget that I can't eat certain foods. They wouldn't forget if I needed a wheelchair or a seeing-eye dog, would they?" Don't hold your anger in, or you could end up exploding and fighting with family or friends about something else entirely simply because you need to vent. Sharing your feelings will help to build a network of family and friends who can be advocates for you at future events.

You can also avoid these situations by being proactive:

- When a get-together with family or friends is being planned, ask to help plan the meal or choose the restaurant. Suggest or select a restaurant that offers gluten-free choices.

- If someone suggests a restaurant you haven't been to before, check its website before you go, or call ahead to find out what choices you can have. (Make sure there are at least two good entrées for you, so that if one isn't available that day, you won't go hungry.) Talk to the manager to make sure the kitchen staff can prevent cross-contamination issues. If your available options include foods you really enjoy, you will be far less likely to get angry.

- If your dining companions want to share their food, don't be afraid to order your own separate appetizer and/or entrée. If need be, explain why, simply and briefly.

- If you are going to a wedding or some other catered event, call the caterer a few days before, explain your dietary limitations, and ask them to create something special for you. Unless the caterer is brand new, they may be familiar with cooking for people who are unable to eat gluten.

Dealing with Culinary Boredom

A lot of my family favorites have ingredients I can't eat. I've learned how to make gluten-free variations of some of those dishes, and I've created a few of my own gluten-free recipes. But, truth be told, I am not that creative a cook. Now that so many of my favorite ingredients are off-limits, I have a hard time making many dishes that I like anymore. There are a few items that I prepare very well, but I can't eat these same few things every day.

Then when I go out to eat, I either can't figure out what's okay to order, or the limited choices I have to pick from the menu are very plain or tasteless. I am just about bored to death. I wish I could find some more interesting foods to eat.

The urge for variety is simply human nature. Discovering that you can't eat gluten does not make this human urge go away! To spice up your plate:

- Start with the recipes in this book, in chapters 4 and 11. You'll be surprised at how creative, delicious, and simple gluten-free eating can be.

- If you don't usually cook and want to find restaurants that offer great gluten-free options, contact your local celiac support groups as members are generally a good source for up-to-date information and reviews and can help you make good choices. (Information on locating celiac support groups can be found in the resources section—located in the back of the book—through the Celiac Sprue Association and The Gluten Intolerance Group of North America.)

- For further gluten-free culinary excitement, go on a gluten-free vacation or take a gluten-free culinary tour. (Yes, there are such things—more of them than you probably realize. And again, some of these can be found in the resources section.)

- Trade recipes with members from the celiac support centers. Other group members will surely have dealt with the same culinary boredom and will be able to offer a variety of tips and solutions.

Dealing with Depressed Feelings

It's no fun going out to eat anymore. Even weddings and parties, which I used to find exciting, have become humdrum, because either I can't eat anything they serve, or they serve me something gluten free that's also dry and taste free.

I try my best, but I'm getting to the point where I'd rather just stay home, watch TV, and make myself something to eat. Staying home can be easier than having to explain my situation to every single person I see, or being served something that tastes like it came out of a hospital kitchen—but it's also lonely, and I feel like I'm missing all the fun.

Many people live their lives accommodating one or more physical challenges. It's not always possible to be cheerful about it, but it's important not to give in to a victim mentality, or to allow yourself to retreat into isolation. Don't be afraid to be assertive. Yes, it's a pain to explain the same thing over and over—but the results will be tastier food and you will enjoy many health benefits by staying on track.

Furthermore, as more and more people ask for gluten-free choices, chefs, caterers, and cooks will catch on. The result will be an ever-wider variety of even tastier gluten-free options.

Remember how just a few years ago, it was hard to find organic food in restaurants and supermarkets? Or, a few years before that, how few vegetarian options there used to be at most restaurants and events? Gluten-free eating is starting to follow the same curve.

Here are some easy ways to be assertive:

- When you are invited to a party, explain your food restrictions and offer to help the host plan the menu. This isn't being pushy—it's being helpful. Chances are your host will feel relieved, because you're making it easier for him or her to accommodate you.

- Feel free to bring some of your favorite foods with you to the gathering. Depending on the circumstances, it might be a little awkward—but if you needed to take medication, you'd bring that with you, wouldn't you?

Understandably, there will still be some times when you feel it's not worth the trouble and would rather stay home, so try to keep some favorites in the freezer so you can just grab-and-go and still have great choices. If you do opt to stay home, make sure you have some of your favorite gluten-free foods available to enjoy.

The trick is to take the lead so that whether you go out or stay home, you get to eat food that's healthy and that you enjoy.

Dealing with Embarrassment

I've never liked to make a big deal out of what restaurant to go to or what to order. For most of my life, if I was given the wrong dressing or side dish, I'd usually just eat it.

I didn't want to be a food prima donna, and it would embarrass me when other people made a fuss if their food wasn't exactly the way they ordered it.

Now that I know I'm gluten intolerant, everything has changed. I need to explain my diet to every waiter, chef, friend, relative, or person who's eating with me. The one thing that hasn't changed is how I feel about it. All that calling attention to myself and all those special requests make me want to crawl under the table. I feel as though everyone around me is looking at me like I have two heads. I get even more embarrassed when I have to explain it all.

The worst is when I'm at an event like a wedding, and the servers are trying to deliver food to 150 people all at once, and I ask, "Does the gravy have flour in it?" If the server doesn't speak a lot of English, I might as well forget about eating at all. It makes me want to just eat whatever everyone else is eating, even if it makes me sick.

Few of us want to be the center of attention when it comes to our health. And who wants to be referred to in the restaurant kitchen as "the pain in the butt at table 4?" If you don't want to make a fuss, that's fine. You don't have to do anything that goes against your nature. Here's how you can be proactive without calling undue attention to yourself:

- Pick restaurants that already have gluten-free choices on the menu. Then it may be a little easier to order.

- Call ahead of time and talk to the manager (try to choose a time when you know that the restaurant isn't too busy) to see what can be done for you.

- Dine out when the restaurant is not as busy so that chefs and cooks will have an easier time accommodating you.

- Print out the dining-out sheets in chapter 12 and carry them with you. (Or, you can download all 14 languages at www .glutenfreehasslefree.com/facts/living/cards.asp and print them out.) These simple pages explain living without gluten in clear, easy-to-understand language, and then list those foods that you can't eat. Simply hand a list to your server, and ask that the chef use it when preparing your meal.

These cards are included in fourteen languages—English, Arabic, Mandarin, French, German, Greek, Hebrew, Hindi, Italian, Japanese, Spanish, Polish, Thai, and Vietnamese—so they can be used in a wide range of ethnic restaurants, as well as with servers who do not speak much English.

Dealing with Hurt Feelings

When I go to a family event, they don't even try to make this easy for me. They just serve whatever foods they please. Doesn't anyone even care? It's like my childhood all over again: I'm invisible and my needs are completely ignored.

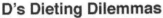

D's Dieting Dilemmas

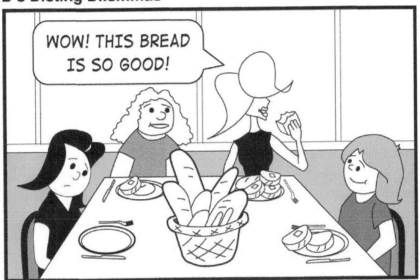

By M. Brown, Ken Brown, and Will Cypser ©

My relatives put out crackers with soft cheese already on them. They toss croutons into the salad, dip the meat in breading, and sprinkle breads crumbs over the vegetables.

When I ask them to just skip the bread crumbs for once, or serve the croutons or crackers separately, they get mad at me. They say, "Just scrape it off," or "Come on, a little won't hurt you. Don't make such a big deal about it, you always ate these foods before." They don't even try to understand. It's like they blame me for making their lives more difficult. It really hurts.

Believe it or not, most people who act this way aren't trying to be hurtful. They just don't understand how important it is that you follow a gluten-free diet at all times. Many simply don't believe that a tiny amount of gluten can harm your health; they just don't get it.

Most people think that celiac disease and non-celiac gluten sensitivity is like diabetes or high blood pressure. Many folks with diabetes can have sugar sometimes, and those with high blood pressure can occasionally have salty food. As a result, a lot of people think that people who don't eat gluten can have a small amount on special occasions. They just assume you're making too big a deal about your dietary restrictions. They may even think you're trying to draw attention to yourself.

You can't always get people to change what they believe, but sometimes you can wake them up by showing them the words of a respected authority. One option is to photocopy "Getting Started Living Gluten Free" in chapter 14, as well as the cover of this book. Give these to your relatives and say, "I brought you this. It explains the whole gluten-free thing much better than I can." If you prefer, send them the web link to "Getting Started Living Gluten-Free"—www.glutenfreehasslefree.com/facts/living/living.asp. Another tip is talking to understanding family members ahead of time so they will speak out on your behalf if others try to bully you.

If that doesn't help, then you may simply need to accept that your family will never change. Whatever their motivations are, you can't make them act differently—so don't try. Some of them may just be clueless. Bring your own foods to family events. If you like, bring gluten-free dishes that anyone would want to eat so your food is the hit. If people make fun of you for eating something different, take your plate into a different room—and, if you can, limit your visits in the future. Overall the best response would be, "You're right. This diet is ridiculous, I hate it, and I really find it very difficult to follow. But the doctor says that if I don't follow it 100 percent of the time I may become ill, so why are you encouraging me not to follow it?"

Dealing with Feeling Overwhelmed

I already have so much to do each day. I can barely keep the house together and get to work on time. I don't have the time to exercise as much as I'd like. Plus, I'd love to catch up on projects I've had on hold for years. I'm already overcommitted, and I feel so tired at the end of each day.

And now this. How can I possibly find the time to plan and cook special meals for myself while taking care of my family, too? I wish I could clone myself so someone else could shop and cook for me.

Most people feel overwhelmed when they first learn they're gluten intolerant. But most of us feel equally overwhelmed when we first begin an exercise program or have our first child or take a new job or go back to school.

So let yourself feel overwhelmed! It's a completely normal and natural feeling.

But remind yourself that this is not the only, the first, or the most difficult challenge that life will throw your way. Also keep in mind that this feeling will go away over time. Once gluten-free living has become a habit, you'll discover that it's not as time-consuming as it is when you first get diagnosed. In fact, because it will greatly improve your health, you'll have more energy and less downtime because of illness. You'll naturally feel less overwhelmed and more able to accomplish everyday tasks, with juice left for your favorite leisure activities.

Part of making a gluten-free lifestyle hassle free is making changes in steps rather than all at once. Start with changes that are easy to make, and make only a few of them at a time. Get familiar with the basic gluten-free foods. Make a gluten-free shopping trip to the supermarket. Start with a few gluten-free recipes and a simple meal plan. Don't try to completely change your life overnight. You'll discover that once you have the first step or two behind you, you'll begin to experience some positive changes, and these in turn will make you excited about incorporating others.

Before you know it, you will find that living a gluten-free life is a lot easier than you thought it would be.

Tips for Living Gluten Free by The Allergic Girl, Sloane Miller, MSW, LMSW, Food Allergy Counselor

Dealing with Anger and Depressed Feelings: After being diagnosed with a medical condition that needs life-long lifestyle management and maintenance, it's normal to have feelings of anger and/or depressed feelings. You may have feelings of loss for your "old" life and those feelings may express themselves as frustration, sadness, hopelessness, or despondency. These are all normal feelings as you adjust to a new lifestyle and help those around you to adjust as well. Be kind to yourself, feel those feelings, talk with a counselor or psychotherapist if you find that those feelings are bleeding into other areas of your life like relationships, work, or recreation.

Dealing with Culinary Boredom: As someone with severe food allergies (tree nuts and fish), each week I add a new, safe-for-me food item to my diet. It could be a new type of vegetable or fruit, or a new safe-for-me treat from a specialty diet food company. As someone with a restricted diet, it's vital to always be expanding your diet in other safe ways. I use this technique with my food allergy counseling clients and encourage them to seek out a registered dietitian, knowledgeable in their dietary needs, for additional support.

Dealing with Embarrassment: Once you fully accept that your dietary needs are just one part of you, embarrassment about advocating for your dietary needs will begin to fall away.

Dealing with Hurt Feelings: It is most important that you understand your medical diagnosis and needs first. Learn how to communicate firmly, factually, and clearly to those around you about your needs. Remember that you never need to apologize for your medical condition. Continue to assert your needs kindly and politely and most people will eventually get on board.

Dealing with Feeling Overwhelmed: It's natural to feel overwhelmed with a medical diagnosis that requires a major lifestyle change. Create manageable, reachable goals and work toward meeting those goals in small, incremental steps. Don't try to do everything at once! And remember, be patient with yourself. Lasting change takes time.

Sloane Miller is the author of *Allergic Girl: Adventures in Living Well with Food Allergies*.

www.allergicgirl.com

STEP II: LIVING GLUTEN FREE

Finding the Hidden Gluten Beyond Food

From Toothpaste to Cosmetics and More

Following a gluten-free diet doesn't just stop with food. Anything that you breathe in or ingest (including vitamins, medications, toothpaste, and lipstick) can contain gluten and can make you ill. Sometimes even the rubber bands used for children's braces are dusted with flour to keep them from sticking together. So knowing where the hidden gluten is can be critical to staying well. Do you know how many lipsticks a typical woman will consume in one year?

So where do you start? Any product that contains gluten that touches your lips or that is in the air you breathe may make you ill, so it's important to check everything you can.

Gluten particles are too large to be absorbed through the skin, but everything that touches your hands has the potential to go into your mouth, so use good handwashing techniques, especially if you use a gluten-containing lotion, shampoo, or sunscreen. Remember, kids will put anything into their mouths, so gluten-free school supplies are a must for a child with celiac disease.

Please note that product formulas change regularly; this list is only a guide. Double-check gluten-free status with each of the manufacturers of the brands you use prior to use.

D's Dieting Dilemmas

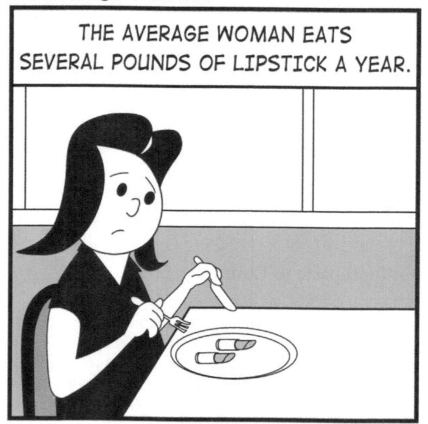

By M. Brown, Ken Brown, and Will Cypser ©

Many common household and personal items can contain gluten, including:

- Lipstick, lip balm, shampoo, soap, cosmetics, and skin lotion (although even if gluten containing it would be unlikely that these products would have more then 20 ppm)

- Mouthwash and toothpaste could possibly contain gluten

- Household products such as cleaning solutions and detergents

- Vitamins and medicines: pills may be dusted in flour, capsules may contain gluten in the oil inside the capsule (glutenfreedrugs. com offers a list of medications that have been checked for gluten)

- Latex or rubber gloves: used to wash dishes and used for food preparation, but may be dusted with wheat or oat flour; be sure to also ask your dentist, doctor, orthodontist, and periodontist to use unpowdered gloves

- School and art supplies such as face paints, markers, glue and glue sticks, paste, tape, hand stamps, Play-Doh, Crayola clay, and Nickelodeon's Floam

- Also some sunscreens and some self-adhesive bandages

- Toothbrushes that are kept in the same holder as those of other family members can get contaminated

TIP Your pharmacist may be able to tell you if your medication is gluten free, but you may need to call the manufacturer or pharmaceutical company to be absolutely sure. Lists of some medications that have been checked for gluten can be found at www.glutenfreedrugs.com.

Some products that are gluten free include:

- **Cosmetics and lip balm:** Lancôme, Chapstick, Blistex (Afterglow Cosmetics has an entire line of gluten-free products)

- **Sunscreens and self-tanners:** Banana Boat children's sunscreen, Lancôme Flash Bronzer Glow 'n Wear Gel, Aveda Sun Source

- **Soaps, shampoos, and laundry detergent:** Arm and Hammer baking soda detergent, Kirkman Labs' Kleen Products soaps and shampoos, Colgate-Palmolive softsoaps, Suave and Dove (gluten ingredients identified on label if present), Pampers Baby Wipes, Purell and Germ-X instant hand sanitizers

- **Dental products:** Aquafresh, Colgate, and Crest toothpaste, Whitestrips, and Night Effects, Gleem toothpaste, Glide dental floss, Polident tablets, Rembrant, Tom's of Maine, Ultrabrite, Anbesol baby, Anbesol Cold Sore Therapy Gel, Oasis moisturizing mouth spray, Oral B Prophy Paste Stages Tooth and Gum Care

- **School Supplies:** Crayola Model Magic modeling material, Model Magic Fusion, Modeling Clay, and Air-Dry Clay, Silly Putty, ColorWonder Fingerpaints, paints, crayons, pencils, markers, modeling clay, glue, glitter glue, and chalk; Elmer's glue, glue sticks, crayons, paints, and watercolors; Roseart stickers, RoseArt crayons, RoseArt markers; Scotch Magic Tape; Palmer Paint; Prang Paints

- **Other:** Johnson and Johnson Band-Aids, Kleenex tissues with lotion and antiviral tissues, Puffs with lotion, Cold-eeze All Natural Lozenges, Country Life vitamins, Freeda Vitamins, Wegman's Chewable Vitamins, Nicorette gum

> **TIP** Always read ingredient lists or check with manufacturer to confirm that a product is gluten free.

How to Gluten-Proof Your Home

In the beginning of this chapter, you learned that gluten can be consumed from nonfood items—just by using everyday products. But these are not the only ways you can accidently take in gluten. It can actually get into your food from hidden sources in your kitchen and around your house. Since most meals are eaten at home, you must gluten-proof your home or at least a food preparation area to prevent contaminating your food choices every day. This is especially important when others are bringing gluten-containing grains into the same areas where you will be having your foods.

Equipment

Using pans and equipment in your kitchen that others use for gluten-containing foods can contaminate your foods.

- Use a separate toaster or protect your food with toaster bags (www.toastitbags.com).

- Protect your food from gluten by having a separate tray for your toaster oven, or make sure you cover the cooking surface with aluminum foil if it is not dedicated gluten free.

- Make sure you don't put food directly on the bottom of the microwave, where gluten can be lurking, without a protective plate.

- Thoroughly clean your grill or cover the surface with aluminum foil.

- Have separate colanders, tongs, spatulas, and sheet pans for your gluten-free cooking. Although tongs and spatulas can be cleaned and then safely used it is difficult to completely clean a colander for safe gluten-free use. Make sure these cooking utensils look different from the others in your house so they don't accidently get mixed up.

Storing Ingredients

It isn't enough to just buy gluten-free foods; you need to store them safely in your home.

- Make sure your condiments are marked separately from those that the rest of the family uses. This includes mayo, mustard, butter, margarine, jam, peanut butter, and any food item you use a spoon or knife to spread. It isn't that you can't use the same condiments as others (most are gluten free), it's that most people double-dip with the knife after using it to touch bread and can cross-contaminate these foods. Having your own spreads and marking them, and using squeeze bottles, helps prevent this from happening.

- Wipe down all cooking surfaces before preparing your gluten-free foods. Some gluten-containing residues, such as flour, can stay in the air for hours and then settle on working surfaces.

- When it comes to storing your gluten-free flours, pastas, crackers, and cereals, keep them in airtight containers stored on upper shelves. Storing them on lower shelves may lead to some gluten-containing ingredients accidently falling in from residues on the shelves above them.

How to Be Gluten Free at Work

Work environments can be tricky because you don't always have the resources and control that you would have at home. You may not have a refrigerator, toaster, and microwave to store and heat your gluten-free foods. There may be meetings, trade shows, and workshops that include set catered menus. You may not have the opportunity to bring in food, so find out what the menu is ahead of time, and ask about the ingredients. It is not only that it may not be easy to control your food here, but in a working business situation it may not always be in your best interest to ask and talk too much about the food. You are conducting business, not out for a good time (as some might put it).

Sometimes asking lots of little questions can be perceived by some business associates as a negative part of your personality, or just being neurotic. They think you are making a big deal about little things. So how do you deal with this? As before, simply plan. Usually business meetings are booked ahead of time, so you can figure on covering your meals for that day. Carry things with you that are easy to bring into your meetings so you can pull out your food when breaks or meals are taken. Some examples include gluten-free bars, fresh fruit, dried fruit

D's Dieting Dilemmas

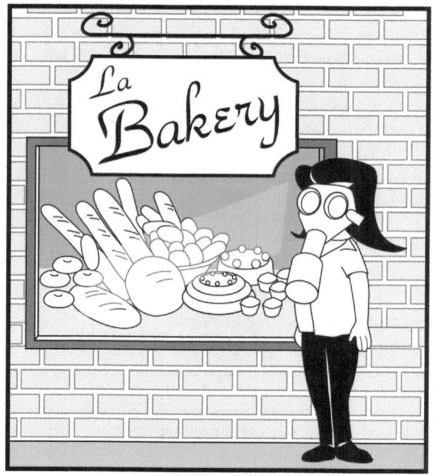

By M. Brown, Ken Brown, and Will Cypser ©

and nuts, yogurt, and gluten-free crackers. In some cases you can even pack a gluten-free sandwich as long as you package the meat and bread separately (it is important to pack the bread separately from the filling, since gluten-free bread can get soggy pretty easily, although cheese sandwiches and nut butters hold up as a sandwich longer). There may be some safe food choices that you can pick up at the meeting, and combining them with the foods you brought with you gives you a complete meal. The most important thing is getting through your meeting while still being able to have safe foods throughout the day.

Gluten in the Air

Gluten can be lurking in places you would never expect, and there have been cases where bakery workers with celiac disease have gotten ill by breathing flour. There is a lot of flour in the air in bakeries and pizzerias where dough is made from scratch. The flour gets puffed into the air, and the particles go everywhere. If you touch something and then your mouth, or if you breathe gluten in (the gluten in the nose will eventually be swallowed), you have then consumed gluten. The amount of gluten consumed is so small that it might not cause a reaction in some people (based on tolerance levels), but others who are extremely sensitive may get sick from being in this environment for even a short time. Also, for those who work in that environment every day the effect can be cumulative, catching up to them in time. There is also a danger if you are gluten free but live in a home where someone bakes with gluten-containing ingredients. Gluten-containing flour may be unavoidable as it gets into the air and spreads so easily. It would be ideal if this family member could learn to bake gluten free.

Eating a Balanced Gluten-Free Diet

Easy Replacements for Missing Nutrients

When you are following a gluten-free diet, you are giving up many foods that have important nutritional value. This means that you are no longer taking in some nutrients that are important for your body. This chapter will explore the nutrients that you are missing and how to get them in other ways, as well as extra supplements that may be beneficial. Lastly, since food intolerances do not occur in a vacuum, this chapter will try to help those of you who are dealing with more than one food intolerance at a time.

In addition, if you have just started a gluten-free diet, you may already have mild nutritional deficiencies due to your intestine's inability to absorb all the nutrients in the foods you were consuming. It is important for you to make up for those losses and rebuild the missing stores in your body. Then, after you have recovered, there are still going to be nutrients that are more difficult to get due to the limitations in the foods you can consume. This is why these nutrients are listed separately. To see the USDA current recommendations for vitamins and nutrients, go to www.nutrition.gov. (Nutrition information in the following charts was obtained from the USDA's National Nutrient Database for Standard Reference, Release 25, Software v.1.2.2, http://ndb.nal.usda .gov/ndb/search/list.)

TIP Use the tables in this chapter to help you make sure you include foods that supply additional healthful nutrients to your meal planning. This is especially important because many with celiac disease may already have nutrient deficiencies.

Vitamin A

Vitamin A is a vitamin that is associated with eye health. A person with celiac disease who has steatorrhea (fatty diarrhea from fat malabsorption) can be deficient in vitamin A. The reason for this is that vitamin A is what is called "fat-soluble." This means that vitamin A likes fat—not water.

Deficiency of this vitamin is rare. If you have or have had steatorrhea, have your doctor check you for a vitamin A deficiency. Correction of this deficiency is usually by supplementation of the vitamin. It is also easy to get vitamin A from your diet since we can make vitamin A from carotinoids. Carotinoids are the yellow, orange, and red colors we see in our fruits and vegetables. This is why carrots are good for your eyes.

Vitamin B1 (Thiamin)

Thiamin or vitamin B1 is found naturally in the hull of grains. In the United States, we started to see deficiencies of this vitamin with the invention of white bread. The process of making bread "white" also stripped off the valuable nutrients hiding in the hull—thiamin, riboflavin, niacin, and fiber, to name a few. The FDA made it a requirement that thiamin be added back into the grain after it was refined. This process is called enrichment. Since mainly wheat and rice are refined, the enrichment program focuses on those grains. Many gluten-free baked products are refined but are currently not enriched, making them very poor sources of many nutrients.

Now if you start putting the pieces together, you see that on a gluten-free diet, with the removal of wheat products, it is very possible to have a thiamin deficiency. Grains that are used as gluten replacements have not been part of the enrichment program in the past. Today, we are seeing many of these manufacturers now including these replacement grains in their enrichment programs—but not all. Getting sufficient amounts of thiamin in your diet, for example, means eating a varied diet.

Generally foods that are a good source of thiamin include beans, soy milk, and pork. The following list includes some other foods and the amount of thiamin in each of the servings listed.

Flours, Grains, Beans, Seeds	Serving Size	Thiamin (mg)
Sunflower seed flour	1 cup	2.0 mg
Corn flour (masa), white or yellow	1 cup	1.7 mg
Soy flour	1 cup	0.7 mg
Rice bran	1 cup	3.2 mg
Rice, white, long-grain, enriched, raw	1 cup	1.1 mg
Rice, white, long-grain, enriched, cooked	1 cup	0.3 mg
Rice, white, medium grain, enriched, raw	1 cup	1.1 mg
Rice, white, medium grain, enriched, cooked	1 cup	0.3 mg
Rice, white, short grain, enriched, raw	1 cup	1.1 mg
Rice, white, short grain, enriched, cooked	1 cup	0.3 mg
Rice, white, long-grain, enriched, raw	1 cup	1.1 mg
Rice, white, long-grain, enriched, cooked	1 cup	0.3 mg
Lentils, raw	1 cup	1.7 mg
Lentils, boiled without salt	1 cup	0.3 mg

(continued)

Flours, Grains, Beans, Seeds (continued)	Serving Size	Thiamin (mg)
Soybeans, mature seeds, raw	1 cup	1.6 mg
Soybeans, mature cooked, boiled	1 cup	0.3 mg
Navy beans, raw	1 cup	1.6 mg
Navy beans, canned	1 cup	0.4 mg
Sesame seeds, whole, dried	1 cup	1.1 mg
Peas, split, raw	1 cup	1.4 mg
Peas, split, boiled	1 cup	0.4 mg
Pinto beans, raw	1 cup	1.4 mg
Pinto beans, cooked	1 cup	0.3 mg
Great northern beans, raw	1 cup	1.2 mg
Great northern beans, boiled	1 cup	0.3 mg
Kidney beans, raw	1 cup	1.0 mg
Kidney beans, boiled	1 cup	0.3 mg
Brazil nuts	1 oz	0.2 mg
Flaxseed, whole	1 Tbsp	0.2 mg
Pistachio nuts	1 oz	0.2 mg
Macadamia nuts	1 oz	0.2 mg
Pecans	1 oz	0.2 mg
Hazelnuts	1 oz	0.2 mg
Meat and Fish		
Pork, tenderloin, roasted	3 oz	0.8 mg
Pompano, cooked, dry heat	3 oz	0.6 mg

(continued)

Meat and Fish (continued)	Serving Size	Thiamin (mg)
Tuna, fresh, bluefin, cooked, dry heat	3 oz	0.2 mg
Vegetables		
Sun-dried tomatoes	½ cup	0.15 mg

Vitamin B2 (Riboflavin)

Riboflavin was once called vitamin B2. It, too, is found in the hulls of grains and is thus part of the enrichment program. Riboflavin is even easier to get than thiamin because it is more common in foods.

Generally, foods that are a good source of riboflavin include meats and dairy. The following list includes some other foods that are good sources of riboflavin.

Flours	Serving Size	Riboflavin (mg)
Soy flour, full fat	1 cup	1.0 mg
Corn flour (masa), white or yellow	1 cup	0.9 mg
Legumes, Nuts, Seeds		
Soybeans, dry roasted	1 cup	0.7 mg
Soybeans, green, boiled	1 cup	0.3 mg
Soybeans, mature, boiled	1 cup	0.5 mg
Almonds	1 oz	0.3 mg
Sesame seed butter, tahini, from roasted and toasted kernels	2 Tbsp	0.1 mg

Meat, Fish	Serving Size	Riboflavin (mg)
Pork, loin, roasted	3 oz	0.2 mg
Mackerel, Atlantic, cooked, dry heat	3 oz	0.4 mg

Milk, Eggs, Cheese, Vegetables		
Milk, whole	1 cup	0.4 mg
Eggs	1 large	0.2 mg
Feta cheese	1 oz	0.2 mg
Roquefort cheese	1 oz	0.2 mg
American cheese	1 oz	0.1 mg
Shitake mushrooms, dried	15 grams (4 mushrooms)	0.2 mg

Vitamin B3 (Niacin)

Niacin was once called vitamin B3. It is a vitamin that we can make in our body, but not in large enough amounts. In order to make it, we need protein foods in our diets that contain an amino acid called tryptophan. Thus, meat, poultry, fish, and dairy foods, all of which contain tryptophan, are good sources. Niacin is also found in the enrichment program, for the same reasons thiamin and riboflavin are. Generally, good sources of niacin are some meats, nuts, and yeasts. The following table lists some good sources of niacin.

Flours, Grains	Serving Size	Niacin (mg)
Peanut flour, defatted	1 cup	16.2 mg
Corn flour (masa), white or yellow	1 cup	11.3 mg
Rice flour, brown	1 cup	10.0 mg

(continued)

Flours, Grains (continued)	Serving Size	Niacin (mg)
Buckwheat flour	1 cup	7.4 mg
Potato flour	1 cup	5.6 mg
Sunflower seed flour	1 cup	4.7 mg
Rice flour, white	1 cup	4.1 mg
Sesame seed flour	1 ounce	3.8 mg
Soy flour, full-fat, raw	1 cup	3.6 mg
Chickpea flour	1 cup	1.6 mg
Millet, raw	1 cup	9.4 mg
Millet, cooked	1 cup	2.3 mg
Rice, long-grain, brown, raw	1 cup	9.4 mg
Rice, long-grain, brown, cooked	1 cup	3.0 mg
Buckwheat groats (kasha), dry	1 cup	8.4 mg
Buckwheat groats (kasha), cooked	1 cup	1.6 mg
Rice, white, long-grain, raw, enriched	1 cup	7.8 mg
Rice, white, long grain, cooked, enriched	1 cup	2.3 mg
Teff, uncooked	1 cup	6.5 mg
Teff, cooked	1 cup	2.3 mg
Corn, white	1 cup	6.0 mg
Cornmeal, whole-grain, white or yellow	1 cup	4.4 mg

(continued)

Flours, Grains (continued)	Serving Size	Niacin (mg)
Rice, wild, raw	1 cup	10.8 mg
Rice, wild, cooked	1 cup	2.1 mg
Beans, Seeds, Nuts, Protein		
Peas, split, raw	1 cup	5.7 mg
Peas, split, boiled	1 cup	1.7 mg
Lentils, raw	1 cup	5.0 mg
Navy beans, raw	1 cup	4.6 mg
Navy beans, boiled	1 cup	1.2 mg
Peanuts, oil-roasted	1 oz	3.9 mg
Kidney beans, raw	1 cup	3.8 mg
Kidney beans, boiled	1 cup	1.0 mg
Black beans, raw	1 cup	3.8 mg
Black beans, boiled	1 cup	0.9 mg
Sunflower seeds, dry roasted	1 oz	2.0 mg
Chickpeas, boiled	1 cup	0.9 mg
Soybeans, green, raw (edamame)	1 cup	4.2 mg
Soybeans, mature seeds, raw	1 cup	3.0 mg
Soybeans, mature seeds, boiled	1 cup	0.7 mg
Peanut butter, smooth	2 Tbsp	4.3 mg
Tuna, light, canned in water, drained	3 oz	8.6 mg
Tuna, skipjack, fresh, cooked using dry heat	3 oz	15.9 mg

(continued)

Beans, Seeds, Nuts, Protein (continued)	Serving Size	Niacin (mg)
Chicken, roasted	1 cup (140 g)	11.0 mg
Veal, loin, lean, roasted	3 oz	8.0 mg
Swordfish, cooked, dry heat	3 oz	7.9 mg
Mackerel, king, cooked using dry heat	3 oz	8.9 mg
Pork, tenderloin, roasted	3 oz	6.3 mg
Salmon, sockeye, cooked using dry heat	3 oz	8.2 mg
Beef, tenderloin, steak, broiled	3 oz	6.0 mg
Turkey, roasted	3 oz	8.1 mg
Halibut, Atlantic and Pacific, cooked using dry heat	3 oz	6.7 mg
Tilapia, cooked using dry heat	1 fillet (87g)	4.1 mg
Haddock, cooked using dry heat	3 oz	3.5 mg
Pompano, cooked using dry heat	3 oz	3.2 mg
Octopus, cooked using moist heat	3 oz	3.2 mg
Crab, dungeness, cooked using moist heat	3 oz	3.1 mg
Clams, cooked using moist heat	3 oz	2.9 mg
Soymilk, enhanced (extra or plus)	1 cup	8.0 mg
Soymilk, unfortified	1 cup	1.2 mg

Vegetables, Fruit	Serving Size	Niacin (mg)
Portabella mushrooms, grilled	1 cup	7.6 mg
Maitake mushrooms, raw	1 cup	4.6 mg
Shitake mushrooms, dried	4 mushrooms (15g)	2.1 mg
Tomatoes, raw	1 cup (chopped)	1.1 mg
White mushrooms, cooked	½ cup	3.5 mg
Potato, white, with skin, baked	1 small	2.1 mg
Peas, green, boiled	1 cup	3.2 mg
Potato, sweet, baked in skin	1 cup	3.0 mg
Sun-dried tomatoes	½ cup	2.5 mg
Tomatillo, raw	1 cup	1.2 mg
Prunes	1 cup	3.3 mg
Apricots, dried, halves	1 cup	3.4 mg

Vitamin B9 (Folate)

Folate, also known as folic acid, is a water-soluble B vitamin that is very important to our health. A deficiency will lead to anemia. Even before a woman knows she is pregnant, folic acid is needed to ensure that the cells of the fetus will divide properly. Since this vitamin is important in the very early stages of pregnancy, the United States added it to the enrichment program of products such as cereal. Folate is easily lost in the cooking process, since it is water-soluble. The best way to get folate is to increase folate-containing foods in your diet. If you are trying to get pregnant or are pregnant, a supplement is recommended, but generally folate can be found in vegetables. The table below provides a list of foods that are good sources of folate.

Flours, Grains, Beans	Serving Size	Folate (mcg)
Chickpea flour	1 cup	402 mcg
Soy flour, full-fat, raw	1 cup	290 mcg
Corn flour (masa), white or yellow	1 cup	382 mcg
Peanut flour, defatted	1 cup	149 mcg
Buckwheat flour, whole-groat	1 cup	65.0 mcg
Cornmeal, degermed, enriched, white or yellow	1 cup	526 mcg
Quinoa, uncooked	1 cup	313 mcg
Quinoa, cooked	1 cup	78 mcg
Rice, white, long grain, parboiled, enriched, cooked	1 cup	215 mcg
Millet, raw	1 cup	170 mcg
Millet, cooked	1 cup	33 mcg
Amaranth, uncooked	1 cup	158 mcg
Rice, wild, raw	1 cup	152 mcg
Rice, wild, cooked	1 cup	43 mcg
Teff, cooked	1 cup	45 mcg
Chickpeas, raw	1 cup	1114 mcg
Chickpeas, boiled	1 cup	282 mcg
Pinto beans, raw	1 cup	1013 mcg
Pinto beans, boiled	1 cup	294 mcg

(continued)

Flours, Grains, Beans (continued)	Serving Size	Folate (mcg)
Lentils, raw	1 cup	920 mcg
Lentils, boiled	1 cup	358 mcg
Great northern beans, raw	1 cup	882 mcg
Great northern beans, boiled	1 cup	181 mcg
Navy beans, raw	1 cup	757 mcg
Navy beans, boiled	1 cup	255 mcg
Kidney beans, raw	1 cup	725 mcg
Kidney beans, boiled	1 cup	230 mcg
Lima beans, raw	1 cup	703 mcg
Lima beans, boiled	1 cup	156 mcg

Seeds, Nuts, Protein, Vegetables, Fruits		
Sunflower seeds	1 cup	318 mcg
Sesame seeds, whole, dried	1 cup	140 mcg
Flaxseeds	1 cup	146 mcg
Peanut butter, smooth style	2 Tbsp	24 mcg
Conch	1 oz	30 mcg
Mussels, cooked using moist heat	3 oz	65 mcg
Crab, dungeness, cooked using moist heat	3 oz	36 mcg
Edamame	1 cup	482 mcg
Brussels sprouts, boiled	1 cup	157 mcg

(continued)

Seeds, Nuts, Protein, Vegetables, Fruits (continued)	Serving Size	Folate (mcg)
Beets, raw	1 cup	148 mcg
Asparagus, boiled	½ cup	134 mcg
Turnip greens, raw	1 cup	107 mcg
Mustard greens, raw	1 cup	7 mcg
Broccoli, cooked	½ cup	84 mcg
Endive, raw	½ cup	36 mcg
Spinach, raw	1 cup	58 mcg
Boysenberries	1 cup	83 mcg
Guava	1 cup	81 mcg
Pineapple juice	1 cup	45 mcg
Orange juice	1 cup	74 mcg
Oranges, Valencia	1 cup, sections	70 mcg
Papaya	1 cup, 1" pieces	54 mcg
Plantains, cooked	1 cup, mashed	52 mcg

Vitamin B12

Vitamin B12 is a very important vitamin for the health and proper functioning of your nervous system. Additionally, when deficient in this vitamin, you can get an anemia. This vitamin is only found in animal products, so vegetarians that exclude all animal products (vegans) need to work on getting this vitamin elsewhere. This vitamin is absorbed in the lower part of the small intestine, and absorption can be affected by damage to the villi in this area. The following table shows some foods that are good sources of vitamin B12.

Fish, Beef, Poultry	Serving Size	Vitamin B12 (mcg)
Clams, cooked using moist heat	3 oz	84.1 mcg
Oysters, Pacific, cooked using moist heat	3 oz	24.5 mcg
Mussels, cooked using moist heat	3 oz	20.4 mcg
Mackerel, Atlantic, cooked using dry heat	3 oz	16.2 mcg
Herring, Atlantic, cooked using dry heat	3 oz	11.2 mcg
Tuna, fresh, bluefin, cooked using dry heat	3 oz	9.3 mcg
Tuna, white, canned in water, drained	3 oz	1.0 mcg
Sardines, canned in oil, drained	1 oz	2.5 mcg
Beef, tenderloin, roasted	3 oz	2.1 mcg
Salmon, sockeye, cooked using dry heat	3 oz	4.8 mcg
Turkey, roasted	3 oz	0.8 mcg
Pork, tenderloin, roasted	3 oz	0.5 mcg
Chicken, roasted	1 cup, chopped or diced (140g)	0.4 mcg
Dairy and Eggs		
Yogurt, plain, low fat	1 cup	1.4 mcg
Milk, whole	1 cup	1.1 mcg
Swiss cheese	1 oz	0.9 mcg

(continued)

Dairy and Eggs (continued)	Serving Size	Vitamin B12 (mcg)
Mozzarella cheese	1 oz	0.7 mcg
Eggs	1 large	0.6 mcg

Vitamin D

Vitamin D is also called the sunshine vitamin, since we make it when we are exposed to sunlight. However, we cannot make it in adequate amounts daily, especially during the colder weather and in northern locations, so we really need to get it from our diets. Vitamin D is so important because it is what makes calcium work in our bodies. Without vitamin D, we can have problems with our bones. This is a common deficiency in individuals with celiac disease, since the small intestine damage leads to a decrease in its absorption—especially with steatorrhea (as is the case with vitamin A).

Even without gluten and digestive tract problems, most of us do not get enough vitamin D. Not many foods have adequate amounts, and with the increased use of sunscreen, vitamin D is produced in even smaller amounts. The best sources are fortified milk and cold water fish. Some other good sources of vitamin D are listed in the following table.

Fish, Dairy, Soy, Fruit	Serving Size	Vitamin D (mcg)
Cod liver oil	1 tsp	11.2 mcg
Herring, Atlantic, cooked using dry heat	3 oz	4.6 mcg
Salmon, sockeye, cooked using dry heat	3 oz	11.1 mcg
Trout, rainbow, farmed, cooked using dry heat	3 oz	16.2 mcg

(continued)

Fish, Dairy, Soy, Fruit (continued)	Serving Size	Vitamin D (mcg)
Catfish, farmed, cooked using dry heat	3 oz	0.3 mcg
Sardines, Atlantic, canned in oil, drained	3 oz	4.2 mcg
Milk, whole, added vitamin D	1 cup	3.2 mcg
Soymilk, with added Ca, A, and D	1 cup	2.7 mcg
Orange juice, fortified with Ca and D	1 cup	2.5 mcg

Vitamin K

Vitamin K is like vitamins A and D in that it is fat-soluble. It is an important vitamin, since its job is to help your blood clot. It also works in the bones, so with a deficiency, bone strength is compromised. Some people with celiac disease will have symptoms of blood-clotting problems and will need to get vitamin K to resolve those issues. Vitamin K is found naturally in many foods, including dark green vegetables and all animal and plant foods.

Calcium

Calcium is a mineral that we need for many functions in the body. The most commonly known need is for bone strength. But it also contributes to proper function of muscle cell contraction and to nerve transmission. The body thinks that this is the most important function and will actually pull calcium from your bones, if there is not enough in the diet, to make sure there is enough for this work. So it is important to consume enough calcium to keep bones strong.

Because of the vitamin D deficiency that accompanies celiac disease, calcium is usually also deficient—remember, vitamin D works to get calcium into your body. Once the intestinal villi return to normal, you should be absorbing calcium like other people, but we all tend to have problems getting enough calcium (and depending how long it took for you to get diagnosed, you may have lost more calcium from your bones then an average person your age).

Calcium is found mainly in milk and dairy products, but can also be found in other foods.

Flours, Grains, Beans, Seeds	Serving Size	Calcium (mg)
Soy flour, full-fat, raw	1 cup	173 mg
Corn flour (masa), white or yellow	1 cup	155 mg
Cornmeal, enriched, white or yellow	1 cup	5 mg
Teff, uncooked	1 cup	347 mg
Amaranth, uncooked	1 cup	307 mg
Soybeans, mature, raw	1 cup	515 mg
Sesame seeds	1 Tbsp	88 mg
Sesame seed paste, tahini, from unroasted kernels	2 Tbsp	40 mg
Navy beans, raw	1 cup	306 mg
Navy beans, cooked	1 cup	126 mg
Great northern beans, raw	1 cup	320 mg
Great northern beans, boiled	1 cup	120 måg
Kidney beans, raw	1 cup	153 mg
Kidney beans, boiled	1 cup	62 mg

Protein, Vegetables, Fruits

	Serving Size	Calcium (mg)
Sardines (with bone)	3 oz	324 mg
Salmon, sockeye, canned (with bone)	3 oz	203 mg
Mackerel, jack, canned	3 oz	204 mg
Shrimp, canned	3 oz	123 mg
Spinach, raw	1 cup	30 mg
Collards, cooked	1 cup	268 mg

(continued)

Protein, Vegetables, Fruits (*continued*)	Serving Size	Calcium (mg)
Kale, raw	1 cup (chopped)	100 mg
Turnip greens, raw	1 cup (chopped)	104 mg
Broccoli rabe, cooked	1 bunch, cooked (437g)	516 mg
Orange juice, calcium fortified	1 cup	349 mg
Dairy		
Milk, whole	1 cup	276 mg
Yogurt, plain, low fat	1 cup	448 mg
Ricotta cheese, part skim milk	½ cup	337 mg
Romano cheese	1 oz	302 mg
Gruyere	1 oz	287 mg
Parmesan cheese	¼ cup	277 mg
Mozzarella, part skim milk	1 oz	207 mg
Cheddar	1 oz	204 mg
Provolone cheese	1 oz	212 mg
Monterey	1 oz	209 mg
Muenster	1 oz	201 mg
Gouda cheese	1 oz	198 mg
Roquefort cheese	1 oz	188 mg
Blue cheese	1 oz	150 mg
Feta cheese	1 oz	140 mg

Iron

Iron is a mineral that is very important in keeping oxygen in your blood. Without enough iron, you will get anemia. Iron deficiency anemia is common in undiagnosed celiac disease. Once the villi in the intestines have healed and the iron deficiency is corrected with supplements, it is important to continue to get enough iron from your diet. First, if you are a woman you lose iron monthly and your needs are greater. Second, iron (along with thiamin, riboflavin, niacin, and folate) is a part of the enrichment program in the United States, but although wheat-containing products will have iron and these other nutrients added, the program does not require enrichment for gluten-free grains.

Iron comes in two forms: heme (from hemoglobin) and nonheme. The body absorbs heme iron—found in red meat, fish, and poultry—more easily. Nonheme iron—mainly found in vegetables, grains, eggs, and fruits—is not as easily absorbed, but we can increase absorption by increasing or decreasing the amounts of certain foods that we eat in meals that contain nonheme sources of iron.

Since nonheme iron can be better absorbed by changing what we eat (or don't eat) with it, we should start there.

- Eat red meat, poultry, or fish with a nonheme (produce form) source of iron. This works because heme iron (such as in meat) improves the absorption of nonheme iron. For example, you might have spinach (nonheme) with steak (heme).

- Have a little vitamin C with your nonheme iron. This works because vitamin C helps the nonheme iron get into your body. For example, you could have your scrambled eggs with orange juice or have a mandarin orange and spinach salad. And in case you were wondering, vitamin C food sources are not only citrus fruits. You can also find vitamin C in kiwi, strawberries, cantaloupe, broccoli, tomatoes, potatoes, peppers, and cabbage.

- Avoid taking non-heme iron foods with coffee or tea, which contain tannins. Foods that contain tannins prevent the absorption of nonheme iron.

- Try to get more iron (heme or nonheme). Here is a short list of some foods that are a good source of iron:

Flours	Serving Size	Iron (mg)
Soy flour, defatted	1 cup	9.7 mg
Sorghum flour	1 cup	3.6 mg
Corn flour, enriched, white or yellow	1 cup	8.5 mg
Buckwheat flour	1 cup	4.9 mg
Chickpea flour	1 cup	4.5 mg
Sunflower seed flour, partially defatted	1 cup	4.2 mg
Rice flour, brown	1 cup	3.1 mg
Grains		
Amaranth, uncooked	1 cup	14.7 mg
Teff, uncooked	1 cup	14.7 mg
Rice, white, enriched, raw	1 cup	8.0 mg
Rice, white, enriched, cooked	1 cup	1.9 mg
Quinoa, uncooked	1 cup	7.8 mg
Quinoa, cooked	1 cup	2.8 mg
Millet, raw	1 cup	6.0 mg
Millet, cooked	1 cup	1.1 mg
Corn, yellow or white	1 cup	4.5 mg
Buckwheat, groats (kasha), dry	1 cup	4.1 mg
Rice, wild, raw	1 cup	3.1 mg
Rice, wild, cooked	1 cup	1.0 mg

(continued)

Beans, Seeds	Serving Size	Iron (mg)
White beans, raw	1 cup	21.1 mg
White beans, boiled	1 cup	5.1 mg
Kidney beans, raw	1 cup	15.1 mg
Kidney beans, boiled	1 cup	5.2 mg
Lima beans, raw	1 cup	13.3 mg
Lima beans, boiled	1 cup	4.2 mg
Lentils, raw	1 cup	14.5 mg
Lentils, boiled	1 cup	6.6 mg
Chickpeas, raw	1 cup	12.5 mg
Chickpeas, boiled	1 cup	4.7 mg
Navy beans, raw	1 cup	11.4 mg
Navy beans, boiled	1 cup	4.3 mg
Great northern beans, raw	1 cup	10.0 mg
Great northern beans, boiled	1 cup	3.8 mg
Pinto beans, raw	1 cup	9.8 mg
Pinto beans, boiled	1 cup	3.6 mg
Flaxseeds, whole	1 Tbsp	0.6 mg
Soybeans, boiled	1 cup	4.5 mg
Pumpkin seeds, dried	1oz	2.5 mg
Sesame seeds	1 Tbsp	1.3 mg

Protein, Vegetables

Oysters, Pacific, cooked using moist heat	3 oz	7.8 mg
Mussels, cooked using moist heat	3 oz	5.7 mg
Beef, tenderloin, roasted	3 oz	2.7 mg
Lamb, loin, broiled	3 oz	1.7 mg
Turkey, dark meat	3 oz	1.2 mg
Turkey, white meat	3 oz	0.6 mg
Spinach, cooked	1 cup	6.4 mg
Tomatoes, sun-dried	1 cup	4.9 mg
Edamame, cooked	1 cup	3.5 mg
Asparagus, raw	1 cup	2.9 mg
Kale, raw	1 cup	1.0 mg
Chard, Swiss, cooked	½ cup	2.0 mg
Peas, cooked	½ cup	1.2 mg

Fruits

Raisins	1 cup	3.1 mg
Apricots, dried	1 cup	3.5 mg

Adding Extras: Fiber, Probiotics, and Omega-3 Fatty Acids

Fiber

Fiber is the part of food that we cannot digest. But just because we cannot digest it doesn't mean we don't need it. Fiber has many health benefits. It not only helps improve bowel function, but it also has been shown to decrease blood cholesterol (associated with heart disease) and improve blood sugar control (important when dealing with prediabetes or diabetes). Fiber may be helpful in preventing cancer, especially cancer of the intestinal tract. Certain kinds of fiber feed the "good" bacteria in your intestine, which also provides a world of health benefits (more on this shortly).

When you remove gluten from your diet, you automatically remove a lot of the fiber you may be consuming. With all the health benefits of fiber, you want to get your daily fiber requirement. Even without eliminating gluten, most people do not get enough fiber. So when you lose the gluten in your diet, you need to be diligent about getting your fiber needs met.

So how do you get that needed fiber without the gluten? Here are some tips:

- Consume whole fruits and vegetables instead of juices, since juice has all the fiber removed. While you're at it, don't remove the peel from those apples, pears, potatoes, or other edible fruit or vegetable skins—that's where much of the fiber is hiding.

- Add beans to many of your dishes. For example, enjoy chickpeas in salad, pinto beans in chili, lentils in soups, and kidney or pinto beans with rice.

- Add nuts and seeds to your meals. For example, enjoy almonds in your cream of rice, sesame seeds in your salad, pumpkin seeds on the tops of breads and muffins, and pecans in your cookies.

- Eat high-fiber snacks such as popcorn, dried fruits (like dried apricots or dried plums), and raw fruits and vegetables.

- Try to use some of the grains and flours that are higher in fiber in your cooking. Look at the next chart for a list of gluten-free foods that are good sources of fiber.

- If you are suffering from constipation and you have attempted to increase the fiber with the tips above, you may need a fiber supplement. However if you take a fiber supplement you must take in a lot of water daily or the fiber can make your more constipated. Some of them are gluten free, such as Benefiber® and Citrucel®.

- Remember to consume an adequate amount of water. This also helps the digestive tract move smoothly.

Flours, Grains	Serving Size	Fiber (g)
Carob flour	1 cup	41 g
Soy flour, defatted	1 cup	18.4 g
Sorghum flour	1 cup	8 g
Buckwheat flour, whole groat	1 cup	12 g
Corn flour (masa), enriched white or yellow	1 cup	7.3 g
Chickpea flour (besan)	1 cup	9.9 g
Peanut flour, defatted	1 cup	9.5 g
Potato flour	1 cup	9.4 g
Rice flour, white	1 cup	3.8 g
Rice flour, brown	1 cup	7.3 g
Arrowroot flour	1 cup	4.4 g
Corn, bran, crude	1 cup	60.0 g
Rice bran, crude	1 cup	24.8 g
Buckwheat, groats (kasha), dry	1 cup	16.9 g
Cornmeal, whole grain	1 cup	8.9 g
Amaranth, uncooked	1 cup	12.9 g
Amaranth, cooked	1 cup	5.2 g
Quinoa, uncooked	1 cup	11.9 g
Quinoa, cooked	1 cup	5.2 g
Rice, brown, long-grain, raw	1 cup	6.5 g
Rice, brown, long-grain, cooked	1 cup	3.5 g

(continued)

Flours, Grains (continued)	Serving Size	Fiber (g)
Rice, wild, raw	1 cup	9.9 g
Rice, wild, cooked	1 cup	3.0 g

Legumes

	Serving Size	Fiber (g)
Soybeans, mature, raw	1 cup	17.3 g
Soybeans, mature, boiled	1 cup	10.3 g
Small white beans, boiled	1 cup	18.6 g
Navy beans, boiled	1 cup	19.1 g
French beans, boiled	1 cup	16.6 g
Kidney beans, boiled	1 cup	11.3 g
Lentils, boiled	1 cup	15.6 g
Peas, split, boiled	1 cup	16.3 g
Pinto beans, boiled	1 cup	15.4 g
Black beans, boiled	1 cup	15.0 g
Miso (Rice)	1 cup	14.8 g
Lima beans, boiled	1 cup	13.2 g
Great northern beans, boiled	1 cup	12.4 g
Refried beans	1 cup	11.4 g
Fava beans, boiled	1 cup	9.2 g
Pink beans, boiled	1 cup	9.0 g

Nuts, Seeds, Vegetables

	Serving Size	Fiber (g)
Coconut meat, dried, unsweetened	1 oz	4.6 g

(continued)

Nuts, Seeds, Vegetables (continued)	Serving Size	Fiber (g)
Sesame seeds	1 Tbsp	1.1 g
Almonds	1 oz	3.5 g
Flax seeds, whole	1 Tbsp	2.8 g
Sunflower seeds, dry roasted	1 oz	3.1 g
Hazelnuts	1 oz	2.7 g
Pine nuts, pinyon, dried	1 oz	3.0 g
Pistachio nuts, dried roasted	1 oz	2.8 g
Pecans	1 oz	2.7 g
Peanut butter, chunky	2 Tbsp	1.8 g
Artichokes, cooked	1 medium	10.3 g
Squash, winter, cooked	1 cup	9.0 g
Parsnips, raw	1 cup	6.5 g
Peas, cooked	½ cup	4.4 g
Edamame, cooked	½ cup	4 g
Mixed vegetables	½ cup	4.0 g
Serrano pepper, raw	1 cup	3.9 g
Spinach, cooked	1 cup	4.3 g
Tomatoes, sun-dried	½ cup	3.3 g
Shitake mushrooms, dried	4 mushrooms (15 g)	1.7 g
Parsnips, cooked	½ cup	2.8 g
Brussels sprouts, cooked	½ cup	2.0 g

(continued)

Nuts, Seeds, Vegetables (continued)	Serving Size	Fiber (g)
Broccoli, cooked	½ cup	2.6 g
Sweet potato in skin	½ cup	3.3 g
Okra, raw	1 cup	3.2 g
Yams, cooked	½ cup	2.7 g
Turnip greens, cooked	½ cup	2.5 g
Carrots, cooked	½ cup	2.3 g
Fruit		
Passion fruit	1 cup	24.5 g
Elderberries	1 cup	10.2 g
Guava	1 cup	8.9 g
Raspberries	1 cup	8.0 g
Blackberries	1 cup	7.6 g
Figs, dried	½ cup	7.3 g
Prunes	½ cup	6.2 g
Blueberries	1 cup	3.6 g
Gooseberries	1 cup	6.4 g
Persimmon	1 medium	6.0 g
Banana	1 cup, mashed	5.8 g
Raisins	½ cup	3.1 g
Cranberries, raw, chopped	1 cup	5.1 g
Prickly pear	1 cup	5.4 g

(continued)

Fruit (continued)	Serving Size	Fiber (g)
Pears, raw (American)	1 small	4.6 g
Plantains, cooked	1 cup, mashed	4.6 g
Apricots, dried	½ cup	4.8 g
Pears, Asian	1 medium	4.4 g
Carambola, starfruit	1 cup	3.7 g
Apple with skin	1 small	3.6 g
Oranges, valencias	1 cup sections	4.5 g
Tangerines	1 cup sections	3.5 g
Cranberries, dried	½ cup	2.3 g
Pomegranates	½ cup	3.5 g
Cherries	1 cup	2.9 g
Apricots	1 cup	3.3 g
Strawberries, sliced	1 cup	3.3 g
Mangos	1 cup	2.6 g
Papayas	1 cup	2.5 g
Peaches	1 large	2.6 g

Probiotics

Probiotics is the term health care professionals use to describe the "healthy" or "good" bacteria in the intestinal tract. These bacteria living in our small and large intestines do marvelous things. They consume some of the food that we cannot digest (fiber known as prebiotics) and produce something known as short-chain fatty acids. These short-chain fatty acids are then used by our gut cells for energy and repair. Also, we believe that these "good" bacteria fight off "bad" bacteria, helping prevent illness like stomach viruses.

When someone does not have enough probiotics in their gut, they are at risk for what is called permeable gut. Our intestinal tract has very special cells designed to allow small molecules of sugar, protein, and fat to enter our body and our bloodstream while preventing waste and pathogens from getting out. When the gut is not healthy, we develop larger "holes" or "gaps" that allow toxins into our body as well, where they can cause illness (like infections) or, as some believe, neurological and autoimmune problems. We will talk a little more about these types of illnesses in Chapter 17. For now, just understand that probiotics help our gut stay healthy and prevent it from becoming "leaky."

So how do you get those "good" bacteria into your body? There are many foods that you probably already eat that contain probiotics. For instance, yogurt is a good source of these "good bugs." Also, many manufacturers have recently begun adding probiotics to foods. Some of these are gluten free, but some are not. Another good source of probiotics is supplements—but you will need to be careful to find probiotics that are gluten free.

Gluten-free probiotic supplements include the following (although formulations change, so double-check these before starting to take them):

- Flora-Q Probiotic

- In-Liven

- Fast-Tract

- NuFerm Organic Whole Foods

- Innergy Biotic-Body Ecology Diet

Omega-3 Fatty Acids

We first learned about omega-3 fatty acids (their chemical makeup gives them their name) from studies into why the Eskimo population had such low heart disease rates. Research found that the Eskimos' diet was high in fish fat, which is high in omega-3 fatty acids. Some of these omega-3 fatty acids work in the body to reduce inflammation and therefore may provide health benefits such as reduced risk of cancer, heart disease, and rheumatoid arthritis (an autoimmune disease). Many studies are currently underway that look at the benefit of these fats on the brain and immune function, and at the time of this writing, they look promising.

Omega-3 fatty acids come in many different forms. The first is what we call essential, meaning that we must get it in our diet. This one is known as alpha-linoleic acid (ALA) for short. The most beneficial forms are known as eicosapentanoic acid (EPA) and docosahexanoic acid (DHA). These forms can be made from ALA by our body, but unfortunately our body does not do this well. It seems that our body only converts 2 to 15 percent of ALA into EPA and only 2 to 5 percent into DHA. The percentage of conversion varies, and women seem to be better at converting than men, but at best it's a very small amount. Fish do a much better job of converting the algae they eat to EPA and DHA, which is why it's recommended that we consume fish two or more times a week.

Bearing in mind that only small amounts are converted, you can still get ALA in your diet. The best sources of ALA are flaxseeds, walnuts, pecans, and hazelnuts. You can also get eggs that are high in ALA omega-3 fatty acids from chickens who have been fed foods that increase the amount in the eggs. Oils that are high in omega-3 fatty acids are flaxseed oil and canola oil.

If you do not eat much fish and still want to make sure you get enough, consider a fish oil supplement. Supplements like cod liver oil or other fish oils will supply you with the EPA and DHA you need. Some people complain that the supplements cause "fish burps"; these can be reduced by refrigerating your supplement.

Where to Find Gluten-Free Products

Gluten-Free Products Are Everywhere

It wasn't very long ago that finding gluten-free foods other than those that are naturally gluten free was next to impossible. Even if you could find them, they were very poor in quality, especially breads and desserts. In taste and consistency they were like eating cardboard. Thankfully, this is no longer the case. Gluten-free products have been getting better and better, and today gluten-free foods are the most rapidly increasing food category being manufactured.

In addition to the variety of choices, changes in food labeling laws are making it easier to identify which foods are gluten free and which are not. Gluten-free foods can now be found in restaurants and fast food establishments as well as in packaged foods. In addition, they are showing up in tasty bakery and dessert options and are working their way onto supermarket shelves.

What's Available

Gluten-free foods are everywhere. Now you can find gluten free:

- Bread, bagels, pancakes, biscuits, coffee cake, waffles
- Pasta, pizza

- Cakes, cookies, pies

- Frozen meals, soups, casseroles

- Options at many chain and private restaurants

The future holds much promise, especially since so many chefs are embracing gluten-free choices in their kitchens.

Where to Find Gluten-Free Items in Stores

Gluten-free foods can be found in supermarkets in the health food and specialties aisle as well as in the freezer case and mixed throughout the store. There are many foods that are gluten free that do not indicate this on their packaging, so learning how to read labels will make it easier to identify more safe choices. There are also many gluten-free shopping guides now available, such as the *Gluten-Free Grocery Shopping Guide*, by Matison & Matison, updated annually, which lists thousands of brand-name products that have already been checked for their gluten-free status.

Health food and specialty stores are the best place to find a large variety of gluten-free products. It is here that you may find more unusual or hard-to-find items. Since everyone has different taste buds, and one product may not appeal to everyone, it may be helpful to try some of the products before purchasing them. You can sample gluten-free foods at some of the many celiac fairs run throughout the country. Find out about events near you by checking with your local celiac organizations. To find a celiac support group in your area, go to www.gluten.net or www.csaceliacs.org.

Where to Find Gluten-Free Items on the Internet

The Internet now provides endless places to find gluten-free foods. Just going to some of the many gluten-free blogs or websites gives you a wonderful variety of products to try. At www.glutenfreeeasy.com you can find a listing of many products for you to review. Also, listed below, you'll find some of the many companies that have great gluten-free choices.

Gluten-Free Grains and Baked Goods Are Available from:

Aleia's
Cookies, breads, bread crumbs, stuffing
www.aleias.com

Aliments Trigone, Inc.
Buckwheat
www.alimentstrigone.com

AltiPlano Gold
Quinoa products
www.altiplano-gold.amazon
webstore.com

Amazake, Grainaissance
Amazake and mochi
www.grainaissance.com

Andean Dreams
Quinoa products
www.andeandream.com

Arrowhead Mills
Grains
www.arrowheadmills.com

Aunt Gussie's Cookies
Cookies
www.auntgussies.com

Authentic Foods
Grains and almond meal, falafel mix, cake mixes (double-check becuase they have both gluten-free and gluten-containing products)
www.Authenticfoods.com

Bakery on Main
Bars and granola
www.bakeryonmain.com

Barbara's Bakery
Baked goods
www.barbarasbakery.com

Barkat
Breads, pastas, and desserts
www.glutenfree-foods.co.uk

The Birkett Mills
Grains and buckwheat products
www.thebirkettmills.com

Bittersweet Bakery
Baked goods
www.bittersweetgf.com

Bob's Red Mill
Grains, mixes, and cereals
www.bobsredmill.com

Breads from Anna
Cake and bread mixes
www.fromanna.com

Bumble Bar Foods
Snack bars
www.bumblebar.com

Casa de Fruta
Mesquite, dried fruits, nuts
www.casadefruta.com

Cause You're Special
Baking mixes
www.causeyourespecial.com

Chebe Bread
Bread mixes
www.chebe.com

Cheecha Krackles
Potato snacks
www.cheecha.ca

Gluten-Free Grains & Baked Goods (continued)

Conte's
Frozen gluten-free pizza, pasta, pierogi
www.contespasta.com

Crave Bakery
Baked goods
www.cravebakery.com

Crunchmaster
Rice crackers
www.crunchmaster.com

Cup4Cup
Gluten-free flour blend
www.cup4cup.com

Dale and Thomas
Popcorn and gourmet kettle corn
www.daleandthomas.com

DeBoles
Pasta
www.deboles.com

Dietary Specialties
Bakery mixes
www.dietspec.com

Domata
Flours, consumer and food service sizes
www.domataglutenfree.com

Dowd & Rogers
Cake mixes, specialty flours
www.dowdandrogers.com/products.html

Ener-G Foods
Bread products, and allergy-safe foods
www.ener-g.com

Enjoy Life Foods
Snack bars and bagels
www.enjoylifefoods.com

Erewhon
Cereal
www.attunefoods.com/products/gluten-free-breakfast

Everybody Eats
Baked goods and fresh pasta; follow their website for Bruce & Pedros special events
www.everybodyeats-inc.com

Expandex
Modified tapioca starch
www.expandexglutenfree.com

Farmer's Kitchen Café
Baked goods
www.farmerskitchencafe.com

Flying Apron Bakery
Baked goods
www.flyingapron.net

Food for Life Baking Company
Breads, corn, and rice tortillas
www.foodforlife.com/about_us/gluten-free-difference

Foods by George
Baked goods, pasta, and pizza
www.foodsbygeorge.com

For Full Flavor
Soups, sauces and gravies
www.forfullflavor.com

French Meadow Bakery
Baked goods
www.frenchmeadow.com

Garden Lites
Muffins, vegetable casseroles
www.gardenlites.com

Gluten-Free Grains & Baked Goods (continued)

General Mills
Rice Chex (more products being developed)
www.generalmills.com

Get Healthy America
Gourmet foods
www.gethealthyamerica.com

Gibbs Wild Rice
Grains and wild rice
www.gibbswildrice.com

Gifts of Nature
Grains
www.giftsofnature.net

Gilbert's Gourmet Goodies
Allergy-friendly cookies and goodies
www.gilbertsgourmetgoodies.com

Gillian's Foods
Baked goods
www.gilliansfoodsglutenfree.com

Gluten Free Creations Bakery
Bakery
www.glutenfreecreations.com

Glutenfreeda Foods
Burritos, granola, oatmeal, pizza wraps, cheesecakes, ice cream sandwiches
www.glutenfreedafoods.com

1-2-3 Gluten Free
Cookie and cake mixes, mixes for other baked goods
www.123glutenfree.com

Gluten-Free Mall
A variety of gluten-free products
www.glutenfreemall.com

Gluten-Free Naturals
Cookie blends, pancake, pizza, and cornbread mixes
www.gfnfoods.com

Gluten Solutions
A variety of products and foods
www.glutensolutions.com

Glutino Food Group
Baked goods
www.glutino.com

GoGo Quinoa
Quinoa and amaranth products
www.quinoa.com

Goldbaums
Cones, chips, pasta
www.goldbaums.com

Good Eatz
Baked goods
www.goodeatz.org

Grainaissance, Inc.
Mochi
www.grainaissance.com

Haley's Corner Bakery
Baked goods
www.haleyscorner.com

Hoi-Grain
Snacks, sauces, and soups
www.conradricemill.com

Island Gluten-Free Bakery
Baked goods
www.islandgfbakery.com

Jennies Gluten-Free Bakery
Macaroons
www.macaroonking.com

Joan's GF Great Bakes
Bagels, muffins, and pizza
(you bake on your own)
www.gfgreatbakes.com

Jubilee Kafe
Baked goods
www.jubileekafe.com

Kathy's Creation
Baked goods
www.kathyscreationsbakery.com

Katz Gluten-Free
Kosher breads and bakery
products
www.katzglutenfree.com

Kays Naturals
Cereals and snacks (protein-
fortified)
www.kaysnaturals.com

Kinnikinnick Foods
Ready-to-eat breads and cakes
www.kinnikinnick.com

Kitchen Table Bakers
Cheese wafer crisps
www.kitchentablebakers.com

La Tortilla Factory
Teff tortillas
www.latortillafactory.com

The Little Aussie Bakery
Baked goods
www.thelittleaussiebakery.com

Lundberg Family Farms
Rice products
www.lundberg.com

Lydia's Organics
Natural sprouted grain, fruit, and
nut products
www.lydiasorganics.com

Manischewitz
Many kosher products
www.manischewitz.com

Maplegrove Gluten Free Foods, Inc.
Pasta
www.maplegrovefoods.com

Mariposa Baking Company
Baked goods
www.mariposabaking.com

Mary's Gone Crackers
Cookies, crackers, crumbs, pretzel
sticks
www.marysgonecrackers.com

Minn-Dak Growers
Buckwheat products
www.minndak.com

Molly's Gluten-Free Bakery
Baked goods
www.mollysglutenfreebakery.com

Moose Lake Wild Rice
Grains and wild rice
www.mooselakewildrice.com

Mr. Ritts
Baked goods
www.mrritts.com

Namaste Foods
Bakery mixes
www.namastefoods.com

Nana's Cookie Company
Cookie bars
www.nanascookiecompany.com

Gluten-Free Grains & Baked Goods (continued)

Northern Quinoa Corporation
Quinoa and other grains and beans
www.quinoa.com

Nu-World Amaranth
Amaranth products
www.nuworldamaranth.com

Outside the Breadbox
Baked goods
www.outsidethebreadbox.com

Pamela's Product
Bakery mixes
www.pamelasproducts.com

Purefit Nutrition
Energy bars
www.purefit.com

Quinoa Corporation
Grains and quinoa products
www.quinoa.net

Rachel Lu
Cookies and muffins
www.rachellugluten freefoods.com

The Really Great Food Company
Bakery mixes
www.reallygreatfood.com

Rice Expressions
Rice mixes
www.riceexpressions.com

Rising Hearts Bakery
Baked goods
risingheartsbakery.com

Rose's Wheat-Free Bakery and Café
Baked goods
www.rosesbakery.com

Russo's
Italian food, Italian dessert shells
www.russosglutenfreegourmet.com

Schär
A variety of pre-made gluten-free
products
www.schar.com

Shiloh Farms
Flours and sorghum
www.shilohfarms.com

The Silly Yak Bakery and Bread Barn
Baked goods
www.freshglutenfree.net

Sinfully Gluten-Free
Baked goods
www.sinfullygf.com

Smart Flour Foods
Flour blends, buns, desserts,
pizza crusts
www.smartflourfoods.com

Strictly Gluten-Free
Gluten-free shopping online
www.strictlyglutenfree.com

Sunny Valley Wheat Free
Baked goods
www.sunnyvalleywheatfree.com

Sweet Christine's Bakery
Gluten-free baked goods
www.sweetchristinesgluten
free.com

Sweet Escape Pastries, LLC.
Baked goods
www.sweetescpastries.com

Sweet 27
Baked goods
www.sweet27.com

Gluten-Free Grains & Baked Goods (continued)

Tate's Bakeshop
Gluten-free baked goods
www.tatesbakeshop.com

The Teff Company
Teff products
www.teffco.com

Three Bakers
Baked goods
www.threebakers.com

Tinkyada
Brown rice pasta
tinkyada.com

Tom Sawyer
Flour blends and gums
www.glutenfreeflour.com

Twin Valley Mills, LLC
Grains and sorghum
www.twinvalleymills.com

Uforia
Triple Delight Gluten-Free Cake
sales@kartikaskitchen.com

Underscores Baked Goods
Cookie dough logs, cookies
www.underscores.goodsie.com

Way Better Snacks
Sprouted chips
www.gowaybetter.com

Wellness Foods
Energy bars, protein chips
www.wellnessfoods.ca

Whole Foods Market Gluten-Free Bakehouse
Baked goods
www.wholefoodsmarket.com

Gluten-Free Oats Are Available from:

Avena Foods
http://avenafoods.com

Bob's Red Mill
www.bobsredmill.com

Cream Hill Estates
www.creamhillestates.com

Gluten-Free Oats
www.glutenfreeoats.com

Holly's
www.hollysoatmeal.com

Only Oats Farm Pure Foods
www.onlyoats.com

Ready-Made Gluten-Free Foods Are Available from:

Allergaroo
Microwavable food
www.allergaroo.com

Alpine Aire Foods
Prepared meals
www.aa-foods.com

Amy's Kitchen
A wide variety of frozen meals
www.amyskitchen.com

Annie's Homegrown
Meals
www.annies.com

Apetito
Textured meals
www.apetito.ca

Caesar's
Frozen meals
www.caesarspasta.com

Ready-Made Gluten-Free Foods (continued)

Celinal Foods
Single-serve mixes and gluten-free starter kits
www.celinalfoods.com

Gluten-Free Café
Frozen meals
www.myglutenfreecafe.com

My Own Meals
Vacuum-sealed meals
www.myownmeals.com

Nu Life Foods
Frozen meals
www.nulifefoods.com

Allergy-Free Gluten-Free Foods Are Available from:

Allergyfree Foods
www.allergyfreefoods.com

Allergaroo
Allergy-friendly foods
www.allergaroo.com

Arico Natural Foods
Chips
www.crisproot.com

Cherrybrook Kitchen
gluten-, dairy-, and egg-free mixes
www.cherrybrookkitchen.com

Dr. Praeger's Sensible Foods
Fish sticks, pancakes,
veggie burgers
www.drpraegers.com

Edward and Sons
Gluten-, dairy-, egg-, and nut-free mixes and dips
www.edwardandsons.com

Gluten-Free Shakes Are Available from:

Boost Shakes
All products except for smoothies
1(800)247-7893
www.boost.com

Ensure Shakes
All products
1(800)986-8501
www.ensure.com

Glucerna Shakes
All products
1(800)227-5767
www.glucerna.com

Nutra Shakes
All products
1(800)654-3691
www.nutra-balance-products.com

Nutren Shakes
All products
1(888)240-2713
www.nestlenutritionstore.com

Gluten-Free Candy Is Available from:

Azure Chocolat
Kosher chocolate
www.azurechocolat.com

Candy Tree
Candy
oliviers.ca/index.php/
candy-home

Gluten-Free Broths and Asian Products Are Available from:

Annie Chun's
Asian foods
www.anniechun.com

Gluten-Free Broths and Asian Products (continued)

Celinal Foods
Individual gluten-free packets
www.celinalfoods.com

Eden Foods
Tamari
www.edenfoods.com

Kari-Out Company
Soy sauce
www.kariout.com

Kettle Cuisine
Frozen soups
www.kettlecuisine.com

Maplegrove Gluten-Free Foods
Broths
www.maplegrovefoods.com

Pacific Foods
Soups
www.pacificfoods.com

Premier Japan
Teriyaki and hoisin sauce
www.edwardandsons.com

San-J International
Tamari and GF Asian sauces
www.san-j.com

Savory Choice
Broths
www.savorychoice.com

Simply Asia Foods
Asian noodles and sauces
www.simplyasia.net

Swiss Chalet
Broths and stocks
www.scff.com

Thai Kitchen
Many Asian products
www.thaikitchen.com

Gluten-Free Bars Are Available from:

Extend Bar
All products, including diabetic energy bar
www.extendbar.com

Larabar
Energy bars
www.larabar.com

Think Products
Bars
www.thinkproducts.com

Other Gluten-Free Products Are Available from:

Celinal Foods
Toaster safety bags
www.toastitbags.com

Traina
Sun-dried tomato ketchup
www.trainafoods.com

Gluten-Free Beer Is Available from:

Anheuser-Busch (Redbridge)
www.anheuser-busch.com

Bard's Tale Beer (Dragon's Gold Gluten-Free Beer)
www.bardsbeer.com

BiAglut
www.biaglut.com/ITA/Prodotti/Birra/default.htm

Gluten-Free Beer (continued)

Green's
www.glutenfreebeers.co.uk

LA Messagere
www.lesbieresnouvellefrance.com

Lakefront Brewery
www.lakefrontbrewery.com

Nick Stafford's Hambleton Ales
www.hambletonales.co.uk

O'Brien Brewing
www.gfbeer.com.au

Schlafly
www.schlafly.com

Silly Yak
www.sillyyak.com.au/beer/faq.html

Sprecher Brewery
www.sprecherbrewery.com/
index.php

TIP   When drinking alcohol, remember that:

- All distilled alcohol (vodka, rum, gin, whiskey, scotch, etc.) is gluten free (the process of distillation will remove gluten). If a flavoring agent is added after distillation then there is a chance that gluten could be present.
- All wine is gluten free, unless a flavoring agent is added.
- Some wine coolers contain gluten; the gluten is not usually listed on the label.
- Most beers and ales are not gluten free because they are usually made from barley.
- Today more and more brands of beer are offering gluten-free alternatives.

Cooking Gluten-Free Dishes with Flair

Making Family Favorites Gluten Free

We all have favorite foods that we have grown up with and enjoy. Learning how to make these favorites gluten free can really make the difference in how you feel about following a gluten-free diet. There may be times when you are unable to find gluten-free foods that you can use as a substitute in a recipe, and sometimes you may need to change the recipe in order to make it work. So to make things easier, start with simple changes; later, as you become more experienced you can work on making substitutions and more complicated recipes. The following examples demonstrate ways how you can modify recipes:

Holiday Green Bean Casserole
Original Recipe: Casserole made with green beans, cream of mushroom soup, and dried onion rings.

Modified Gluten-Free Recipe: In a casserole dish, combine green beans and gluten-free cream soup with sliced mushrooms. In place of the dried onion rings, sauté thin onion slices in olive oil until brown, crumble in gluten-free cereal or bread crumbs, add salt and pepper, and mix into green bean mixture and bake.

Chicken Cutlet Parmesan
Original Recipe: Breaded and fried cutlets topped with mozzarella and tomato sauce and served with pasta.

Modified Gluten-Free Recipe: Toast gluten-free bread and process in food processor; add garlic, onion powder, Italian herbs, (or buy gluten-free bread crumbs) and parmesan cheese. Dip chicken in beaten eggs, then use bread crumbs to coat the cutlets. Fry cutlets in large frying pan in olive oil, place in casserole dish, top with sauce and cheese, and bake. Serve with gluten-free brown rice or quinoa pasta and tomato sauce.

Butter Cookies

Original Recipe: Made with butter, sugar, egg yolk, salt, baking powder, vanilla extract, and all-purpose flour.

Modified Gluten-Free Recipe: Check baking powder to see if it is gluten free, use an all-purpose gluten-free flour mixture (as found in chapter 5), add a little extra gluten-free flour to achieve the same texture, and continue to finish the recipe as usually prepared.

As you can see, if you are modifying recipes to make them gluten-free, you need to start by making small changes. On occasion, you will find a recipe that may require ingredients that are hard to find a gluten-free alternate for, such as puff pastry and phyllo dough. In these cases, you may need to modify the recipe a lot more to suit the ingredients you have available (as I did in my spinach feta pie recipe later in this chapter). More and more gluten-free products are on the horizon, so increasingly you will be able to find good substitutes for your ingredients; but, for now, we can work with what is available in order to make the best possible alternatives. And I'd like to share with you some fabulous gluten-free recipes from my own collection.

ALLERGY INFORMATION: All recipes in this book are gluten-free but since people often have multiple allergies I have placed an allergy guide for each recipe using the following codes by the Tips: GF = gluten free, MF = milk free, SF = soy free, EF = egg free, NF = nut free, PF = peanut free, FF = fish free, SFF = shellfish free, V = vegetarian, VG = vegan.

If a recipe can be modified to remove the allergen, this information is also included.

**Note that some cooking sprays have soy oil. For soy free recipes make sure you, use soy-free oil spray or vegetable oil.

Every care has been made to try to accurately list allergens and provide allergy recommendations, but since products and ingredients often change, please always double-check the label and call manufacturers on any questionable products.

The Gluten-Free Gourmet: Best Recipes

Breakfast:

- Amaranth and Apricot Granola
- Pumpkin Pancakes/Waffles
- Blueberry Crumb Muffins
- Italian Frittata
- Pancakes with Cream Cheese Filling
- Banana Chocolate Chip Bread
- Blueberry Buckwheat Corncakes
- Corn Muffins

Amaranth and Apricot Granola   Serves 6

This is great served on top of yogurt, as a cereal, or as a snack mix. It is easy to prepare, and any dried fruit or nuts can be substituted in this recipe.

Gluten-free cooking spray (or vegetable oil)
⅓ cup whole amaranth grain
2 cups gluten-free Rice Chex cereal
½ cup dried apricots, chopped
¼ cup dried cranberries
½ cup hazelnuts, chopped
½ cup sugar
3 Tb water
½ tsp cinnamon
¼ tsp nutmeg
1 tsp vanilla

1. Preheat oven to 325 degrees F. Line a baking sheet with aluminum foil and spray with cooking spray.

2. Heat a small nonstick frying pan over medium-high heat until very hot. Pop the amaranth by adding a teaspoon at a time to the pan, then cover and shake until grain pops. Pour out onto a plate and repeat with remaining amaranth.

3. In a large bowl, mix the popped amaranth with the Rice Chex, apricots, cranberries, and hazelnuts.

4. In a medium skillet, heat sugar, water, cinnamon, nutmeg, and vanilla to a boil. Boil for about 2 minutes, until sugar is dissolved.

5. Pour sugar mixture over amaranth in bowl. Stir gently to coat.

6. Spread mixture in a single layer on baking sheet. Bake in preheated oven for 15 minutes.

7. Remove from oven, cool slightly. Break granola apart to serve (about 1 cup per serving).

Nutritional information per serving: 270 calories, 3.6 grams protein, 47 grams carbohydrates, 7.5 grams fat, 3 grams fiber, 0 milligrams cholesterol, 89 milligrams sodium, 76 milligrams calcium, 3.6 milligrams iron.

Tip: The amaranth grain burns easily when popping. Be careful!

** Allergy Tip: This recipe is GF, MF, EF, SF, PF, FF, SFF, V, VG. To keep this recipe soy free, use soy-free vegetable oil in place of the cooking spray. To make nut free, omit the hazelnuts.

Pumpkin Pancakes/Waffles   Serves 3
(Makes 6 Pancakes or 3 Waffles)

Pumpkin pancakes are all the rage in the fall, but they are just as yummy as a special treat any time.

Dry Ingredients:
1 cup gluten-free all-purpose flour blend (see chapter 5 or buy store brand)
1 tsp baking powder
1 tsp salt
1 tsp cinnamon
¼ tsp nutmeg
⅛ tsp ginger
⅛ tsp cloves
2 Tb brown sugar
2 Tb granulated sugar
1 tsp xanthan gum

Wet Ingredients:
1 Tb butter, melted
1 egg or 3 egg whites
2 Tb low-fat buttermilk (optional)
½ cup pumpkin purée
¾ cup skim milk
1 tsp vanilla extra
Gluten-free cooking spray or vegetable oil

1. Mix dry ingredients together.

2. Beat all wet ingredients together and pour into dry. Mix until just combined.

3. Spray a large skillet with cooking spray and heat until hot. Lower flame and pour in pancake batter to make 4-inch pancakes. (If making waffles, spray the waffle iron with cooking spray and follow manufacturer's directions for making waffles.)

4. Brown on both sides. Serve with maple syrup or jam. Looks great sprinkled with confectioner's sugar and berries.

Nutritional information: 162 calories, 4.3 grams protein, 29.5 grams carbohydrates, 3.4 grams fat, 41 milligrams cholesterol, 487 milligrams sodium, 1.6 grams fiber, 96 milligrams calcium, 1.1 milligrams iron.

Tips: This is also delicious with sliced bananas and chocolate chips. To make without the pumpkin, omit the pumpkin, cinnamon, nutmeg, ginger, and cloves. Reduce the amount of milk to ½ cup. (Makes 2 jumbo waffles or four 4-inch pancakes.) If you like crisp waffles, leave in the waffle iron a few minutes longer.

** Allergy Tip: This recipe is GF, SF, NF, PF, FF, SFF, V. To keep soy free, use soy-free vegetable oil in place of cooking spray; double-check the flour blend to make sure it is soy free; and use soy-free margarine if you opt for margarine over butter. To make nut free, make sure flour blend doesn't contain nuts or peanuts. To make milk free, use dairy-free products in place of the butter (such as margarine) and milk and buttermilk (such as rice or soy milk or coconut butter). To make egg free, use any gluten-free eggless egg substitute. To make vegan, use gluten-free alternatives for the buttermilk, milk, butter, and egg.

Blueberry Crumb Muffins   Serves 12

Light and delicious, the perfect breakfast. Freeze extras so you can take them out when you need them. Any berry can be used in this recipe.

½ cup white rice flour
½ cup brown rice flour
½ cup tapioca starch
½ cup sorghum flour
¼ cup granulated sugar
2 tsp baking powder
½ tsp baking soda
1 tsp xanthan gum
¼ tsp salt
1 tsp lemon zest
2 eggs
½ cup plain low-fat yogurt
1 cup low-fat 1% milk
4 Tb melted butter, divided in half
2 cups fresh or frozen blueberries
2 Tb brown sugar
¼ cup almond flour
¼ cup white rice flour
¼ tsp nutmeg

1. Preheat oven to 400 degrees F. Line a 12-cup muffin tin with paper muffin cups.

2. Mix all dry ingredients (white rice flour through lemon zest) in a large mixing bowl.

3. In a separate bowl, beat together eggs, yogurt, milk, and 2 Tb of the melted butter.

4. Make a well in the center of the dry ingredients. Pour in wet ingredients and stir until just combined.

5. Stir in blueberries. Divide batter evenly among the 12 prepared muffin cups.

6. In a small bowl, use a fork to mix together brown sugar, almond flour, white rice flour, nutmeg, and remaining 2 Tb of melted butter.

7. Sprinkle crumb mixture evenly over the 12 muffins.

8. Bake for 25 minutes or until a toothpick inserted in the middle comes out clean.

Nutritional information per serving: 209 calories, 4.6 grams protein, 36 grams carbohydrates, 6 grams fat, 47 milligrams cholesterol, 174 milligrams sodium, 72 milligrams calcium, less than 1 milligram iron.

Tips: These muffins are best served warm with butter or jelly. Freeze unused muffins so you can have delicious muffins whenever you want them.

** Allergy Tip: This recipe is GF, SF, PF, FF, SFF, V. To keep soy free, check egg substitute for soy and use a soy-free cooking spray or oil. To make egg free, use any gluten-free eggless egg substitute. To make milk free, use a dairy-free yogurt and milk (such as rice milk) and margarine in place of the butter. To make vegan, use vegan substitutes for the yogurt, milk, butter, and eggs.

Italian Frittata   Serves 4

Viva l'Italia! This is rich delicious breakfast that tastes a lot like a crustless quiche. It is great served as a breakfast or a brunch treat.

Gluten-free cooking spray or vegetable oil
1 medium onion, sliced thin
½ cup baby spinach
2 cups Egg Beaters
1 tsp gluten-free Dijon mustard
2 Tb 2% milk
½ tsp salt
¼ tsp pepper
2 Tb brown rice flour, or use a premade gluten-free flour blend
4 oz low-fat shredded Swiss cheese

1. Preheat oven to 350 degrees F

2. Spray a medium skillet with cooking spray and sauté onion until light brown, stirring occasionally. Add baby spinach and sauté spinach until wilted and any additional liquid in the pan evaporates.

3. Spray a 10-inch casserole pan with cooking spray.

4. Whisk together Egg Beaters with Dijon mustard, 2% milk, salt, and pepper, and pour in casserole dish. Top with spinach mixture. Mix Swiss cheese with flour and sprinkle over the top.

5. Bake for 35–45 minutes until set through; cut into quarters and serve.

Nutritional information: 151 calories, 21.6 grams protein, 11.3 grams carbohydrates, 1.8 grams fat, 10.5 milligrams cholesterol, 499 milligrams sodium, 1 gram fiber, 360 milligrams calcium, 3.2 milligrams iron.

Tips: Egg whites or other egg substitute can be used in place of the Egg Beaters. Also, chopped cooked broccoli works well in place of the spinach, and low-fat cheddar in place of the Swiss.

** Allergy Tip: This recipe is GF, SF, NF, PF, FF, SFF, V. To keep soy free, check egg substitute for soy and use a soy-free cooking spray or oil. To make milk free, use dairy-free milk and cheese (if you are also soy free, make sure the cheese alternative does not contain soy).

Pancakes with Cream Cheese Filling   Serves 6

A bit like cheese blintzes, and terrific served with a side of sour cream and strawberry jam.

Cream Cheese Filling

4 Tb light cream cheese
¾ cup 1% gluten-free cottage cheese
1 Tb granulated sugar
1 cup skim milk
1 tsp vanilla extract
2 eggs
2 Tb butter, melted
1½ cups gluten-free flour blend (see chapter 5 or use premade blend)
2 Tb sugar
2 tsp baking powder
1 tsp baking soda
½ tsp salt
½ tsp xanthan gum
Gluten-free cooking spray or olive oil
1 Tb powdered sugar

Optional fruit fillings: strawberries, blueberries, bananas, or all-fruit preserves.

1. Blend together cream cheese filling ingredients and set aside.

2. In a medium bowl, mix all remaining ingredients together (skim milk through butter).

3. In a large bowl, mix all dry ingredients together (gluten-free flour blend through xanthan gum) and set aside.

4. Fold wet ingredients into dry.

5. Heat a flat skillet and spray with cooking spray.

6. Drop batter by scant ¼ cupfuls onto hot griddle.

7. Brown pancakes on both sides.

8. Meanwhile, warm cream cheese filling in the microwave for about 30 seconds.

9. Fill each pancake with cream cheese filling and fruit if desired. Fold in half to serve. If using fruit preserves, spread pancake with preserves, then cream cheese filling, then fold.

10. Sprinkle pancakes with powdered sugar.

Nutritional information: 332 calories, 10.8 grams protein, 53.5 grams carbohydrates, 8.4 grams fat, 87.7 milligrams cholesterol, 596 milligrams sodium, 1 gram fiber, 132 milligrams calcium, 1.5 milligrams iron.

Tip: Ricotta cheese works well in place of cottage cheese in this recipe.

** Allergy Tip: This recipe is GF, SF, NF, PF, FF, SFF, V. To keep soy free, use a soy-free cooking spray or vegetable oil and double-check the gluten-free flour blend to make sure it is soy free. To keep nut free, double-check the flour blend to make sure it is nut free. To make egg free, use any gluten-free eggless egg substitute.

Banana Chocolate Chip Bread   Yield 1 Loaf (14 Servings)

Gluten-free nonstick cooking spray
2 cups gluten-free all-purpose flour blend (see chapter 5 or buy)
1 tsp xanthan gum
¾ tsp baking soda

½ tsp salt
¼ cup salted butter (softened)
1 cup sugar
2 large eggs
1½ cups mashed ripe banana (about 3)
⅓ cup plain fat-free Greek yogurt
1 tsp vanilla extract
1 cup gluten-free chocolate chips (such as Nestles or Hersheys)

1. Preheat oven to 350 degrees F. Coat a 8½ in. × 4½ in. loaf pan with gluten-free cooking spray.

2. Sift gluten-free flour blend, xanthan gum, baking soda, and salt into a bowl.

3. Place sugar and butter into a large mixing bowl and beat at medium speed until well blended (about 1 minute). Add the eggs, one at a time, beating well after each addition. Add banana, yogurt, and vanilla. Beat until blended.

4. Add the flour mixture and beat at low speed just until moist. Stir in chocolate chips.

5. Spoon batter into prepared pan. Bake for 1 hour or until wooden pick inserted in center comes out clean. Cool for 10 minutes in pan; remove from pan and cool completely on wire rack.

Nutritional Information: 254 calories, 4.8 grams protein, 44 grams carbohydrates, 8.7 grams fat, milligrams 48 cholesterol, 214 milligrams sodium, 4.3 milligrams fiber, 25.2 milligrams calcium, 1.47 milligrams iron.

Tips: Add pecans or walnuts for additional texture and flavor. Can also be made into 12 muffins. Decrease cooking time to 20–25 minutes.

** Allergy Tip: This recipe is GF, FF, SFF, V. To make egg free, use any gluten-free eggless egg substitute. To make nut free, omit the nuts in the tip and check the flour blend and chocolate chips for nuts.

Blueberry Buckwheat Corncakes   **Serves 8 (2 Pancakes Each)**

A delicious satisfying breakfast that is sure to get your day started well.

½ cup 100% buckwheat flour
½ cup cornmeal
½ tsp gluten-free baking powder

¼ tsp baking soda
1 ½ Tb agave nectar
1 Tb distilled white vinegar
¼ cups unsweetened gluten-free almond milk
1 cup fresh or frozen blueberries
Gluten-free nonstick cooking spray or olive oil

1. Stir the buckwheat flour, cornmeal, baking powder, and baking soda together in a mixing bowl.

2. In a separate bowl, combine the agave nectar, vinegar, and 1 cup of the almond milk.

3. Combine the liquid and dry ingredients and stir until just combined. The batter should be pourable. If it is too thick, add the remaining almond milk. Fold in blueberries.

4. Preheat a nonstick skillet or griddle and spray with cooking spray. Pour small amounts of the batter onto the heated surface and cook until the top bubbles. Turn with spatula and cook the other side until golden brown. Serve immediately.

Nutritional information per serving: 72 calories, 3.4 grams protein, 12.3 grams carbohydrates, 1 gram fat, 1.9 gram fiber, 0 milligrams cholesterol, 100 milligrams sodium, 17 milligrams calcium, less than 1 milligram iron.

Tips: Buckwheat adds a hearty, earthy quality to any gluten-free blend. Add some pecans and apples to this recipe for an extra special treat. Serve topped with agave nectar, maple syrup, applesauce, or blueberry preserves.

** Allergy Tip: This recipe is GF, MF, EF, SF, PF, FF, SFF, V, VG. To keep soy free, use a soy-free cooking spray or vegetable oil. To make nut free, substitute rice milk for the almond milk.

Corn Muffins   Serves 18

Theses corn muffins are so good you will never think you missed a thing when you went gluten free.

1 stick butter, softened
¾ cup sugar
2 eggs

1 cup buttermilk

1 tsp vanilla extract

½ cup gluten-free all-purpose flour blend (see chapter 5, or buy any gluten-free flour blend)

½ cup tapioca starch

⅔ cup cornmeal

1 tsp xanthan gum

1 tsp salt

½ tsp gluten-free baking powder

½ tsp baking soda

Cooking spray or olive oil

1. Preheat oven to 375 degrees F

2. Mix together butter and sugar, add eggs, buttermilk, and vanilla extract.

3. Combine other dry ingredients, slowly beat into wet ingredients for about 3 minutes until creamy.

4. Pour into cupcake cups and bake, or spray 12 in. × 9 in. × 3 in. cake pan with cooking spray and pour batter in.

5. Bake muffins about 20 minutes until golden, cake about 25 minutes until golden.

Nutritional information per serving: 138 calories, 2 grams protein, 19 grams carbohydrates, 6 grams fat, 1 grams fiber, 35 milligrams cholesterol, 207 milligrams sodium, 41 milligrams calcium, less than 1 milligram iron.

Tip: Serve with jam, honey butter, or apple butter.

** Allergy Tip: This recipe is GF, SF, NF, PF, FF, SFF, V To keep soy free, use a soy-free cooking spray or vegetable oil and double-check the flour blend to make sure it is soy free. For nut free, check the flour blend for nuts and peanuts. To make milk free, use any milk-free product in place of the buttermilk (such as rice milk) and the butter (such as margarine). To make egg free, use any gluten-free eggless egg substitute. To make vegan, use gluten-free vegan alternatives for the butter, buttermilk, and eggs.

Breads:

- Broccoli and Cheese Calzones

- Mediterranean Pizza

- Potato Flat Bread

- Italian Pizza

- Hamburger Rolls

- Pretzel Nuggets

- Basic Crêpes

- English Muffins

- Gluten-Free Challah Bread

Broccoli and Cheese Calzones   Serves 4

Serve with tomato sauce, or wrap in aluminum foil and take with you as a great packed lunch choice to go.

Dry Ingredients:
1 package rapid-rise yeast
½ cup tapioca starch
⅓ cup chickpea flour
⅓ cup sorghum flour
1 tsp xanthan gum
½ tsp salt
1 tsp unflavored gelatin
1 tsp sugar
1 tsp garlic powder
¼ cup water
½ cup low-fat 1% milk
2 Tb olive oil
½ cup frozen, chopped broccoli, defrosted
½ cup part-skim ricotta cheese
½ cup part-skim mozzarella cheese
¼ tsp black pepper
1 tsp dried basil
1 egg white
1 Tb Parmesan cheese

1. In a large bowl, sift together dry ingredients.

2. Heat water, milk, and olive oil in a small saucepan over medium heat until just simmering.

3. Add milk mixture to dry ingredients. Stir to combine. Dough should hold together. If too dry, add more milk; if too wet, add more white rice flour.

4. Put dough into a clean bowl that was sprayed with cooking spray; cover and let rest for 10 minutes.

5. Preheat oven to 400 degrees F.

6. Mix broccoli, ricotta cheese, mozzarella cheese, black pepper, and basil together in a small bowl.

7. Divide dough into 4 equal-sized pieces. Press each piece into a 4-inch circle. Place about 2 Tb of broccoli mixture onto one half of each dough circle.

8. Fold dough in half and press with tines of a fork to seal edges. Brush each calzone with egg white and sprinkle with Parmesan cheese.

9. Bake for 20 minutes, until crust is browned and filling is bubbly.

Nutritional information per serving: 316 calories, 16 grams protein, 37 grams carbohydrates, 13 grams fat, 20 milligrams cholesterol, 481 milligrams sodium, 3 grams fiber, 233 milligrams calcium, 2 grams iron.

Tips: Serve with a marinara sauce for dipping. Don't worry if the dough rips as you are trying to fill the calzones—just patch them back together and continue to wrap shut.

** Allergy Tip: This recipe is GF, SF, NF, PF, FF, SFF. To make egg free, use any gluten-free eggless egg substitute in place of the egg whites.

Mediterranean Pizza   Serves 2

This is so easy to prepare, and so full of flavor, that you'll be tempted to polish off the whole pizza yourself. You don't feel like you're missing anything when you make this delicious treat.

1 small individual gluten-free pizza dough (such as from Udis or Kinnikinnick)
2 Tb prepared gluten-free hummus
1 tomato, sliced
¼ tsp salt
¼ tsp oregano
1½ oz crumbled feta cheese

2 thin slices of red onion
2 Tb olives, chopped
1 tsp olive oil
¼ tsp garlic powder

1. Preheat oven to 350 degrees F.

2. Cook pizza crust in oven on a cookie sheet that has been coated with aluminum foil until it starts to toast lightly.

3. Spread hummus on pizza crust and top with sliced tomato. Sprinkle with salt and oregano. Sprinkle with feta; top with onions, olives, olive oil, and garlic powder.

4. Turn oven up to broil and place pizza on a cookie sheet and cook for about 3 minutes, until cheese starts to melt.

5. Serve with a crisp green salad.

Nutritional information: 222 calories, 5.5 grams protein, 22.7 grams carbohydrates, 12.2 grams fat, 18.9 milligrams cholesterol, 750 milligrams sodium, 2.9 grams iron, 133 milligrams calcium, 1.3 milligrams iron.

Tip: This is delicious with any cheese or flavored bean dip—a real winner!

** Allergy Tip: This recipe is GF, SF, NF, PF, FF, SFF, V. When you buy prepared crusts, double-check to make sure that the crusts are nut free, peanut free, and soy free if you have any of these allergies.

Potato Flat Bread   **Serves 6**

Potatoes have long been used throughout the world as a staple food. They are inexpensive and provide good flavor, and can be used as an alternative in some traditional dishes.

1 large russet potato, ¾ pound
1 tsp salt
¼ stick butter or margarine, melted
1 egg
2 tsp sugar
½ cup gluten-free flour blend (see chapter 5) or use brown rice flour
1 cup potato starch
2 tsp xanthan gum
½ tsp baking powder

2 Tb milk or buttermilk or rice milk
Rice flour for rolling
Gluten-free cooking spray or olive oil

1. Boil potato until just cooked; cool and peel. (You can cut up the potato and cook in the microwave in a small amount of water as well.)

2. Combine, gluten-free flour, potato starch, and xanthan gum.

3. Peel potato and process in a food processor with salt until smooth.

4. Meanwhile, in a large bowl, cream butter with egg and sugar; mix in potato mixture, then add gluten-free flour, potato starch, xanthan gum, baking powder, and milk. Process together until smooth.

5. Work dough into ½-cup balls. If too sticky, add additional flour blend or potato starch. If too stiff, add a little of the water you used to boil or cook the potato to loosen it.

6. On wax paper that has been dusted with rice flour, roll out each dough ball to make a ¼-inch-thick disk.

7. Spray skillet with cooking spray or vegetable oil, then heat.

8. Cook each disk until brown and bubbling on each side. Serve warm.

Nutritional information: 237 calories, 3.8 grams protein, 47 grams carbohydrates, 4 grams fat, 35 milligrams cholesterol, 478 milligrams sodium, 2.2 grams fiber, 50.6 milligrams calcium, less than 1 milligram iron.

Tips: Great with dips or served as an open-face sandwich. Delicious when made with added seasoning such as garlic and onion powder. If made ahead of time and kept refrigerated, microwave for about 30 seconds before using. Lots of appetizer options as well:

Garlic Knots: Make small balls of dough and roll into rope and shape into knots. Bake in oven then sauté with garlic, oil, and Parmesan cheese.

Cheese Puffs and Mini Knishes: Make small balls of dough, fill with cheese or mashed potatoes, and bake or pan sauté.

Pigs in a Blanket: Make small ropes of dough, flatten, wrap around gluten-free mini hot dogs and bake. Or make small, 1 in. dough balls (about ping-pong size), push the mini hot dog though the dough ball, and roll to flatten a little.

** Allergy Tip: This recipe is GF, SF, NF, PF, FF, SFF, V. To keep soy free, use a soy-free cooking spray or vegetable oil and soy-free margarine or butter and double-check that the gluten-free flour blend and mini hot dogs (for pigs-in-a-blanket) are soy free. To make egg free, use any gluten-free eggless egg substitute. To make milk free, use any gluten-free dairy alternative for the milk (such as rice milk or potato water) and margarine in place of the butter (note most margarine contains soy). To make vegan, use an eggless egg substitute, and a milk-free alternative for the butter and buttermilk.

Italian Pizza   **Serves 12 (1 Large Pizza, 4 Small)**

This pizza is just fabulous—take care to follow the instructions for letting it rise, and you will have a pizza that tastes the way pizza should.

1½ packets rapid yeast
1 Tb sugar or molasses
1 Tb cider vinegar
½ cup buttermilk
½ cup warm water
¼ tsp salt
1½ cups gluten-free all-purpose flour blend (see chapter 5 or buy)
1½ cups potato starch
½ cup cornmeal
2 tsp xanthan gum
1 tsp salt
⅓ cup olive oil
½ cup cornmeal
2 cups tomato sauce
1 tsp dried Italian herbs
½ tsp garlic powder
½ tsp onion powder
1½ cups part skim mozzarella cheese
¼ cup Parmesan cheese

1. Combine yeast, sugar, vinegar, buttermilk, water, and ¼ tsp salt (let sit at room temperature about 15 minutes until bubbling).

2. Combine flour blend, potato starch, ¼ cup cornmeal xanthan gum, and 1 tsp salt.

3. Combine yeast mixture with flour mixture until dough forms a ball, if too wet add a little additional gluten-free flour blend. Add 2 Tb olive oil and let rest in warm place until doubled in bulk.

4. Roll dough either into one large ball or 4 smaller balls and shape into pizza rounds, sprinkle pizza pans with remaining cornmeal and place rounds on pans. (Let sit for about 30 minutes before par baking them.)

5. Preheat oven to 450 degrees F. If you have baking stones, place them in the oven.

6. Drizzle each pizza with olive oil and bake in the oven for about 5–8 minutes to set a little. Remove from oven.

7. Top pizza with tomato sauce, Italian herbs, garlic powder, onion powder, mozzarella cheese, and Parmesan cheese. Bake for about 10–15 minutes until golden.

8. Slice with a pizza cutter and serve.

Nutritional information: 323 calories, 7.3 grams protein, 53 grams carbohydrates, 9 grams fat, 11 milligrams cholesterol, 583 milligrams sodium, 2.0 grams fiber, 151 milligrams calcium, 1.1 milligrams iron.

Tips: Add extra cheese or favorite toppings such as fresh herbs (such as basil or oregano), grilled eggplant or zucchini, pepperoni, sausage, sliced grilled chicken, shrimp, olives, shallots, roasted garlic, roasted peppers, grilled onions, anchovies, and more. Try a sesame seed pizza crust: sprinkle sesame seeds on the pizza pan and press the pizza dough on top of them. A great flour blend for pizza is ⅓ parts cornstarch, ⅓ parts 100% buckwheat flour, and ⅓ parts millet flour.

** Allergy Tip: This recipe is GF, EF, SF, NF, PF, FF, SFF, V. To keep soy free, check flour blend for soy. To keep nut free and peanut free, check the flour blend for nuts. To make milk free and vegan, use dairy-free alternatives in place of buttermilk (such as rice milk) and cheeses (if you are also soy free, make sure these alternatives do not contain soy).

Hamburger Rolls   Serves 8

This recipe can be used to make either hamburger or hot dog rolls. Delicious fresh out of the oven, or toasted on the barbecue.

¼ cup lukewarm water (105 degrees F)
1 package rapid-rise yeast

½ cup mashed potatoes
¾ cup potato water
⅓ cup sugar
4 Tb butter
1 tsp salt
1½ cups brown rice flour
1 cup tapioca flour
1 cup quinoa or soy flour
½ cup dry milk powder
2 tsp xanthan gum
2 eggs
2 Tb sesame seeds

1. Combine water and yeast in a small bowl and let sit for 5 minutes.

2. Combine fresh hot mashed potatoes with potato water, sugar, butter, and salt. Whisk together until smooth. Let cool to lukewarm.

3. Combine flours with milk powder and xanthan gum.

4. Add 1 egg to potato mixture.

5. Mix yeast, water, 2 cups of flour mixture, and potato blend, mix until well-combined.

6. Stir in remaining flour to make a stiff dough.

7. Form dough into 8 round balls. Place on cookie sheet that has been lined with parchment paper. Flatten slightly.

8. Beat remaining egg. Brush on top of rolls and sprinkle with sesame seeds.

9. Let rise in a warm place for about 1 hour.

10. Bake at 400 degrees F for 15–20 minutes, or until browned.

Nutritional information: 347 calories, 12 grams protein, 52 grams carbohydrates, 10.6 grams fat, 69 milligrams cholesterol, 418 milligrams sodium, 5 grams fiber, 150 milligrams calcium, 2.4 milligrams iron.

Tips: The oven is a good place for this dough to rise. Set oven at 175 degrees F for 5 minutes. Turn off oven, put in hamburger rolls, and let rise for about 1 hour. To make potato water, boil potatoes in about 1½ cups of water until cooked. Mash potatoes and save water for potato water. Also, if you want a hot dog roll, shape each dough ball into a small log and follow the recipe as indicated for hamburger rolls.

** Allergy Tip: This recipe is GF, SF, NF, PF, FF, SFF, V. For soy free, use quinoa flour. To make egg free, use any gluten-free eggless egg substitute.

Pretzel Nuggets   Makes 36 Pieces

A nice treat for those late-night munchies or for a party snack.

2 packages rapid-rise yeast
1 Tb brown sugar
1 tsp salt
2 Tb butter, melted
2¾ cups gluten-free all-purpose flour blend (see chapter 5 or buy)
1 cup lukewarm water (105 degrees F)
5 tsp baking soda
4 cups water
2 tsp kosher salt

1. In a large bowl, combine yeast, sugar, salt, butter, and 1 cup flour mixture. Add water and stir until smooth and well-blended.

2. Add remaining flour and stir until mixed in and dough is stiff.

3. Spray a large cookie sheet with nonstick cooking spray, or line with parchment paper.

4. Break dough into 1½-inch pieces (nuggets) and place on cookie sheet.

5. Let sit, covered with a towel, for 1 hour.

6. Bring baking soda and water to a boil in a deep stainless steel pot.

7. Place pretzel nuggets a few at a time into the boiling water. Let boil for 1½ minutes. Remove with a slotted spoon, drain, and place on greased cookie sheet.

8. Preheat oven to 475 degrees F.

9. Sprinkle with salt and bake for 9–10 minutes until golden brown.

Nutritional information (per pretzel): 52 calories, less than 1 gram protein, 10.5 grams carbohydrates, less than 1 gram fat, 1.7 milligrams cholesterol, 336 milligrams sodium, less than 1 gram fiber, 2.8 milligrams calcium, less than 1 milligram iron.

Tips: This dough falls apart easily, so it works best in nugget shape rather than traditional pretzel shape. These pretzels are best warm from the oven.

** Allergy Tip: This recipe is GF, EF, SF, NF, PF, FF, SFF, V. Double-check flour blend to make sure it doesn't contain any nuts or soy. To make milk free, use margarine in place of the butter (if you are also soy free make sure you select a soy-free margarine). To make vegan, substitute margarine for butter.

Basic Crêpes   Serves 4

Terrific filled with seafood or chicken and some shredded cheese. Works great as an appetizer entrée or as a dessert crêpe.

⅔ cup sorghum flour
⅓ cup potato starch
2 eggs
1 cup low-fat milk
½ tsp salt
2 Tb butter, melted
Gluten-free cooking spray or olive oil

1. In a large mixing bowl, whisk together flour, potato starch, and eggs. Add milk, and stir to combine.

2. Beat in salt and butter. Continue to mix until smooth.

3. Heat a medium-size nonstick skillet over medium-high heat. Spray with cooking spray.

4. Pour ¼ cup batter onto a nonstick skillet pan. Tilt pan back and forth so that the batter coats the surface evenly.

5. Cook for about 1 minute, until the bottom starts to brown. Flip crêpe with spatula and cook the other side for about 30 seconds.

6. Remove to platter and cover to keep warm.

7. Fill as desired and serve.

Nutritional information: 272 calories, 8.8 grams protein, 40 grams carbohydrates, 9.8 grams fat, 124 milligrams cholesterol, 395 milligrams sodium, 2 grams fiber, 96.6 milligrams calcium, 1.8 milligrams iron.

Tips: Add a tablespoon of sugar or sprinkle with sugar to make a dessert crêpe. Can be made ahead, refrigerated and wrapped until ready to heat and serve. Batter doesn't hold well refrigerated.

** Allergy Tip: This recipe is GF, SF, NF, PF, FF, SFF, V. To keep soy free, use a soy-free cooking spray or vegetable oil. To make milk free, use a dairy-free product, such as rice milk in place of the milk, and margarine in place of the butter (if you are also soy free, make sure you select a soy-free margarine). To make vegan, use margarine in place of butter and alternatives for the egg and milk.

English Muffins   Makes 6

Millet gives a nice texture and flavor to this English muffin—perfect toasted with jam and butter.

Gluten-free cooking spray or olive oil

Dry Ingredients:

¼ cup gluten-free cornmeal
¾ cup millet flour
1 cup white rice flour
¼ cup potato starch
¼ cup tapioca starch
1 tsp cream of tartar
1 package rapid-rise yeast
½ cup dry milk powder
½ tsp salt
1 Tb sugar
1 cup lukewarm seltzer (105 degrees F)
1 egg, beaten
2 Tb butter, melted

1. Grease 6 hamburger bun/muffin cups (available online, or see tip below) with cooking spray and dust lightly with cornmeal.

2. Mix all dry ingredients in a large bowl.

3. Mix seltzer, egg, and butter into the flour mixture. Stir until smooth and well-combined.

4. Pour into prepared cups. Let sit for 1 hour in a warm place, until doubled in size.

5. Preheat oven to 375 degrees F.

6. Cook muffins for 15–20 minutes, or until a toothpick inserted into the middle comes out clean. (Muffins will not be browned; if you would like them browned on top, brush each with egg yolk before putting in the oven.)

7. Let cool for 5 minutes in pan before removing. Cut in half and serve warm, or toast before eating.

Nutritional information: 265 calories, 6.6 grams protein, 47 grams carbohydrates, 5.7 grams fat, 46 milligrams cholesterol, 265 milligrams sodium, 2 grams fiber, 79 milligrams calcium, 1.5 milligrams iron.

Tip: If you do not have a hamburger muffin pan, 6-oz tuna cans that have been cleaned and had the label removed work just fine—or order an English muffin pan from a cooking supply company.

** Allergy Tip: This recipe is GF, SF, NF, PF, FF, SFF, V. To keep soy free, use a soy-free cooking spray or vegetable oil. To make egg free, use any gluten-free eggless egg substitute.

Gluten-Free Challah Bread   Serves 20

¾ cup skim milk
2/3 cup sugar
2 packets of rapid yeast
5–5½ cups GF flour blend (* see tip)
½ cup super fine rice flour
2 tsp. kosher or sea salt
2 tsp. xanthan gum
6 eggs
1 stick (8 Tb.) of butter melted (at room temperature) (margarine or oil can be used if desired)
1 cup of yellow raisins (optional)
2 Tb. olive oil

Gluten-Free cooking spray or olive oil
2 tsp. poppy seeds (optional)

1. Warm milk until lukewarm, and then add 2 Tb. sugar and 2 packets of yeast. Let it sit about 5 minutes until foamy.

2. Meanwhile, combine flours, salt, xanthan gum, and remaining sugar.

3. Beat 5 eggs, and mix together with the melted butter. Combine with foaming yeast mixture.

4. Mix wet and dry ingredients until well combined. It should feel like modeling clay. The dough should not be sticky. If needed, add more gluten-free flour until you achieve the right texture (see *tip). If adding raisins, mix into dough now. Shape dough into a ball.

5. Coat a clean bowl with 2 Tb. of oil and place dough ball in the middle, rolling to coat with oil. Cover bowl and place in warm place. Let rise for 2- 2 1/2 hours until doubled in bulk.

6. Punch down dough. It will be a bit crumbly. Work it until it stays together.

7. Gluten-free dough isn't as easy to shape as regular challah dough here are a few options:

   a. Place dough into an oil-coated molded cake, Bundt, or loaf pan. Reserve a little dough to shape a design on the top.

   b. Shape the dough into a round and place on a cookie sheet that has been coated with olive oil.

   c. Carefully form the dough into 3 logs and braid. Be sure to squeeze together any dough that crumbles apart and place it on an olive oil–coated pan.

   d. Make a long rope and circle it into a round on a cookie sheet that has been coated with olive oil.

8. Cover and let dough rise for an hour until doubled in bulk. Beat remaining egg and brush over loaf, sprinkle with poppy seeds.

9. Preheat oven to 375 degrees F and bake for about 35-45 minutes until golden and the bread sounds hollow when it is tapped.

Nutritional Information: 283 calories, 4.4 grams protein, 49 grams carbohydrates, 7.6 grams of fat, 1.9 grams fiber, 68 milligrams cholesterol, 319 milligrams sodium, 56 milligrams calcium, 1 milligram iron.

*Tip: Different gluten-free flour blends will soak up liquids more then others, and you may need to add up to a cup of additional flour. When mixing, dough will be right when it is almost the texture of play dough, just a little wetter.

**Allergy Tip: GF, SF, NF, PF, FF, SFF, V. To keep soy free, use olive oil and double-check gluten-free flour blend. To make milk free, use margarine in place of butter and a milk substitute.

Starters & Small Plates:

- Eggplant Dip

- Super Bean Dip

- Salmon Salad

- Chicken Satay

- Beets with Blue Cheese

- Albanian Meatballs (Quofte)

- Chicken Fingers with Apricot Sauce

- Hushpuppies

- Shrimp Scampi Wrapped in Bacon

- Grilled Stacked Eggplant and Mozzarella Tower

- Buffalo Chicken Wings

- Honey–Soy Glazed Chicken Wings

- Polenta Cups with Avocado and Mango Salsa

- Gluten-Free Capellini Fritti

Also see the appetizer ideas in the tip section of the potato flat bread recipe earlier in this chapter (p. 248).

Eggplant Dip   **Serves 8**

This is a terrific dip, delicious on gluten-free crackers, corn tortillas, or rice cakes, or served with a vegetable platter.

Gluten-free cooking spray or olive oil
1 Tb olive oil
4 Tb garlic, minced
1 medium onion, finely chopped
2 green zucchini, cut into ½-inch pieces
1 green pepper, cut into ½-inch pieces
1 small eggplant, peeled and cut into ½-inch pieces
1 cup tomato sauce
1 tsp onion powder
½ tsp black pepper
1 tsp Italian seasoning
1 Tb sugar
1 Tb balsamic vinegar
2 Tb parmesan cheese

1. Spray skillet with cooking spray; add olive oil and sauté garlic, then add onion and sauté until translucent.

2. Add zucchini, green pepper, and eggplant; sauté until cooked through (add water if pan starts to dry out).

3. Add to pan 1 cup tomato sauce, onion powder, pepper, Italian seasoning, sugar, vinegar, and Parmesan cheese. Cover and simmer for about 10–20 minutes (until vegetables are soft and tomato sauce is cooked down).

4. Refrigerate overnight to allow flavors to combine. Serve eggplant with gluten-free lentil or brown rice crackers.

Nutritional information: 67 calories, 2.3 grams protein, 11 grams carbohydrates, 2.3 grams fat, 1.1 milligrams cholesterol, 27 milligrams sodium, 3.5 grams fiber, 38 milligrams calcium, less than 1 milligram iron.

Tips: You can add more veggies to this dish and add extra garlic, onion powder, pepper, and Italian seasoning if you like. Gluten-free hot sauce is also great added to this dip if you want it spicier—season to taste.

** **Allergy Tip:** This recipe is GF, EF, SF, NF, PF, FF, SFF, V. To keep soy free, use a soy-free cooking spray or vegetable oil. To make milk free and vegan, omit the cheese or use a vegan gluten-free cheese substitute.

Super Bean Dip   Serves 8

This bean dip is high in fiber and loaded with flavor. Why not toast up a mini gluten-free pizza crust and spread bean dip on top and sprinkle with mozzarella cheese?

15-oz can chickpeas (garbanzo beans), drained
15-oz can kidney beans, drained
15-oz can black beans, drained
1 Tb garlic, minced
4–5 Tb lemon juice
⅓–½ cup water (for desired texture)
3 Tb tahini (sesame seed paste)
1 tsp cumin
½ tsp paprika
1 tsp salt
1 tsp pepper
½ cup parsley, chopped
½ cup green onions, chopped

1. Purée all ingredients together in a food processor.

2. Add extra water as needed to achieve desired texture.

3. Add additional spices to suit your taste.

4. Refrigerate until ready to use.

Nutritional information: 165 calories, 8.6 grams protein, 25 grams carbohydrates, 3.9 grams fat, 0 milligrams cholesterol, 506 milligrams sodium, 7.3 grams fiber, 56 milligrams calcium, 2.2 milligrams iron.

Tip: Most canned beans are gluten-free, but on occasion some companies have added gluten-containing products, so be sure to check your labels.

** **Allergy Tip:** This recipe is GF, MF, EF, SF, NF, PF, FF, SFF, V, VG.

Salmon Salad   **Serves 4**

Serve this as part of an impressive salad platter, or rolled into a gluten-free wrap.

1 lb salmon fillets
2 Tb low-fat mayonnaise
2 Tb nonfat plain yogurt
1 tsp lemon juice
½ cup celery, chopped
1 Tb capers (optional)
1 tsp dried dill weed or 1 Tb fresh dill, chopped
1 tsp dried tarragon or 1 Tb fresh tarragon, chopped
¼ tsp black pepper
4 large lettuce leaves

1. Cook salmon fillets until just cooked (poach, grill, or broil) and cool to room temperature.

2. Mix remaining ingredients (except lettuce leaves) in a large bowl.

3. Flake salmon and stir into mixture.

4. Serve over lettuce leaves

Nutritional information per serving: 211 calories, 19.6 grams protein, 2.3 grams carbohydrates, 13 grams fat, 56.5 milligrams cholesterol, 190 milligrams sodium, less than 1 gram fiber, 46 milligrams calcium, less than 1 milligram iron.

Tips: Great served with other veggies such as sliced tomatoes, or roasted peppers. Before cooking check to make sure there are no bones in the salmon by running your hand across the top of the salmon and feeling for bones. Use needle nosed pliers to pull out any you find.

** Allergy Tip: This recipe is GF, NF, PF, SFF. To make egg free, use an egg-free mayonnaise. To make soy free, use a soy-free mayonnaise. To make milk free, omit the yogurt and double up on the mayonnaise or eliminate the mayonnaise and double up on a milk-free yogurt.

Chicken Satay   **Serves 4**

This is an impressive appetizer that is sure to delight your guests. Serve as the perfect finger food, or as part of an appetizer platter.

1 lb chicken tenders, cleaned
½ cup coconut milk
1 tsp curry powder
1 tsp ginger
1 clove garlic, minced
Gluten-free cooking spray or olive oil
2 Tb creamy peanut butter
2 Tb tahini (sesame seed paste)
1 Tb gluten-free soy sauce (such as La Choy, or San-J)
1 Tb brown sugar
½ cup (4 oz) gluten-free chicken broth
1 Tb lime juice
1 Tb red curry paste

1. Place chicken tenders, coconut milk, curry powder, ginger, and gar-lic in a 1-gallon zipper bag. Mix well and place in refrigerator to marinade for 1–2 hours.

2. Soak 4 wooden skewers in water for 30 minutes.

3. In a small saucepan, mix peanut butter, tahini, soy sauce, sugar, chicken broth, lime juice, and curry paste. Heat over low heat, stir-ring until smooth and well-combined.

4. Heat stove top grill pan or outdoor grill. Remove chicken from mar-inade.

5. Thread chicken onto skewers, distributing chicken evenly.

6. Grill chicken for 3–5 minutes per side, until cooked through. Serve with peanut sauce.

Nutritional information per serving: 248 calories, 30 grams protein, 7 grams carbohydrates, 11 grams fat, less than 1 gram fiber, 66 milligrams cholesterol, 378 milligrams sodium, 34 milligrams calcium, 1.5 milligrams iron.

Tip: Use beef, pork, or shrimp in place of chicken.

** Allergy Tip: This recipe is GF, MF, EF, NF, FF, SFF. Coconut is techni-cally considered a nut but most with tree nut allergies can consume them, if you have a nut allergy you should check with your allergist and doctor.

Beets with Blue Cheese   Serves 4

This was inspired by the classic recipe often served in many top steak houses.

16-oz jar pickled beets, drained
4 oz blue cheese
4 Tb gluten-free bread crumbs
4 cups mesculin greens, washed and dried
4 Tb shaved parmesan cheese

Dressing

2 Tb olive oil
2 Tb lemon juice
2 tsp sugar
Dash of salt
Dash of oregano
Dash of pepper
¼ cup white wine

1. Whisk together dressing ingredients.

2. Place beets on a cookie sheet and top with crumbling of bleu cheese and sprinkle with bread crumbs.

3. Turn oven to broil and place beets under broiler.

4. Arrange greens on 4 plates and top with dressing.

5. As soon as cheese starts to melt on the beets, remove from oven and arrange over greens.

6. Sprinkle with parmesan cheese and serve.

Nutritional information: 278 calories, 7.8 grams protein, 27 grams carbohydrates, 15.2 grams fat, 18.6 milligrams cholesterol, 785 milligrams sodium, 4.2 grams fiber, 204 milligrams calcium, 1 milligrams iron.

Tip: No time to make homemade dressing? Mix some gluten-free Italian dressing and squeeze in a little lemon juice.

** Allergy Tip: This recipe is GF, EF, SF, NF, PF, FF, SFF, V. Check beets, and gluten-free bread crumbs for soy, and double the bread crumbs to make sure they don't contain nuts, or eggs.

Albanian Meatballs (Quofte)   Serves 8

These Mediterranean meatballs are lighter than the typical Italian meatballs. They can be served plain but are especially delicious with yogurt sauce.

1 lb ground beef sirloin
1 large Spanish onion, finely minced
1½ tsp dried mint
½ tsp pepper
1½ tsp salt
2 eggs
2 Tb water
¼ cup brown rice flour (or gluten-free flour blend)
½ cup additional brown rice flour (or gluten-free flour blend) for coating
Gluten-free cooking spray or olive oil

1. Preheat oven to broil, and spray a baking sheet with cooking spray.

2. Mix meat, onion, spices, eggs, water, and ¼ cup flour together thoroughly. Mixture should be fairly wet; if not, add a little more water.

3. Shape meat into an oval shape with 2 tsp and roll in flour. It should resemble the shape of ⅓ of a cigar, a little bumpy.

4. Place meatballs on the prepared baking sheet.

5. Spray meatballs lightly with cooking spray and place in oven.

6. Broil until brown on both sides.

7. Serve with garlic yogurt sauce (see sauces).

Nutritional information: 174 calories, 15.6 grams protein, 13.4 grams carbohydrates, 6 grams fat, 84 milligrams cholesterol, 506 milligrams sodium, 1 gram fiber, 19 milligrams calcium, 1.8 milligrams iron.

Tips: Traditionally these meatballs are made with a higher-fat meat and deep-fried. This recipe cuts down the fat and calories. I find these just as delicious as the traditional version. Other meats can be mixed with these meatballs. Dried currants and nuts make a nice addition as well.

** Allergy Tip: This recipe is GF, MF, SF, NF, PF, FF, SFF. To keep soy free, use a soy-free cooking spray or vegetable oil. To make egg free, use an egg-free egg substitute.

Chicken Fingers with Apricot Sauce   Serves 4

Both kids and adults will love these delicious, easy-to-make chicken fingers. They can be served with any sauce.

16 oz skinless boneless chicken breast
2 Tb gluten-free cornmeal
2 Tb seasoned gluten-free bread crumbs
2 Tb crushed pecans
2 tsp garlic powder
1 tsp onion powder
8 egg whites
Gluten-free cooking spray or olive oil
4 Tb apricot preserves
2 Tb gluten-free light mayonnaise
1 dash of gluten-free hot sauce (optional)

1. Preheat oven to 350 degrees.

2. Clean and pound chicken cutlets. Cut into chicken fingers 3–4 inches long and 2–3 inches wide.

3. Toss cornmeal, bread crumbs, pecans, garlic powder, and onion powder together in a medium bowl.

4. Dip chicken in egg whites and then coat in cornmeal mixture.

5. Spray baking sheet with cooking spray, put coated chicken on baking sheet and spray top with cooking spray.

6. Cook until brown on one side; turn, spray again with cooking spray, and bake until just cooked through and crispy and brown on the outside.

7. Mix together apricot preserves, light mayo, and hot sauce and serve with chicken fingers.

Nutritional information: 280 calories, 34.5 grams protein, 21 grams carbohydrates, 6.7 grams fat, 68 milligrams cholesterol, 247 milligrams sodium, less than 1 gram fiber, 29 milligrams calcium, 1.3 milligrams iron.

Tip: If gluten-free bread crumbs are not available, toast 1 slice of gluten-free bread and process in a food processor with ¼ tsp Italian seasoning and ¼ tsp salt and a dash of pepper

** Allergy Tip: This recipe is GF, MF, PF, FF, SFF. To keep milk free, make sure bread crumbs do not contain milk. To make soy free, use a soy-free cooking spray or vegetable oil and mayonnaise and check the bread crumbs. To make egg free, use any gluten-free eggless egg substitute in place of the egg whites and mayonnaise and check the bread crumbs.

Hushpuppies   Serves 12

Put these in a basket, sprinkle with powdered sugar, and watch them disappear.

1 cup buttermilk
1 egg
2 cups gluten-free cornmeal
½ cup gluten-free flour blend (see chapter 5 or buy)
¼ cup frozen corn kernels, defrosted
4 Tb granulated sugar
1 tsp salt
½ tsp gluten-free baking soda
½ tsp gluten-free baking powder
1 tsp xanthan gum
¼ cup corn oil for frying
4 Tb powdered sugar (for garnish)

1. Beat together buttermilk and egg.

2. Combine egg mixture with all other ingredients except corn oil and powdered sugar, and stir to combine.

3. In a large skillet, heat corn oil a little at a time until hot.

4. Spoon a few tablespoons of cornmeal mixture at a time into the hot oil.

5. Pan fry until golden. Remove from skillet and drain on paper towels if greasy.

6. Sprinkle with powdered sugar and serve warm.

Nutritional information: 210 calories, 3.5 grams protein, 38.6 grams carbohydrates, 7 grams fat, 18 milligrams cholesterol, 290 milligrams sodium, less than 1 gram fiber, 39 milligrams calcium, less than 1 milligram iron.

Tip: For spicier hushpuppies, add cayenne pepper and skip the powdered sugar.

✶✶ Allergy Tip: This recipe is GF, SF, NF, PF, FF, SFF, V. For nut free and soy free, check the flour blend for nuts, peanuts, and soy. To make milk free, use any dairy-free milk substitute, such as rice milk, in place of the buttermilk. To make egg free, use any gluten-free eggless egg substitute. To make vegan, use gluten-free alternatives for the buttermilk and egg.

Shrimp Scampi Wrapped in Bacon   Serves 4

This classic recipe never goes out of style.

12 oz jumbo shrimp, shells removed
6 pieces of gluten-free bacon
Olive or canola oil gluten-free cooking spray
2 Tb butter or margarine
2 Tb garlic, minced
½ tsp salt
1 Tb lemon juice
¼ cup white wine
2 Tb parmesan cheese

1. Preheat oven to 350 degrees F.

2. Lightly cook bacon in microwave until just cooked, but still soft.

3. Cut each piece of bacon in half and wrap around shrimp, secure with a toothpick.

4. Spray a cooking sheet with cooking spray, and place shrimp on the sheet.

5. Mix together butter, garlic, salt, lemon juice, and wine and heat in microwave, just to melt butter.

6. Pour mixture over shrimp on baking sheet and cook until shrimp are just cooked (pink).

7. Sprinkle with parmesan cheese and serve.

Nutritional information: 220 calories, 21.4 grams protein, 2.2 grams carbohydrates, 12.4 grams fat, 158 milligrams cholesterol, 714 milligrams sodium, less than 1 gram fiber, 77 milligrams calcium, 2.1 milligrams iron.

Tips: Scallops or chicken can be used in this recipe in place of the shrimp as well. Garnish with chopped scallions and lemon wedges.

** Allergy Tip: This recipe is GF, SF, EF, NF, PF, FF. For soy free, use a soy-free cooking spray or vegetable oil and butter or a soy-free margarine and double-check the bacon for soy. To make milk free, omit the cheese and use margarine in place of the butter (if you are also soy free make sure you select a soy-free margarine).

Grilled Stacked Eggplant and Mozzarella Tower   Serves 6

This makes an impressive appetizer, layered and served on individual plates.

1 large eggplant peeled and sliced into ½-inch round slices
2 Tb garlic, minced
½ tsp salt
½ tsp pepper
2 Tb olive oil
6 slices gluten-free bread
2 Tb olive oil
1 tsp garlic powder
2 Tb parmesan cheese
2 roasted red peppers sliced
2 tomatoes, sliced thin
6 oz fresh mozzarella, sliced thin (if you are following a low-fat diet, substitute skim mozzarella)
4 Tb fresh basil, finely chopped

1. Mix eggplant slices with garlic, salt, pepper, and 2 Tb olive oil, and then grill in a George Foreman–type countertop grill until just cooked.

2. Meanwhile, preheat your oven to broil, and toast all 6 pieces of bread.

3. Using a coffee cup or a muffin cutter, cut a circle in the middle of each piece of toast, brush the top of each round with olive oil, sprinkle with garlic powder and parmesan cheese, and broil on a baking sheet until cheese melts.

4. Layer garlic crouton, eggplant, roasted peppers, tomatoes, and mozzarella on 6 small plates.

5. Garnish with fresh chopped basil and serve.

Nutritional information: 257 calories, 8.5 grams protein, 22 grams carbohydrates, 15.6 grams fat, 24 milligrams cholesterol, 483 milligrams sodium, 2.6 grams fiber, 222 milligrams calcium, 1.5 milligrams iron.

Tips: This recipe works well without the garlic crouton, if desired. It is best prepared with fresh roasted peppers. To roast peppers, preheat your oven to 450 degrees F, place aluminum foil on a baking sheet, and cook peppers until they just start to blacken. Take out of the oven and wait until peppers cool, then peel, and pop out seeds. Can be made ahead and kept in the refrigerator in a glass jar for a few days.

** Allergy Tip: This recipe is GF, EF, NF, PF, FF, SFF, V. To keep nut free, peanut free and egg free, double-check that the bread does not contain nuts or eggs. To make soy free, use a soy-free bread.

Buffalo Chicken Wings   Serves 16

Settle down with a crowd of friends to watch the football game and polish off a bucket of chicken wings—add hot sauce to taste.

5 lbs chicken wings, separated into winglet and drumlet
½ cup brown rice flour
1 tsp salt
½ tsp pepper
½ cup vegetable oil
6 Tb lite butter
1 Tb gluten-free hot sauce or to taste
½ cup gluten-free blue cheese salad dressing
8 celery stalks, sliced long, then quartered

1. Mix together brown rice flour, salt, and pepper.

2. Wash and dry chicken wings, and dredge into flour mixture.

3. Heat vegetable oil in a saucepan and fry wings in hot vegetable oil until golden; discard remaining oil.

4. In a small saucepan, melt butter and mix with hot sauce.

5. Preheat oven to broil.

6. Toss wings with butter mixture, and place on a cookie sheet that has been covered with aluminum foil.

7. Cook under the broiler until the wings are crispy.

8. Serve with blue cheese dressing and celery sticks.

Nutritional information: 422 calories, 25 grams protein, 4.7 grams carbohydrates, 34 grams fat, 125 milligrams cholesterol, 370 milligrams sodium, less than 1 gram fiber, 18.4 milligrams calcium, 1.77 milligrams iron.

Tip: To make your own blue cheese dressing, in a food processor combine 4 oz blue cheese, 1 cup light mayonnaise, ½ cup light gluten-free sour cream (such as Friendship), 2 Tb lemon juice, ½ tsp garlic powder, 1 Tb grated onion, and salt and pepper to taste.

** Allergy Tip: This recipe is GF, SF, NF, PF, FF, SFF. For soy free, make sure the salad dressing does not contain soy and use a soy-free vegetable oil.

Honey-Soy Glazed Chicken Wings   Serves 8

This Chinese favorite is cooked until the chicken practically falls off the bone.

2 lbs chicken wings
4 Tb vegetable oil
⅓ cup light gluten-free soy sauce (such as La Choy or San-J)
4 Tb honey
2 Tb sherry
1 tsp garlic, minced
½ tsp fresh ginger, minced
2 stalks scallions chopped
1 Tb brown sugar
1 Tb vinegar
4 Tb scallions, chopped

1. Separate each wing into 2 pieces.

2. In a large skillet, heat oil and stir fry chicken wings in small batches until lightly browned.

3. Drain on paper towels.

4. Mix together all remaining ingredients (except the scallions) and heat in a medium-sized sauté pan.

5. Cook chicken wings in sauce mixture for about 30 minutes, until chicken is soft.

6. Garnish with additional chopped scallions if desired.

Nutritional information: 358 calories, 21.7 grams protein, 11 grams carbohydrates, 25 grams fat, 87 milligrams cholesterol, 610.8 milligrams sodium, less than 1 gram fiber, 27 milligrams calcium, 1.6 milligrams iron.

Tip: Gluten-free tamari works well in this recipe as an alternate to the soy sauce.

** Allergy Tip: This recipe is GF, MF, EF, NF, PF, FF, SFF.

Polenta Cups with Avocado and Mango Salsa   Servings 24

A light, refreshing appetizer that is sure to be a hit. Registered dietitian Cathie Brittan loves these because they are delicious while being low in calories and fat.

For the Salsa

1 can (14-oz) diced tomatoes with green chiles
1 green pepper, finely chopped
1 red onion, finely chopped
1 clove garlic, minced
1 avocado, chopped
1 small mango, chopped
¼ cup fresh cilantro, finely chopped
2 Tb red wine vinegar
1 Tb olive oil
1 Tb lime juice

For the Polenta

4 cups water
½ tsp kosher salt
1 cup yellow cornmeal
1 tsp minced fresh cilantro
¼ tsp black pepper
Gluten-free nonstick cooking spray or olive oil

1. Combine the salsa ingredients in a small bowl and refrigerate.

2. In a large saucepan, bring water and salt to a boil. Keeping water at a gentle boil, slowly whisk in cornmeal. Cook and stir for 15 to 20 minutes until polenta is thickened and pulls away from the sides of the pan. Remove from heat and stir in cilantro and pepper.

3. Coat a miniature muffin pan with gluten-free nonstick cooking spray. Spoon heaping tablespoons of polenta into muffin cups. Using the back of a spoon, make an indentation in the top center of each polenta cup. Cover and chill until set.

4. Unmold polenta and place on serving tray. Top each with a tablespoon of salsa.

Nutritional information per serving: 49 calories, 1 gram protein, 9 grams carbohydrates, 1 gram fat, 1.1 grams fiber, 0 milligrams cholesterol, 115 milligrams sodium, 8.7 milligrams calcium, less than 1 milligram iron.

** Allergy Tip: This recipe is GF, MF, EF, SF, NF, PF, FF, SFF, V, VG. To keep soy free, use a soy-free cooking spray or vegetable oil.

Gluten-Free Capellini Fritti   **Serves 20**

A fabulous new appetizer from Vincent Barbieri of Café Formagio in Carle Place, New York, who is always creating extraordinary new gluten-free recipes for his many restaurants and stores.

10 oz gluten-free capellini (angel hair) pasta
2 cups corn oil
1 lb. ricotta cheese
½ cup chopped Italian parsley
1 cup grated Romano cheese
½ lb gluten-free low-sodium deli ham, chopped fine
4 oz. heavy cream
1 lb shredded mozzarella
6 eggs, beaten
16 oz seasoned gluten-free bread crumbs
Pinch white pepper
Pinch onion powder

1. Boil pasta according to directions on box. Drain and leave pasta sitting in colander for 30 minutes to dry.

2. In large mixing bowl combine ricotta, parsley, ham, grated cheese, and shredded mozzarella and mix thoroughly.

3. Add pasta to mix and again mix thoroughly.

4. Add pinch white pepper and onion powder for taste.

5. Add heavy cream, and mix well. The mix should have a paste-like consistency. If too wet, add a little more mozzarella or if dry add a little more heavy cream to moisten.

6. Form a patty with your hands in the shape of a small hockey puck approximately ½ inch thick by 3 inches round.

7. Dip patties in eggs and then in gluten-free flavored bread crumbs, coating completely.

8. Heat corn oil and place patties in frying pan with hot oil and cook until golden brown on each side by turning over.

9. Serve with your favorite tomato sauce on side for dipping.

Nutritional information per serving: 364 calories, 18 grams protein, 28 grams carbohydrates, 19.8 grams fat, 1.1 grams fiber, 102 milligrams cholesterol, 1017 milligrams sodium, 2.74 milligrams calcium, 1.1 milligrams iron.

** Allergy Tip: This recipe is GF, SF, NF, PF, FF, SFF. For soy free, double-check the bread crumbs and the ham.

Soups and Salads:

- Cranberry Quinoa Salad

- French Onion Soup

- Beef Stew

- Swiss Chard and White Bean Soup

- Crispy Chopped Chicken Salad

- Pear, Gorgonzola Cheese, and Walnut Mixed Green Salad

- Sautéed Spinach Salad

- Butternut Squash and Apple Soup

- Gluten-Free Butternut Bisque

Cranberry Quinoa Salad   **Serves 6**

This tasty salad is great as a side or tossed with slices of grilled chicken as an entrée.

1 cup whole quinoa, rinsed two to three times
2 cups gluten-free chicken or vegetable broth (such as Pacific)
2 tsp olive oil
1 medium yellow onion, chopped
½ cup frozen peas, defrosted and drained
¼ cup dried cranberries
¼ cup walnuts, chopped
2 Tb fresh parsley, roughly chopped

1. Cook quinoa in gluten-free broth for 15–20 minutes, or until cooked.

2. In separate skillet, heat oil; then, add onion and cook until soft.

3. Add cooked onion and peas, dried cranberries, walnuts, and parsley to cooked quinoa.

4. Can be served hot or cold.

Nutritional information: 197 calories, 6.6 grams protein, 29 grams carbohydrates, 6.6 grams fat, 0 milligrams cholesterol, 166 milligrams sodium, 4.2 grams fiber, 35 milligrams calcium, 1.9 milligrams iron.

Tip: Unless you buy prerinsed quinoa, it is important to rinse it several times to remove the bitter outer coating. Quinoa is cooked when a little tail pops out of each grain.

** Allergy Tip: This recipe is GF, MF, EF, SF, PF, FF, SFF. To keep soy free, make sure the broth is soy free. To make nut free, omit the walnuts. To make vegetarian and vegan, use gluten-free vegetable broth.

French Onion Soup   **Serves 4**

This rich, flavorful soup can stand alone as a meal. If you want to make it really decadent, sprinkle extra shredded cheese on top of the soup before broiling.

2 Tb vegetable oil

1 Tb unsalted butter

2 sweet onions (such as Vidalia), thinly sliced

1 Tb cornstarch

1 tsp dried thyme leaves

1 qt (32 oz) gluten-free beef stock (such as Kitchen Basics)

4 slices gluten-free bread

2 tsp olive oil

4 tsp shredded parmesan cheese

1. Place vegetable oil and butter in a large (4-qt) saucepan and heat over medium heat until butter is melted.

2. Add onions and cook for 10–15 minutes until softened and golden brown.

3. Stir in cornstarch and thyme until well blended with onions.

4. Add beef stock and bring to a boil. Reduce heat and simmer for 20 minutes.

5. Preheat broiler.

6. Using a cookie cutter, cut a 2-inch round circle from the center of each slice of bread.

7. Brush with olive oil and sprinkle with cheese.

8. Place bread under broiler for 2–3 minutes until cheese is melted.

9. Pour soup into 4 bowls and top with bread croutons and serve.

Nutritional information: 289 calories, 4 grams protein, 26.4 grams carbohydrates, 18 grams fat, 16 milligrams cholesterol, 797 milligrams sodium, 1.8 grams fiber, 84 milligrams calcium, 1.6 milligrams iron.

Tip: Swiss or provolone cheese works great in this recipe when melted over the top of the soup.

** Allergy Tip: This recipe is GF, EF, SF, NF, PF, FF, SFF. To keep soy free, make sure the broth and bread are soy free. To keep egg free, make sure the bread is egg free. To make milk free, use margarine in place of the butter and use a milk-free cheese substitute (may contain soy). To make vegetarian, use margarine and gluten-free vegetable broth in place of the beef broth. To make vegan, follow directions to make this recipe vegetarian, check the bread for egg, and omit the cheese or use vegan cheese (may contain soy).

Beef Stew   Serves 10

Beef stew is a satisfying standalone meal. Serve with toasted gluten-free English muffins to soak up the extra juices.

1½ lbs beef chunks for stew
2 Tb gluten-free rice flour
Gluten-free cooking spray or olive oil
3 Tb garlic, minced
1 medium onion, chopped
2 tsp Italian seasoning
1 tsp salt
1 tsp pepper
1 cup baby carrots
6 small potatoes cut into 2-inch pieces
8 oz button mushrooms
1 large can crushed tomatoes
10-oz package frozen green beans
48-oz low-sodium gluten-free beef broth (such as Pacific)

1. Toss beef with rice flour.

2. Spray a large pot with cooking spray and sauté beef in batches until browned.

3. Set beef on the side. To the pot add a few tablespoons water, garlic and onion, and cook until onion is translucent.

4. Add Italian seasoning, salt, pepper, baby carrots, potatoes, mushrooms, tomatoes, and green beans and heat for about 10 minutes.

5. Add beef, broth, and 2 cups of water and simmer for about 1½–2 hours, until beef is soft and veggies are cooked.

Nutritional information: 220 calories, 21.5 grams protein, 21.8 grams carbohydrates, 6 grams fat, 33 milligrams cholesterol, 432 milligrams sodium, 3.7 grams fiber, 66.3 milligrams calcium, 3.3 milligrams iron.

Tips: If stew gets too thick when cooking, add some water as needed. Any kind of leftover veggies work well added to the beef stew.

** Allergy Tip:** This recipe is GF, MF, EF, SF, NF, PF, FF, SFF. To keep soy free, use a soy-free cooking spray or vegetable oil and make sure the broth is soy free.

Swiss Chard and White Bean Soup   Serves 6

This classic Italian favorite is easy to make and delicious. If you like it really garlicky, add extra garlic to taste.

2 Tb olive oil
2 large onions, chopped into medium-sized pieces
1 cup carrots, chopped
4 stalks celery, chopped
4 Tb garlic, chopped
1 large bunch fresh Swiss chard, thoroughly washed and chopped into
     medium pieces
48 oz low-sodium gluten-free chicken broth or vegetable broth (such
     as Pacific)
½ tsp salt
1 tsp pepper
2 Tb fresh oregano, finely minced
1 19-oz can white beans (cannelloni beans) drained and rinsed
2 tsp sugar
1 Tb balsamic vinegar
4 Tb parmesan cheese

1. Heat olive oil and sauté onion, carrots, celery, and chopped garlic
   until the onions start to brown.

2. Add Swiss chard; heat until wilted.

3. Add chicken broth salt, pepper, oregano, beans, sugar, and balsamic
   vinegar.

4. Cook 40 minutes until all flavors are incorporated and the Swiss
   chard is soft.

5. Sprinkle with Parmesan cheese and serve.

Nutritional information: 208 calories, 12.9 grams protein, 27.9 grams carbohydrates, 7 grams fat, 2.9 milligrams cholesterol, 485 milligrams sodium, 6.5 grams fiber, 134.6 milligrams calcium, 2.6 milligrams iron.

Tip: Escarole works nicely in this recipe in place of the Swiss chard.

** Allergy Tip: This recipe is GF, EF, SF, NF, PF, FF, SFF. To keep soy free, make sure the broth is soy free. To make milk free, omit the cheese. To make vegetarian, use vegetable broth. To make vegan, omit the cheese and use vegetable broth.

Crispy Chopped-Chicken Salad   Serves 4

This is an amazing salad—when you are making it, be sure to make extra breaded chicken breasts, which are great for quick meals.

12 oz skinless, boneless chicken breast
1 egg, beaten
¼ cup seasoned gluten-free bread crumbs (see tip)
Gluten-free cooking spray or olive oil
6 cups romaine lettuce, chopped
2 oz blue cheese crumbled
1 apple, peeled and chopped
1 cup tomato, chopped
1 cup cucumber, chopped
1 cup red pepper, chopped
1 cup carrots, chopped

1. Clean chicken breasts and pound until 1 inch thick (if you get thin chicken breasts, you can skip this step).

2. Preheat oven to 350 degrees F.

3. Dip chicken in egg and then bread crumbs.

4. Spray a baking sheet with cooking spray and place chicken on it, then spray the top of chicken lightly with cooking spray.

5. Bake chicken until it starts to brown on one side, then turn, spray top again with cooking spray, and bake until golden brown and cooked through.

6. Slice chicken into 2-inch pieces. Mix in large bowl with all other ingredients and serve with favorite gluten-free salad dressing or balsamic vinegar.

Nutritional information: 251 calories, 26.8 grams protein, 18.7 grams carbohydrates, 8.1 grams fat, 112.8 milligrams cholesterol,

328 milligrams sodium, 5.5 grams fiber, 152 milligrams calcium, 2.3 milligrams iron.

Tips: Grilled chicken or shrimp can be used in place of the crispy chicken as well. To make seasoned gluten-free bread crumbs, process gluten-free bread in a food processor until you have crumbs; mix with a little garlic, onion powder, and Italian seasoning.

** Allergy Tip: This recipe is GF, SF, NF, PF, FF, SFF. To keep soy free, use soy-free cooking spray or vegetable oil and check bread crumbs for soy. To keep nut and peanut free, check bread crumbs for nuts and peanuts. To make milk free, omit the cheese and check bread crumbs for milk. To make egg free, use any gluten-free eggless egg substitute.

Pear, Gorgonzola Cheese, and Walnut Mixed Green Salad   Serves 6

Serve this salad at the beginning of a holiday meal for an impressive start.

2 pears, sliced, cored, and sectioned into ¼-inch pieces
1 Tb lemon juice
Gluten-free cooking spray or olive oil
¼ cup walnuts, chopped
2 Tb sugar
½ tsp cinnamon
3 oz gorgonzola cheese crumbled
6 cups mixed greens, chopped
1 cup cherry tomatoes
1 cup shredded carrots
1 cup, sliced and peeled cucumbers
¾ cup gluten-free, fat-free Italian dressing (as needed)

1. Toss pears with lemon juice until ready to combine with salad.

2. Spray a skillet with cooking spray and heat. Give the nuts a quick spray with cooking spray and heat about 2 minutes. Add sugar and cinnamon, remove from heat, and set aside to cool.

3. Drain pears.

4. Combine all ingredients and serve.

Nutritional information: 167 calories, 5.5 grams protein, 22.2 grams carbohydrates, 7.7 grams fat, 22 milligrams cholesterol, 516 milligrams sodium, 4.2 grams fiber, 120 milligrams calcium, less than 1 milligram iron.

Tip: Try using mandarin orange sections or cranberries in place of the pears for delicious alternatives.

** Allergy Tip: This recipe is GF, EF, SF, PF, FF, SFF, V. For soy free, make sure you use a soy-free cooking spray or olive oil and salad dressing. To make milk free, omit cheese or use gluten-free dairy-free cheese alternative. To make nut free, omit the nuts. To make vegan, omit the cheese or add a dairy-free cheese alternative.

Sautéed Spinach Salad   **Serves 4**

This showstopping recipe is always a hit.

1 slice white gluten-free bread, crust removed and cut into 1-inch pieces
Gluten-free cooking spray or olive oil
⅛ tsp garlic and onion powder
1 red pepper
5 scallions, chopped
1 cup mushrooms, sliced
2 tomatoes, cut into small wedges
½ cup cucumber, peeled, sliced, and cut into half-moons
4 Tb gluten-free, fat-free balsamic salad dressing
2 Tb balsamic vinegar
1 7-oz bag baby spinach
4 oz drained mandarin oranges
1½ Tb parmesan cheese

1. Preheat oven to 450 degrees F.

2. Spray a baking sheet with cooking spray and place bread cubes on it; sprinkle with garlic and onion powder.

3. Bake until light brown and set aside.

4. Place red pepper in oven on a pan covered with aluminum foil and bake until black on the outside about 30 minutes (taking care not to burn).

5. Set red pepper aside to cool, then peel and remove seeds and skin. Cut into 1-inch strips.

6. Spray sauté pan with cooking spray and heat pan.

7. Sauté scallions in sauté pan about 4 minutes.

8. Add mushrooms to pan and sauté until they start to soften.

9. Add tomatoes, cucumber, and roasted pepper with salad dressing and vinegar and heat for several minutes until well-combined.

10. Add baby spinach and heat about 1–2 minutes (do not wilt spinach).

11. Toss everything together in a large salad bowl with Mandarin oranges and top with parmesan cheese, then with gluten-free croutons.

Nutritional information: 71.6 calories, 3.8 grams protein, 12.3 grams carbohydrates, 1.2 grams fat, 1.5 milligrams cholesterol, 249 milligrams sodium, 2.7 grams fiber, 70 milligrams calcium, 1 milligrams iron.

Tip: This is a crowd-pleasing salad, great with an Italian meal of gluten-free pasta and meat sauce.

** Allergy Tip: This recipe is GF, SF, NF, PF, FF, SFF, V. To keep soy free, use a soy-free cooking spray or vegetable oil, and check the salad dressing and bread for soy. To make milk free, omit the cheese or use a gluten-free dairy-free substitute (note that this may contain soy), and double-check the bread for milk. To make egg free, use eggless salad dressing and eggless gluten-free bread. To make vegan, use vegan salad dressing and omit the cheese and check the bread for milk or eggs.

Butternut Squash and Apple Soup   Serves 8

All I can say is: creamy, sweet, satisfying, delicious.

3 Tb butter
1 onion, minced
½ tsp nutmeg
1 tsp fresh ginger, chopped
1 tsp cinnamon
1 Tb garlic, chopped
2 apples, peeled, cored, and chopped
½ cup apple juice
5 cups low-sodium gluten-free chicken or vegetable stock (such as Pacific blend)
2 lbs butternut squash, peeled, seeded, and cut into 1-inch cubes

1 tsp salt

1 tsp pepper

½ cup fat-free half-and-half

1 cup light sour cream (such as Friendship)

1. Melt butter in large pot over a medium heat and sauté onion until it starts to brown.

2. Add nutmeg, ginger, cinnamon, garlic, apples, apple juice, chicken stock, and squash. Bring to a boil.

3. Lower heat to a simmer and cook uncovered about 30–45 minutes, until apple and squash are tender.

4. Purée in small batches in a blender until smooth, and return to pot. Add salt and pepper.

5. Fold in ½ cup fat-free half-and-half.

6. Serve with sour cream garnish.

Nutritional information: 191 calories, 5.8 grams protein, 27.3 grams carbohydrates, 8.2 grams fat, 20.6 milligrams cholesterol, 411.6 milligrams sodium, 3.7 grams fiber, 123.6 milligrams calcium, 1.4 milligrams iron.

Tip: You can use pumpkin in place of the butternut squash in this recipe if so desired.

** Allergy Tip: This recipe is GF, EF, SF, NF, PF, FF, SFF, V. To keep soy free, make sure the broth is soy free. For vegetarian, use vegetable broth.

Gluten-Free Butternut Bisque   **Serves 8**

Roasting the vegetables brings out an intense flavor. From Christopher Singlemann, certified executive chef.

1 lb butternut squash peeled, seeded and chopped into ½ in. cubes

¼ lb fresh carrots, peeled and cut into ½ in. dice

1 large white onion diced

3 Tb olive oil

1 medium sweet potato, peeled and cut into ½ in. pieces

1 Tb minced garlic

1 tsp salt

Pepper to taste

2 bay leaves
5 cups reduced sodium gluten-free chicken or vegetable broth
10 oz half-and-half

1. Preheat oven to 375 degrees F.

2. Toss all vegetables with olive oil, salt, and pepper. Spread everything evenly in a roasting pan and roast for about 45 minutes, stirring occasionally until soft and golden brown. The vegetables will be starting to caramelize.

3. Place roasted vegetables into a large pot and cover with chicken broth, add bay leaves, and bring to a boil. Lower heat and simmer covered for approximately 30 minutes, vegetables should be soft and falling apart.

4. Remove bay leaves and puree the soup. If you are using a standing blender wait to let soup cool a little first.

5. Stir in the half-and-half, return to a medium heat, check seasonings. If too thick, add a little chicken stock to obtain the desired consistency.

Nutritional information per serving: 240 calories, 7 grams protein, 25.4 grams carbohydrates, 13.1 grams fat, 2.7 grams fiber, 21 milligrams cholesterol, 564 milligrams sodium, 85 milligrams calcium, 1.2 milligrams iron.

Tip: Can be made with acorn squash or pumpkin if desired.

** Allergy Tip: This recipe is GF, EF, SF, NF, PF, FF, SFF, V. To keep soy free, make sure the broth is soy free. For vegetarian, use vegetable broth (note that this may contain soy).

Entrees:

- Beer-Battered Shrimp

- Roasted Chicken Breasts with Caramelized Onions

- Veggie Stir Fry

- Shrimp Teriyaki

- Chicken Cutlet Francese

- Lasagna

- Gluten-Free Fresh Pasta

- Crescent-Shaped Ravioli

- Chicken Enchiladas

- Grouper Piccata

- Walnut-Crusted Chicken Breast in Mustard Sauce

- Parmesan Gnocchi

- Chicken Vegetable Curry with Mango Chutney

- Chicken and Spinach–Stuffed Crêpes

- Basic Gluten-Free Crêpes

- Pierogies with Potato Cheese Filling

- Chili

- Gluten-Free White Bean and Turkey Chili

- Chicken Cutlet Parmesan

- Unstuffed Cabbage

- Spinach Feta Pie

- Annie Brown's Sweet and Sour Pepper Steak

Beer-Battered Shrimp   Serves 4

These shrimp are best deep-fried. The gluten-free beer gives them a light crispy coating.

1 lb large raw shrimp (shells removed except tail)
1 egg separated (room temperature)
½ Tb olive oil
½ cup gluten-free all-purpose flour blend (see chapter 5 or buy)
1 tsp xanthan gum
½ tsp salt
½ cup gluten-free beer
Corn oil for frying
Gluten-free cocktail or tartar sauce

1. Mix together egg yolk, olive oil, gluten-free flour, xanthan gum, salt, and gluten-free beer until smooth.

2. Beat egg white until stiff peaks form and fold into batter.

3. Spray a nonstick skillet and heat until hot.

4. Dip shrimp one at a time in batter and place in skillet; use a teaspoon to put a little extra batter on top.

5. Heat corn oil in a fryer or a medium pot and fry shrimp until golden brown; remove shrimp with a slotted spoon, and drain on paper towels.

6. Keep shrimp warm until all are cooked; serve with gluten-free cocktail sauce or tartar sauce.

Nutritional information: 307 calories, 26 grams protein, 19.6 grams carbohydrates, 12.7 grams fat, 225 milligrams cholesterol, 496 milligrams sodium, 1 gram fiber, 95 milligrams calcium, 3.4 milligrams iron.

Tips: Make sure you use a fryer dedicated to gluten-free frying. If you prefer not to fry shrimp, you can spray a skillet with cooking spray and cook shrimp on both sides until golden. They will be a little flat in shape but still delicious. This batter also works well for onion rings.

** Allergy Tip: This recipe is GF, MF, SF, NF, PF, FF. Make sure you check the flour blend to be sure it is free of soy, milk, nuts, or peanuts. If soy free, select cocktail sauce instead of tartar sauce. To make egg free, use any gluten-free eggless egg substitute and use the cocktail sauce.

Roasted Chicken Breasts with Caramelized Onions   Serves 4

A real family favorite, this is great with any sides on any occasion.

16 oz (four 4-oz) bone-in chicken breasts with skin
½ tsp salt
½ tsp pepper
Gluten-free cooking spray or olive oil
4 yellow or white onions
1 Tb olive oil
1 Tb butter
2 Tb sugar
1 Tb red wine vinegar

1. Preheat oven to 375 degrees F. Place chicken on baking sheet and season with salt and pepper. Bake for 40–45 minutes or until chicken is cooked.

2. Peel and thinly slice onions.

3. In large skillet, heat olive oil and butter over medium-high heat. Add onions and stir to coat. Reduce heat to medium, and cook onions for 8–10 minutes, stirring frequently; if pan is too dry, add a little water.

4. Stir in sugar. Continue to cook for 15–20 minutes, until golden brown in color, stirring occasionally.

5. Remove from heat; stir in vinegar.

6. Remove skin from chicken and serve covered with onions.

Nutritional information: 327 calories, 25 grams protein, 20 grams carbohydrates, 11 grams fat, 90 milligrams cholesterol, 395 milligrams sodium, 3 grams fiber, 81.2 milligrams calcium, 1.8 milligrams iron.

Tip: If you use sweet onions, such as Vidalia, you do not need to add any sugar.

** Allergy Tip: This recipe is GF, EF, MF, SF, NF, PF, FF, SFF. To keep soy free, use a soy-free cooking spray or vegetable oil. To keep milk free, substitute margarine for the butter (note that most margarine contains soy).

Veggie Stir Fry   Serves 4

Restaurant stir fries include gluten from soy sauce, but you can make a gluten-free version at home. This recipe can be prepared with chicken, pork, or beef and served over brown rice as a complete meal.

¼ cup (2 oz) gluten-free vegetable broth (such as Pacific)
2 Tb gluten-free soy sauce (such as La Choy or San-J)
1 tsp cornstarch
1 tsp brown sugar
½ tsp fresh ginger, chopped
¼ tsp red pepper flakes

2 sp vegetable oil
1 cup sugar snap peas
2 cups bok choy, washed and cut into small pieces
1 cup carrots, sliced
1 cup mushrooms, sliced
4 green onions, sliced
1 red pepper, sliced
1 clove garlic, minced
½ cup water chestnuts, drained

1. Whisk together broth, soy sauce, cornstarch, brown sugar, ginger, and red pepper flakes in a small bowl and set aside.

2. Heat oil in a large wok or skillet. Add vegetables (peas through red pepper).

3. Stir fry vegetables 1–4 minutes, until vegetables start to soften. Add garlic and water chestnuts and continue to cook for 1 more minute.

4. Add sauce and sauté for 1–2 minutes, until sauce thickens.

Nutritional information: 96 calories, 4 grams protein, 15 gram carbohydrates, 3 grams fat, less than 1 milligram cholesterol, 430 milligrams sodium, 4.4 grams fiber, 80.5 milligrams calcium, 1 milligram iron.

Tip: Use any combination of vegetables you wish.

** Allergy Tip: This recipe is GF, MF, EF, NF, PF, FF, SFF, V, VG. To make soy free, use olive oil, a soy-free vegetable broth, and omit the soy sauce. Add ½ tsp salt and 2 Tb additional vegetable broth instead.

Shrimp Teriyaki   Serves 4

The teriyaki sauce in this recipe is perfect for salmon, beef, chicken, or scallops.

16 oz raw shrimp, cleaned and shelled
2 tsp garlic, minced
½ tsp onion powder
¼ cup low sodium gluten-free soy sauce (such as San-J)
2 Tb honey
1 Tb white vinegar

½ tsp dried ginger
½ tsp sesame oil
4 scallions, chopped
¼ cup red pepper, chopped

1. Preheat oven to 350 degrees F.

2. Mix together minced garlic, onion powder, gluten-free soy sauce, honey, vinegar, ginger, and sesame oil; pour over shrimp in an oven-safe casserole dish.

3. Arrange scallions, and chopped red pepper over the top of shrimp. Bake about 15 minutes, until shrimp are pink, and serve.

4. Great with brown rice or quinoa and steamed broccoli.

Nutritional information: 184 calories, 25 grams protein, 14 grams carbohydrates, 26 grams fat, 172 milligrams cholesterol, 699 milligrams sodium, less than 1 gram fiber, 75 milligrams calcium, 3.1 milligrams iron.

Tip: This recipe works well with salmon or tuna steaks.

** Allergy Tip: This recipe is GF, MF, EF, NF, PF, FF.

Chicken Cutlet Francese   **Serves 4**

This dish is so easy to prepare that you'll want to make it over and over again.

1 lb boneless, skinless chicken breasts, cleaned and sliced thin or pounded
    gluten-free cooking spray or olive oil
1 Tb garlic, minced
2 scallions, chopped
2 eggs, lightly beaten
½ cup brown rice or chickpea flour
2 Tb butter or olive oil
1 cup mushrooms, sliced
½ tsp salt
½ tsp pepper
1 tsp Italian seasoning
½ cup white wine
½ Tb lemon juice
2 Tb scallions, chopped (for garnish)

1. Spray a skillet with cooking spray. Sauté garlic and scallions for a few minutes.

2. Dip chicken in egg, then flour.

3. Add chicken to pan and brown on both sides. Add butter, mushrooms, salt, pepper, Italian seasoning, white wine, and lemon juice to the pan and continue cooking until chicken is cooked through, mushrooms are soft, and sauce thickens.

4. If needed, add a little extra white wine.

5. Garnish with scallions and serve.

Nutritional information: 295 calories, 31.8 grams protein, 17.7 grams carbohydrates, 10.3 grams fat, 186.7 milligrams cholesterol, 445 milligrams sodium, 1.5 grams fiber, 41.2 milligrams calcium, 2 milligrams iron.

Tip: Egg substitutes can be used in place of whole eggs if so desired.

** Allergy Tip: This recipe is GF, MF, SF, NF, PF, FF, SFF. To keep soy free, use olive oil instead of cooking spray. To keep milk free, use olive oil in place of butter. To make egg free, use a gluten-free eggless egg substitute.

Lasagna   Serves 16

This is perfect for when you have company and want a one-dish meal that you can serve to everyone. For a smaller lasagna, cut this recipe in half.

Gluten-free lasagna noodles (two 10-oz boxes gluten-free lasagna noodles or use the pasta recipe following this recipe)
2 Tb olive oil
3 Tb garlic, minced
2 large onions, chopped
2½ lb ground sirloin
3 tsp Italian seasoning
1 tsp salt
1 tsp pepper
3 quarts marinara sauce
3 cups part-skim ricotta cheese
⅓ cup parmesan cheese
1½ lb shredded skim mozzarella

1. Cook lasagna noodles until just cooked.

2. In a large pot, heat olive oil; sauté garlic 2 minutes.

3. Add onions to oil mixture and sauté until onions start to brown; add a little water to pan if needed to keep onions from sticking.

4. Add sirloin to the pot and sauté until brown; then add Italian seasoning, salt, and pepper.

5. Preheat oven to 350 degrees F.

6. Pour some sauce over the bottom of a lasagna pan. Cover with 3 lasagna noodles, pour half of meat mixture, some sauce, and 1½ cups ricotta cheese spread across, 5 Tb parmesan cheese, and ½ lb mozzarella cheese.

7. Start again with another layer, then finish with another layer of noodles, sauce, Parmesan, and mozzarella cheese. Reserve about 2 cups of the sauce to serve on the side.

8. Place the lasagna pan on top of a baking sheet.

9. Cover with aluminum foil and bake for about 30–45 minutes, until cheese is bubbling.

Nutritional information: 626 calories, 38 grams protein, 66.7 grams carbohydrates, 21.5 grams fat, 90.6 milligrams cholesterol, 1172 milligrams sodium, 5.9 grams fiber, 531 milligrams calcium, 3.5 milligrams iron.

Nutritional information (reduced-fat version): 505 calories, 37 grams protein, 66 grams carbohydrates, 8 grams fat, 56 milligrams cholesterol, 1171 milligrams sodium, 5.9 grams fiber, 452 milligrams calcium, 2 milligrams iron.

Tips: To reduce the fat in this recipe, use fat-free ricotta and fat-free mozzarella cheese and reduce the mozzarella to only 1 lb; you can also use white meat ground turkey in place of the sirloin. Lasagna can be made ahead and frozen until you are ready to use.

** Allergy Tip: This recipe is GF, EF, SF, NF, PF, FF, SFF. To keep egg free make sure the pasta is egg free. To keep gluten free, make sure the shredded cheese does not contain wheat as an anticaking agent. To make vegetarian, omit the sirloin.

Gluten-Free Fresh Pasta   **Serves 16**

If you want to make delicious homemade gluten-free pasta or lasagna noodles, this recipe is a sure winner.

1 cup sorghum flour
½ cup brown rice flour
1½ cups tapioca flour
1⅓ cups potato starch
⅔ cup cornstarch
2 tsp xanthan gum
4 eggs, beaten
4 Tb olive oil
2 tsp salt
⅔ cup water
Brown rice flour (about ½ cup, for rolling)

1. In a large bowl, combine dry ingredients except for extra brown rice flour for rolling.

2. Add eggs and oil to the dry ingredients and blend in (by hand or with a food processor).

3. Work in water a little at a time, until the dough has a nice consistency. Cover dough until ready to use.

4. Sprinkle some rice flour on parchment paper.

5. Break off tennis-ball-size pieces of dough and roll into oval logs.

6. Press dough into parchment paper, sprinkle the top with rice flour, and roll out into a ⅛-inch thick and 6-inch wide rectangular noodle.

7. Trim off edges so it makes a clean-looking rectangle and cover with a damp dish cloth.

8. Leave as a lasagna noodle or cut into desired pasta shape.

9. Boil a large pot of water with ½ tsp salt and 1 Tb olive oil.

10. Add pasta noodles and cook until desired doneness is achieved (undercook a little for al dente pasta).

11. Rinse noodles under cool water in a colander before using.

Nutritional information: 217 calories, 40.4 grams carbohydrates, 3.3 grams protein, 5 grams fat, 52.8 milligrams cholesterol, 336 milligrams sodium, 2.3 grams fiber, 55 milligrams calcium, 1.8 milligrams iron.

Tips: This pasta recipe can be used to make tortellini, ravioli, or any favorite noodle. To make noodles, cut into ¼-inch strips. To make tortellini, roll into marble-sized balls and flatten into half-dollar-size disks, fill with ricotta cheese, fold in half and seal shut by pinching ends together (refrigerate or freeze until ready to use). For ravioli, lay the long pieces of rolled pasta over a ravioli pan; fill with desired filling, top with another piece of pasta, and cut using the top of the ravioli pan.

** Allergy Tip: This recipe is GF, MF, SF, NF, PF, FF, SFF, V. To make egg free and vegan, use any gluten-free eggless egg substitute.

Crescent-Shaped Ravioli   Serves 6

This pasta recipe gives a nice texture to all those recipes that call for a pasta with a little more chew that holds up to many sauces.

4 eggs, beaten
4 Tb olive oil
2 tsp salt
⅓ cup water
¾ cup brown rice flour
½ cup tapioca flour
½ cup potato starch
¼ cup cornstarch
2 tsp xanthan gum
Brown rice flour (for dusting)
1 cup part skim ricotta
¼ cup parmesan cheese
1 tsp Italian seasoning

1. Beat together 2 eggs, ⅓ cup water, and 3 Tb olive oil.

2. In a bowl combine brown rice flour, tapioca flour, potato starch, cornstarch, xanthan gum, and 1 tsp salt.

3. Either by hand or in a food processor, work in wet ingredients until they become a well-incorporated dough; add extra rice flour if needed.

4. Mix together skim ricotta, parmesan, Italian seasoning, and remaining eggs.

5. On parchment paper dusted with brown rice flour, take tennis-ball-size balls of dough and roll to about 1/8 inch thick. Use a biscuit cutter to cut small round circles. Roll again so the surface of each circle is doubled in size.

6. Use a tablespoon to portion out 1 spoon of ricotta filling to fill each circle, then fold in half and shut by crimping the edges with a fork.

7. Boil a large pot of water. Add 1 tsp of salt and 1 Tb of olive oil. Add ravioli and cook for about 10 minutes until desired texture is achieved.

8. Rinse in a colander with warm water.

9. Serve with favorite pasta sauce.

Nutritional information: 346.7 calories, 10.5 grams protein, 44.7 grams carbohydrates, 14 grams fat, 121.4 milligrams cholesterol, 562 milligrams sodium, 2.6 grams fiber, 221 milligrams calcium, 2 milligrams iron.

Tip: You can mix a variety of fillings in these ravioli—try folding in some spinach with the cheese filling, or some sun-dried tomatoes.

** Allergy Tip: This recipe is GF, SF, NF, PF, FF, SFF, V. To make egg free, use any gluten-free eggless egg substitute.

Chicken Enchiladas   Serves 4

This delicious Mexican dish goes great with rice and beans and is easy on your budget as well.

2 whole bone-in chicken breasts with skin
¼ tsp black pepper
2 Tb olive oil
2 Tb water
2 Tb cornstarch
2 Tb chili powder
1 (8-oz) can tomato sauce
1½ cups water

½ tsp cumin

½ tsp garlic powder

Gluten-free cooking spray or olive oil

½ cup onions, chopped

½ cup gluten-free low-fat cream cheese

1 can (4 oz) diced green chili peppers

8 gluten-free corn tortillas, warmed until they are just starting to soften

½ cup shredded Monterey jack cheese (check to make sure it is gluten-free as some shredded cheese is tossed with wheat)

1. Sprinkle chicken with black pepper and bake at 375 degrees F for 40–45 minutes, until cooked through. Remove, and set aside to cool slightly.

2. Remove skin and bone from chicken. Using 2 forks, shred chicken and set aside.

3. Heat oil in a medium saucepan over medium-high heat. Add cornstarch and chili powder. Decrease heat to medium and cook for 3–4 minutes until light brown, stirring constantly.

4. Stir in tomato sauce, water, cumin, and garlic powder. Continue to cook for 5–10 minutes, until slightly thickened. Add additional water if sauce is too thick.

5. Spray a large nonstick skillet with cooking spray and heat over medium-high heat.

6. Add onions and cook for 3–4 minutes, until softened. Add cream cheese and chili peppers. Stir to combine. Continue to cook until cream cheese starts to melt. Add chicken and 1 cup of the enchilada sauce. Stir to combine. Remove from heat.

7. Preheat oven to 350 degrees F. Spray a 9 in. × 13 in. pan with cooking spray.

8. Spread ¼ cup enchilada sauce on bottom of pan.

9. Divide filling among 8 tortillas. Roll up and place seam-side down in pan.

10. Cover with remaining sauce and sprinkle with cheese.

11. Bake for 25 minutes, until hot and bubbly.

Nutritional information per serving: 450 calories, 29 grams protein, 38 grams carbohydrates, 20 grams fat, 78 milligrams cholesterol, 575 milligrams sodium, 6 grams fiber, 216 milligrams calcium, 3 milligrams fiber.

Tips: Serve with shredded lettuce and tomatoes.

** Allergy Tip: This recipe is GF, EF, SF, NF, PF, FF, SFF. To keep soy free, use a soy-free cooking spray or vegetable oil and double-check the cream cheese. To make vegetarian, omit chicken and double up on the cheese.

Grouper Piccata   Serves 2

Grouper is a delicious fish, especially when served with the capers, olives, and tomato sauce.

8 oz grouper
2 Tb brown rice flour
1 Tb olive oil
1 Tb butter or margarine
4 Tb white wine
1 Tb capers
1 tomato, chopped
¼ cup black olives, sliced
2 Tb lemon juice

1. Dredge fish in brown rice flour.

2. Heat olive oil in a skillet over medium-high heat

3. Place fish in skillet and brown fish slowly on both sides. Remove from pan and set aside.

4. To pan, add butter, wine, capers, tomatoes, and olives, heating until the mixture begins to simmer.

5. Add fish back to the pan with the sauce, and heat until cooked through.

6. Add lemon juice and serve.

Nutritional information: 309 calories, 23.6 grams protein, 13.5 grams carbohydrates, 15.9 grams fat, 57.2 milligrams cholesterol, 379 milligrams sodium, 1.9 gram fiber, 37 milligrams calcium, 2 milligrams iron.

Tip: Any fish works well in this recipe, including catfish, cod, orange roughy, flounder, and tilapia.

** Allergy Tip: This recipe is GF, EF, SF, NF, PF, SFF. To make milk free, substitute margarine for the butter (note that most margarine contains soy).

Walnut-Crusted Chicken Breasts with Mustard Sauce   Serves 4

This fabulous chicken dish can be served plain but is great with any sauce. The walnut coating makes a great cutlet.

1 lb (4 [4-oz]) boneless, skinless chicken breasts
Gluten-free cooking spray or olive oil
¼ cup crushed walnuts
4 Tb gluten-free cornmeal
½ tsp salt
1 tsp garlic powder
1 tsp onion powder
1 tsp paprika
½ tsp pepper
¼ tsp cinnamon
¼ tsp nutmeg
1 egg, beaten

Mustard Sauce

1 Tb olive oil
1 shallot, chopped
1 tsp garlic, chopped
2 Tb brown mustard
1 Tb wine vinegar
½ tsp oregano
4 Tb fat-free half-and-half

1. Preheat oven to 350 degrees F.

2. Mix walnuts and all spices together.

3. Lightly toast walnut spice mixture in sauté pan about 2–3 minutes, then remove from heat.

4. Dip chicken breasts in egg, then coat chicken breasts in walnut spice mixture.

5. Spray cooking spray in a large skillet over medium heat.

6. Brown chicken on both sides and cook through.

7. To make sauce, heat olive oil in a sauté pan over medium heat. Add shallots and garlic and sauté about 5 minutes, until softened.

8. Add mustard, vinegar, and oregano, and heat for several minutes.

9. Add fat-free half-and-half and heat through.

10. Serve chicken with mustard sauce over the top.

Nutritional information: 268 calories, 30.4 grams protein, 12.3 grams carbohydrates, 9.4 grams fat, 119.3 milligrams cholesterol, 585.3 milligrams sodium, 2.1 grams fiber, 48.6 milligrams calcium, 1.8 milligrams iron.

Tip: Shrimp or pork loin can be used in this recipe in place of the chicken breasts.

** Allergy Tip: This recipe is GF, SF, PF, FF, SFF. To keep soy free, use a soy-free cooking spray or vegetable oil. To make milk free, use a dairy-free product, such as rice milk, for the half-and-half. To make egg free, use any gluten-free eggless egg substitute.

Parmesan Gnocchi   **Serves 4**

These gnocchi taste just like the classic version. Serve with vodka sauce and fresh peas or with olive oil and Parmesan cheese, as below.

2 large russet potatoes
2 eggs
2 tsp salt
2 cups gluten-free all-purpose flour blend (see chapter 5 or buy)
1 tsp xanthan gum
2 Tb olive oil
¼ cup parmesan cheese

1. Bake potatoes; cool and peel skin.

2. Mash potatoes in a food processor, adding eggs, salt, flour blend, and xanthan gum; process until smooth.

3. Boil a large pot of water.

4. Take out dough in baseball-sized pieces, one at a time, and roll into a log of cigar thickness. Cut into ½-inch pieces; add extra flour blend if too sticky. Keep the rest of the dough covered with plastic wrap.

5. Cook gnocchi in small batches, taking care not to overcrowd the pot. Cook for about 8 minutes; then remove with a slotted spoon, place in a colander, and rinse with warm water.

6. When gnocchi are done, drizzle with olive oil and sprinkle with parmesan cheese.

Nutritional information: 481 calories, 11.8 grams protein, 84 grams carbohydrates, 12.3 grams fat, 110 milligrams cholesterol, 1301 milligrams sodium, 2.7 grams fiber, 111 milligrams calcium, 2.7 milligrams iron.

Tip: Gnocchi is also delicious with tomato, vodka sauce or pink sauce, or pesto sauce, or with roasted garlic and olive oil as well.

** Allergy Tip: This recipe is GF, SF, NF, PF, FF, SFF, V. To keep soy free and nut free, make sure the gluten-free flour blend you select is free of soy and nuts. To make milk free, omit the cheese and check that the flour blend is milk free. To make egg free, use any gluten-free eggless egg substitute. To make vegan, omit the cheese and use a gluten-free eggless egg substitute.

Chicken Vegetable Curry with Mango Chutney   Serves 4

Bursting with the flavors of curry and sweet potatoes, you will want to make this savory dish time and time again.

½ lb boneless, skinless chicken breast
2 Tb olive oil
1 small yellow onion, chopped

2 cloves garlic, minced
1 tsp fresh ginger, minced
½ tsp ground cumin
½ tsp turmeric
½ tsp cinnamon
1 Tb curry powder
½ tsp salt
2 tomatoes, chopped
2 cups gluten-free low sodium chicken broth
1 medium sweet potato, peeled and cut into ½-inch cubes
1 medium russet potato, peeled and cut into ½-inch cubes
½ cup plain nonfat yogurt
1 tsp garam masala
2 cups frozen cauliflower, defrosted

1. Cut chicken into bite-sized pieces. Heat oil in a large nonstick skillet. Add chicken and cook until browned.

2. Remove chicken from pan. Add onion, garlic and ginger. Sauté for 2–3 minutes, until softened.

3. Add cumin, turmeric, cinnamon, curry, and salt, and stir for 1–2 minutes, until curry becomes fragrant—be careful not to burn.

4. Add tomatoes, broth, chicken, and potatoes, then cover and simmer over low heat for about 45 minutes, until chicken is cooked and potatoes are tender.

5. Stir in yogurt, garam masala, and cauliflower, then cook for about 5 more minutes, until heated through.

6. Serve with mango chutney (see sauces and seasoning section) and brown rice.

Nutritional information: 266 calories, 21 grams protein, 27 grams carbohydrates, 9 grams fat, 33.5 milligrams cholesterol, 430 milligrams sodium, 5.2 grams fiber, 139.5 milligrams calcium, 2.7 milligrams iron.

Tip: Garam masala is an aromatic North Indian spice blend that can be used in everything from flat breads to soups.

** Allergy Tip: This recipe is GF, EF, SF, NF, PF, FF, SFF. To keep soy free, make sure the broth does not contain soy. To make milk free, omit the yogurt.

Chicken and Spinach–Stuffed Crêpes   **Serves 4**

The crêpes in this recipe can be stuffed with any filling and served for any occasion, from breakfast to appetizers to desserts. A simple recipe that yields amazing results.

1 Tb vegetable oil
1 shallot, finely chopped
12 oz boneless, skinless chicken breast tenders, cut into bite-sized pieces
2 cups fresh spinach, chopped
1 Tb butter
2 Tb cornstarch
1 cup milk
¾ cup gluten-free, low-sodium chicken broth (such as Pacific)
¼ tsp salt
¼ tsp white pepper
⅛ tsp nutmeg
    A basic crêpes recipe follows the recipe for this chicken filling.

1. Heat vegetable oil in a large nonstick skillet over medium-high heat. Add shallot and cook for 2–3 minutes, until softened.

2. Add chicken and continue to cook until chicken is cooked through. Add spinach and remove from heat.

3. In a medium saucepan, melt butter. Stir in cornstarch until smooth.

4. Add milk, chicken broth, salt, pepper and nutmeg. Whisk until smooth. Bring to a boil, stirring constantly, until sauce starts to thicken. Remove from heat.

5. Return chicken to medium heat. Stir in 1 cup of the sauce. Remove from heat.

6. Use filling for crêpes. Spoon remaining sauce over the crêpes to serve (basic crêpe recipe follows).

Basic Gluten-Free Crêpes   **Serves 4**

⅔ cup sorghum flour
⅓ cup potato starch
2 eggs
1 cup low-fat milk
½ tsp salt

2 Tb butter, melted
Gluten-free cooking spray or olive oil

1. In a large mixing bowl, whisk together sorghum flour, potato starch, and eggs. Add milk, and stir to combine.

2. Beat in salt and butter. Continue to mix until smooth.

3. Heat a medium nonstick skillet over medium-high heat. Spray with cooking spray.

4. Pour ¼ cup of batter onto pan. Tilt pan back and forth so that the batter coats the surface evenly.

5. Cook for about 1 minute, until the bottom starts to brown. Flip crêpe with spatula and cook the other side for about 30 seconds.

6. Remove to platter and cover to keep warm.

Nutritional information for Chicken and Spinach Crêpes: 515 calories, 35 grams protein, 52 grams carbohydrates, 20 grams fat, 188 milligrams cholesterol, 760 milligrams sodium, 5.6 grams fiber, 324 milligrams calcium, 4.5 milligrams iron.

Tip: Asparagus would also work well in this dish.

Nutritional information for Crêpes: 272 calories, 8.8 grams protein, 40 grams carbohydrates, 9.8 grams fat, 124 milligrams cholesterol, 395 milligrams sodium, 2 grams fiber, 96.6 milligrams calcium, 1.8 milligrams iron.

Tip: Add a tablespoon of sugar to make a dessert crêpe

** Allergy Tip: This recipe is GF, SF, NF, PF, FF, SFF. To keep soy free, use a soy-free cooking spray or vegetable oil and double-check that the chicken broth is soy free. To make milk free, substitute the milk for a dairy-free alternative, such as rice milk, and the butter for margarine (note that most margarine contains soy). To make egg free, use any gluten-free eggless egg substitute.

Pierogies with Potato and Cheese Filling   **Serves 8**

Serve with melted butter and sautéed onions, with sour cream on the side.

Filling

2 Tb vegetable oil
1 cup onion, finely chopped
2 cups hot mashed potatoes
1 cup sharp cheddar cheese, shredded

Dough

2 cups gluten-free flour blend (see recipe below)
2 tsp xanthan gum
½ tsp salt
3 Tb vegetable oil
2 eggs
⅓ cup plain seltzer water
Brown rice flour (for rolling)

Gluten-Free Flour Blend

¾ cup brown rice flour
½ cup tapioca flour
½ cup potato starch
¼ cup cornstarch

1. Heat oil in a medium skillet. Add onions and sauté for 3–4 minutes until softened.

2. Mix onions and cheese with mashed potatoes. Stir to combine and make sure cheese melts. Set aside to cool.

3. In a large bowl, combine the flour blend, xanthan gum, and salt. Make a well in center.

4. In a separate bowl, combine vegetable oil, eggs and seltzer. Pour into well in flour mixture. Stir to combine and form a stiff dough. Add extra flour blend if too wet.

5. Cut dough into 4 pieces. Roll out the first ball about ¼ -in. thick, using additional brown rice flour for dusting. Using a biscuit cutter, cut out individual pierogi. Repeat with remaining three dough pieces.

6. Take each individual circle and roll out until double in size.

7. Take 1 teaspoon of filling and place on one half of each circle. Fold over, wet edges, and press edges together with fork tines.

8. Place pierogis on two large cookie sheets and freeze for 1–2 hours before cooking.

9. Bring large pot of water to boil. Cook pierogi in batches of 10. Boil for 6–8 minutes, until they rise to the top. Cook for an additional 1–2 minutes. Remove with a slotted spoon and serve immediately.

Nutritional information: 364 calories, 9.2 grams protein, 45.6 grams carbohydrates, 17 grams fat, 68 milligrams cholesterol, 368 milligrams sodium, 2.7 grams fiber, 155.6 milligrams calcium, 1.7 milligrams iron.

Tips: Pierogi can be cooked and frozen. To serve, defrost and sauté in butter or drop into boiling water for 3–4 minutes.

** Allergy Tip: This recipe is GF, SF, NF, PF, FF, SFF, V. To keep soy free make sure you use a soy-free vegetable oil. To make milk free, use dairy-free cheese (if you are also soy free, make sure the cheese alternative does not contain soy). To make egg free, use any gluten-free eggless egg substitute.

Chili   Serves 8

This chili is great as a main course and can also be stuffed into a pepper, a potato, or a corn tortilla with melted cheddar.

2 Tb olive oil
3 Tb garlic, chopped
1 large onion, chopped
2 green or red peppers, chopped
1 lb sirloin, chopped
½ tsp cumin
1 tsp paprika
¼ tsp pepper
¼ tsp chili powder
1 tsp oregano
½ tsp cinnamon

2 Tb brown sugar

1 Tb balsamic vinegar

2 15.5-oz cans cooked kidney beans

28 oz can crushed tomatoes

½ can water

Gluten-free hot sauce to taste

1. Heat olive oil. Sauté garlic, onions, and peppers.

2. Add beef, seasonings, and balsamic vinegar.

3. Add beans, tomatoes, and water, then cook at least 30 minutes for all flavors to merge.

4. Add hot sauce and additional seasoning to taste.

Nutritional information: 285 calories, 19.4 grams protein, 31.7 grams carbohydrates, 9.8 grams fat, 36.8 milligrams cholesterol, 455.8 milligrams sodium, 9.1 grams fiber, 87.2 milligrams calcium, 4.3 milligrams iron.

Tips: Any kind of bean can be used in this recipe; you can easily use ground chicken or turkey in place of the beef.

** Allergy Tip: This recipe is GF, MF, EF, SF, NF, PF, FF, SFF. To make vegetarian and vegan, omit the sirloin.

Gluten-Free White Bean and Turkey Chili   Serves 8

White beans give a different texture and flavor to chili. Recipe from Christopher Singlemann, certified executive chef.

2–2½ pounds uncooked ground turkey breast

2 Tb olive oil

3 Tb minced garlic

8 cloves

2 red peppers diced into ¼ in. pieces

1 green pepper diced into ¼ in. pieces

2 small chipotle peppers seeded and diced

1 large white onion diced into ¼ in. pieces

4 plum tomatoes ½ in. dice

1 Tb gluten-free soy sauce

2 bay leaves

2 Tb chili powder
2 tsp cumin powder
1 tsp salt
2–15.5 oz cans white great northern beans, rinsed and drained
32 oz gluten-free low-sodium chicken broth

1. Heat large pot on medium-high heat. Add olive oil and turkey and sear until turkey meat is golden brown.

2. Add garlic, onion, and peppers to the browned turkey. Stir in bay leaves, chili powder, salt, and cumin. Continue to sauté for approximately 3–5 minutes.

3. Add tomatoes and chicken stock. Bring to a simmer and add beans. Continue to simmer uncovered for an additional 45 minutes, stirring occasionally. Remove bay leaves, ladle into warm chili bowls and serve.

Nutritional information per serving: 266 calories, 26.3 grams protein, 27 grams carbohydrates, 6 grams fat, 7.7 grams fiber, 49 milligrams cholesterol, 1177 milligrams sodium, 84.5 milligrams calcium, 2.8 milligrams iron.

Tips: Add other spices to turn your chili into you own signature dish. To lower the sodium in this recipe use low-sodium soy sauce, and omit salt (substitute Mrs Dash).

** Allergy Tip: This recipe is GF, MF, EF, NF, PF, FF, SFF. To make soy free, omit soy sauce, and make sure the chicken broth is soy free.

Chicken Cutlet Parmesan   Serves 4

This same basic recipe can be used to make shrimp parmesan, veal parmesan, or eggplant parmesan.

Gluten-free cooking spray or olive oil
1 cup gluten-free bread crumbs
1 tsp garlic powder
1 tsp onion powder
½ tsp oregano
⅛ tsp pepper
½ tsp salt
3 Tb parmesan cheese

1 egg
1 lb boneless, skinless chicken breasts
1 cup marinara sauce
½ tsp garlic powder
1 cup shredded mozzarella

1. Spray a cookie sheet with cooking spray

2. Mix bread crumbs, garlic powder, onion powder, oregano, pepper, salt, and 2 Tb parmesan cheese.

3. Beat egg, then dip chicken in egg and then in breadcrumb mixture. Coat on both sides.

4. Spray top of chicken with cooking spray and place on cookie sheet.

5. Set oven to broil and cook chicken until brown on both sides.

6. Pour ⅓ sauce in casserole dish. Top with chicken, then with rest of the sauce, 1 Tb Parmesan cheese, and mozzarella cheese.

7. Turn oven to 350 degrees F and bake chicken for about 20 minutes until bubbling and the cheese is melted.

Nutritional information: 401.4 calories, 38.6 grams protein, 24.7 grams carbohydrates, 15.9 grams fat, 138 milligrams cholesterol, 986 milligrams sodium, 4 grams fiber, 324.6 milligrams calcium, 2.2 milligrams iron.

Tip: If gluten-free bread crumbs are not available, crush 1½ cups of gluten-free cornflakes as a substitute.

** Allergy Tip: This recipe is GF, SF, NF, PF, FF, SFF. To keep soy free, use soy-free cooking spray or vegetable oil and check the bread crumbs for soy. For nut free and peanut free, double-check the bread crumbs. To make milk free, use dairy-free cheese (if you are also soy free, make sure the cheese alternative does not contain soy) and check the bread crumbs for milk. To make egg free, use any gluten-free eggless egg substitute.

Unstuffed Cabbage   Serves 8

A delicious classic that never goes out of style or demand.

1 head cabbage, shredded
1½ lbs lean ground beef

1½ tsp kosher salt
3 Tb ketchup
¼ cup gluten-free bread crumbs
1 egg
5 Tb cooked rice
24 oz ginger ale
2 Tb brown sugar
4 Tb honey
1 can (14-oz) diced tomatoes

1. Combine ground beef, salt, ketchup, GF bread crumbs, egg, and rice in a large bowl. Form into 1-in. round meatballs.

2. Bring ginger ale, brown sugar, honey, and diced tomatoes to a boil in a large pot. Reduce heat to simmer. Add cabbage and meatballs. Cover and simmer for 2 hours.

Nutritional information per serving: 206 calories, 16 grams protein, 29 grams carbohydrates, 3 grams fat, 1.9 grams fiber, 56 milligrams cholesterol, 668 milligrams sodium, 40 milligrams calcium, 2.4 milligrams iron.

Tips: The biggest part of the work making stuffed cabbage is the wrapping and rolling; this unstuffed cabbage gives you the taste without all the extra work. This can be served over hot cooked rice.

** Allergy Tip: This recipe is GF, MF, SF, NF, PF, FF, SFF. To keep allergen safe check the bread crumbs for milk, soy, and nuts. To make egg free, use an eggless egg substitute.

Spinach and Feta Pie   Serves 12

Do you love Mediterranean spinach pie but miss it since phyllo dough contains gluten? Well, you will love this recipe: intense flavor and a light crust without the fuss of working with phyllo. This is a gluten-free version of my grandma Ruthie's classic spinach bodek.

Crust

1½ cups chick pea (garbanzo bean) flour
1½ cups water
1 Tb olive oil
¼ tsp salt
¼ tsp pepper

1 Tb minced dried onions
Gluten-free cooking spray or olive oil

Filling

1 large Spanish onion (finely chopped)
10-oz bag baby spinach, washed, drained, and dried
2 lb 2% large-curd cottage cheese
⅓ lb crumbled feta cheese
½ tsp salt
¼ tsp pepper
2 eggs
4 Tb rice or gluten-free flour blend.
4 Tb olive oil

1. Mix together chick pea flour, water, 1 Tb olive oil, salt, pepper, and dried onions. Let the batter sit for about 30 minutes at room temperature. (Mixture will resemble a thick cream)

2. Preheat oven to 375 degrees F.

3. Prepare filling. Spray a large sauté pan with cooking spray and heat.

4. Sauté onions until golden brown, fold in spinach until just wilted.

5. Meanwhile, in a large bowl, combine cottage cheese, feta cheese, eggs, salt, pepper, rice flour, and mint.

6. In a 12 in. × 9 in. × 3 in. rectangular pan, drizzle 2 Tb olive oil, pour half of the chick pea batter in the pan, and use a spatula to coat the bottom. Put in the oven for 10 minutes until set and starting to get crisp. Then spread spinach filling in pan. Top with remaining batter and try to evenly spread over the top of the spinach filling. Place in the oven for about 30 minutes until set.

7. Drizzle remaining olive oil over the top, and turn the oven up to broil, cooking it for another 10 minutes until golden brown. If the casserole is still too liquid, lower heat to 350 degrees F and let cook until the casserole is set.

Nutritional Information: 223 calories, 16.2 grams protein, 13.8 grams carbohydrate, 11.4 grams fat, 29.4 milligrams cholesterol, 617 milligrams sodium, 2.3 grams fiber, 141 milligrams calcium, 1.7 milligrams iron

Tip: Any filling can be used to make a great pie. If you like a thicker crust, double up the batter recipe. If you like a lighter crust, replace half of the chick pea flour with sweet (gluten-free glutenous) rice flour. Cook it on a pizza pan with a rim to make it even lighter and crispier. Make sure the spinach is dry before you combine it or the recipe might be watery.

** Allergy Tip: This recipe is GF, SF, NF, PF, FF, SFF, V. To keep soy free, use a soy-free cooking spray or olive oil. To make egg free, use any gluten-free eggless egg substitute.

Annie Brown's Sweet and Sour Pepper Steak   Serves 4

My mom was always a hit whenever she served her pepper steak.

1 Tb olive oil
1 Tb minced garlic
2 large onions, peeled and sliced
2 large sliced red peppers
14-oz lean steak cut into 2-in. long slices (cut across the grain, easier to
    cut when slightly frozen)
½ cup pineapple chunks in their own juice, drained
2 Tb molasses
1 Tb lemon juice
¼ cup gluten-free beef broth
1 Tb cornstarch mixed with 2 Tb water
2 Tb light gluten-free soy sauce
Pepper to tastes
Chopped scallions to garnish

1. Heat oil and brown garlic.

2. Add onions and peppers and sauté until onions are translucent.

3. Add beef, molasses, lemon juice, beef bouillon, and soy sauce. Cover and simmer about 20 minutes.

4. Stir in pineapple and cornstarch mixture, heat through 5 minutes uncovered until thickened and serve garnished with scallions.

Nutritional information per serving: 280 calories, 18.3 grams protein, 30.6 grams carbohydrates, 9.3 grams fat, 4.2 grams fiber, 33 milligrams cholesterol, 302 milligrams sodium, 58 milligrams calcium, 2.7 milligrams iron.

Tips: If you like it a little sweeter, add extra molasses. It's great served over rice or quinoa.

** Allergy Tip: This recipe is GF, MF, EF, NF, PF, FF, SFF.

Sides:

- Black Beans and Rice

- Red Potatoes and Bacon

- Steamed Broccoli in Garlic Sauce

- Quinoa with Sautéed Onions and Lima Beans

- Wild Rice and Pecan Pilaf

- Escarole and White Beans

- Spicy Baked Sweet Potato Fries

- Stuffed Tomatoes

- Kasha Varnishkes

- Creamed Spinach

Black Beans and Rice **Serves 4**

This is a great Spanish side dish that works well with almost any entrée.

1 cup brown rice
2 cups (16 oz) water or gluten-free chicken or veggie broth (such as Pacific)
½ tsp salt
1 tsp olive oil
1 small red onion, finely chopped
¾ cup gluten-free salsa
16-oz can black beans, drained and rinsed
1 Tb lime juice
¼ cup cilantro, roughly chopped

1. Cook brown rice in salted water or gluten-free broth for 45–50 minutes until cooked through.

2. Heat oil in bottom of a skillet. Add red onion, and cook 2–3 minutes. Add salsa, black beans, and lime juice and heat through.

3. Combine black bean salsa mixture with cooked brown rice. Before serving, toss in cilantro. If desired, top with guacamole, sour cream, and cheese.

Nutritional information per serving: 283 calories, 10 grams protein, 56 grams carbohydrates, 2.6 grams fat, 0 milligrams cholesterol, 762 milligrams sodium, 7.2 grams fiber, 64.8 milligrams calcium, 2.2 milligrams iron.

Tips: If you like it spicy, add gluten-free hot sauce, extra salsa, and cilantro. You can add guacamole, sour cream, or cheese, if desired.

** Allergy Tip: This recipe is GF, MF, EF, SF, NF, PF, FF, SFF, V, VG. To keep soy free, check that the chicken broth does not contain soy. To make vegetarian or vegan, use a vegan vegetable broth.

Red Potatoes and Bacon   Serves 4

Serve this with roasted chicken and steamed vegetables for a satisfying and delicious meal.

1½ lb red potatoes
2 tsp olive oil
½ tsp dried thyme leaves
½ tsp dried parsley
¼ tsp salt
⅛ tsp black pepper
4 slices turkey bacon, diced

1. Fill a large pot with water and add potatoes. Bring to a boil and cook for 5–6 minutes, until just fork tender.

2. Drain and cool slightly.

3. Preheat oven to 400 degrees F.

4. Cut potatoes into ½-inch cubes and place in a 2-qt baking dish.

5. Add oil, thyme, parsley, salt, and pepper. Toss until potatoes are coated.

6. Top with bacon.

7. Bake for 40 minutes, until bacon is crisp and potatoes are browned. Add a little water if the pan is too dry.

Nutritional information: 212 calories, 8 grams protein, 34 grams carbohydrates, 5 grams fat, 15 milligrams cholesterol, 326 milligrams sodium, 4 grams fiber, 37.3 milligrams calcium, 2.1 milligrams iron.

Tip: Using the red potatoes gives this dish a nice look—I like the small red potatoes because they taste so sweet.

** Allergy Tip: This recipe is GF, MF, EF, SF, NF, PF, FF, SFF. For gluten free, make sure that the turkey bacon is gluten free. For soy free, make sure the turkey bacon does not contain soy. To make vegetarian and vegan, omit the turkey bacon.

Steamed Broccoli in Garlic Sauce **Serves 4**

Steaming the broccoli saves a lot of calories over sautéing.

1 medium head garlic
½ tsp olive oil
1 Tb butter
1 Tb cornstarch
½ cup fat-free milk
½ cup gluten-free chicken or veggie broth (such as Kitchen Basics)
¼ tsp salt
⅛ tsp pepper
2 cups broccoli florets
½ cup water

1. Preheat oven to 400 degrees F. Slice off top of garlic head: drizzle with olive oil and wrap in foil. Bake for 45–50 minutes, until very soft. Cool.

2. Melt butter in small saucepan over medium heat. Stir in cornstarch, until well-blended.

3. Using a wire whisk, add milk and broth. Bring to a boil, stirring constantly until thickened. Reduce heat.

4. Remove the garlic cloves from the skin and stir into the sauce. Remove from heat and season with salt and pepper.

5. In a large skillet, place broccoli and water. Cover and cook for 5–6 minutes until tender.

6. Drain broccoli. Serve with sauce.

Nutritional information: 74 calories, 3 grams protein, 7.5 grams carbohydrates, 4 grams fat, 11 milligrams cholesterol, 243 milligrams sodium, 1.2 grams fiber, 67 milligrams calcium, less than 1 milligram iron.

Tip: This garlic sauce is nice on any vegetable, such as asparagus, spinach, zucchini, and yellow squash.

** Allergy Tip: This recipe is GF, EF, SF, NF, PF, FF, SFF, V. To keep soy free, double-check the broth, and if you opt for margarine instead of butter make sure it is soy free. To keep vegetarian, use vegetable broth. To make milk free, use margarine and a dairy-free milk substitute in place of the butter and the fat-free milk. To make vegan, use vegetarian broth and use vegan substitutes for the butter and milk (may contain soy).

Quinoa with Sautéed Onions and Lima Beans   Serves 4

This recipe is high in protein and fiber and loaded with flavor.

2 tsp olive oil
½ cup diced onion
1 tsp turmeric
½ tsp ground coriander
¼ tsp ground cinnamon
¼ tsp allspice
1 cup quinoa (if not prerinsed, rinse two to three times)
2 cups (16 oz) gluten-free vegetable broth (such as Pacific or Kitchen Basics)
1 cup precooked lima beans

1. Heat oil in a large saucepan over medium-high heat. Add onions and sauté for 3–4 minutes until softened.

2. Add spices and quinoa and stir to coat.

3. Add broth and bring to a boil. Reduce heat and simmer for 10–15 minutes.

4. Stir in lima beans and continue to simmer for another 5–10 minutes, until quinoa is tender and liquid is absorbed.

Nutritional information: 259 calories, 9.4 grams protein, 44.5 grams carbohydrates, 5 grams fat, 0 milligrams cholesterol, 261 milligrams sodium, 6 grams fiber, 51 milligrams calcium, 3.6 milligrams iron.

Tips: Millet and brown rice work nicely in this recipe as well. If you use brown rice, a little additional liquid may be needed in the recipe.

** **Allergy Tip:** This recipe is GF, MF, EF, SF, NF, PF, FF, SFF, V, VG. To keep soy free, make sure the broth is soy free.

Wild Rice and Pecan Pilaf   **Serves 4**

Wild rice and pecans add a nutty texture to this wonderful rice dish.

1 cup wild rice, uncooked
1 Tb butter or olive oil
½ cup red onions, chopped
4 Tb raisins
2 cups gluten-free chicken or vegetable broth (such as Pacific)
4 Tb pecans, coarsely chopped

1. In saucepan toast rice for about 2–4 minutes, then add butter, onions, and raisins. Heat for about 5 minutes, until onions are translucent.

2. Add chicken broth and bring to boil. Stir, lower heat, and cover.

3. Cook for about 45–50 minutes until rice is done.

4. Fold in pecans and serve.

Nutritional information per serving: 270 calories, 9.5 grams protein, 40.4 grams carbohydrates, 8.9 grams fat, 7.6 milligrams cholesterol, 413 milligrams sodium, 3.8 grams fiber, 28 milligrams calcium, 1.4 milligrams iron.

Tip: Wild rice is much denser than regular rice. If too chewy, add some water or broth and cook a little longer.

** **Allergy Tip:** This recipe is GF, MF, EF, SF, PF, FF, SFF, V, VG. To keep soy free, make sure the broth does not contain soy. To keep peanut free, make sure the pecans are not contaminated with peanuts. To make milk free, select oil in place of butter. To make nut free, omit the pecans. To make vegetarian or vegan, use a vegan vegetable broth.

Escarole and White Beans   **Serves 4**

This Italian classic is a perfect side to your gluten-free pasta dinner.

1 head of escarole, washed, drained, and chopped
½ cup (4 oz) gluten-free chicken or vegetable broth (such as Pacific)

1 Tb olive oil
½ head fresh garlic, chopped
½ large onion, chopped
15.5-oz can white navy beans, drained
½ tsp salt
½ tsp pepper
1 Tb balsamic vinegar
1 tsp sugar
1 Tb lemon juice

1. In a large pot, cook escarole in chicken broth until cooked (if broth evaporates, add additional broth or water).

2. Place olive oil in skillet over medium heat. Sauté garlic and onions for about 5 minutes, until softened.

3. Add beans, salt, pepper, and balsamic vinegar to garlic and onions.

4. Add sugar and lemon to cooked escarole.

5. Add escarole and broth to bean mixture and cook for about 10 minutes, then serve.

Nutritional information: 127 calories, 7.7 grams protein, 21.5 grams carbohydrates, 4.1 grams fat, 0 milligrams cholesterol, 590 milligrams sodium, 7.2 grams fiber, 91 milligrams calcium, 1.9 milligrams iron.

Tip: To peel garlic: cut head in half, microwave in small bowl with a little water about 30 seconds, peel off cloves and chop.

** Allergy Tip: This recipe is GF, MF, EF, SF, NF, PF, FF, SFF, V, VG. To keep soy free double-check the broth. For vegetarian and vegan, make sure you use a gluten-free vegetarian, vegan vegetable broth.

Spicy Baked Sweet Potato Fries   Serves 4

These potatoes are so easy to make and are truly a treat. Baking these fries saves a lot of fat over traditional deep-fried fries.

2 medium sweet potatoes, cut into thin French fries
1 tsp onion powder
1 tsp garlic powder

2 tsp paprika
1 tsp salt
½ tsp cinnamon
½ tsp pepper
Gluten-free cooking spray or olive oil

1. Preheat oven to 375 degrees F.

2. Mix all spices together in a large bowl.

3. Toss sweet potatoes with the spices.

4. Spray a cookie sheet with cooking spray and place sweet potato mixture on tray.

5. Spray tops of sweet potato fries with cooking spray.

6. Bake until crisp on the outside and cooked through, turning frequently, and spraying again with cooking spray if too dry. Bake for 35–40 minutes.

Nutrition Information: 64.5 calories, 1.4 grams protein, 15 grams carbohydrates, less than 1 gram fat, 0 milligrams cholesterol, 618 milligrams sodium, 2.7 grams fiber, 28.2 milligrams calcium, less than 1 milligram iron.

Tips: Other spices can work well in this recipe, too. If you like your sweet potato fries plain, skip the spices and proceed from step 4 on. If you want, you can fry the potatoes, but baking this way reduces the fat drastically. Many gluten-free foods are often very high in fat, so it helps to cut back when you can.

** Allergy Tip: This recipe is GF, MF, EF, SF, NF, PF, FF, SFF, V, VG. To keep soy free, use a soy-free cooking spray or vegetable oil.

Stuffed Tomatoes   Serves 2

This recipe is perfect for barbecues, or served up with a steak, chicken, or hamburger.

2 large tomatoes
1 Tb olive or canola oil
1 small onion, chopped
2 Tb garlic, chopped

1 tsp Italian seasoning
1 Tb capers
½ tsp salt
¼ tsp pepper
½ cup seasoned gluten-free bread crumbs (see cooking tips)
2 Tb parmesan cheese
¼ cup white wine

1. Preheat oven to 350 degrees F.

2. Cut off top of tomato; remove pulp and place in small bowl.

3. Heat a medium skillet and add oil.

4. Sauté onion in skillet until translucent; add garlic and sauté 2–3 minutes.

5. Add tomato pulp, Italian seasoning, capers, salt, pepper, and gluten-free bread crumbs and heat a few minutes.

6. Stuff mixture into tomatoes, place in casserole dish, and sprinkle with parmesan cheese.

7. Pour wine into casserole dish.

8. Bake for about 25 minutes, until tomatoes start to soften.

Nutritional information: 257 calories, 5 grams protein, 25.9 grams carbohydrates, 13 grams fat, 4.4 milligrams cholesterol, 894 milligrams sodium, 4.7 grams fiber, 130 milligrams calcium, 1.1 milligrams iron.

Tip: If gluten-free bread crumbs are not available, toast gluten-free bread and put through a food processor with some Italian seasoning, garlic, onion powder, and a little salt.

** Allergy Tip: This recipe is GF, EF, SF, NF, PF, FF, SFF, V. Make sure the bread crumbs do not contain eggs, milk, soy, nuts, and peanuts. To make milk free and vegan, omit the cheese and make sure the bread crumbs do not contain milk.

Kasha Varnishkes   Serves 8

This is a terrific side dish that can be served just as easily with scrambled eggs as with a piece of chicken or steak.

6 oz spiral brown rice or quinoa pasta
3 Tb olive oil

1 Tb garlic, minced

1 large Spanish onion, chopped into ½-inch pieces

2 cups mushrooms, sliced

1½ tsp salt

½ tsp pepper

1 cup whole kasha (buckwheat groats)

1 egg, beaten

2 cups gluten-free chicken or vegetable broth (Pacific)

1. Cook and drain pasta.

2. While pasta is cooking, heat olive oil in a skillet over medium heat and sauté garlic and onion.

3. When onion is starting to brown, add about 2 Tb water, mushrooms, salt, and pepper. Cover and continue to cook until mushrooms are soft.

4. Drain pasta and place in a large bowl. Stir in onion and mushroom mixture.

5. In a separate medium pot, put on a high heat and add buckwheat groats. When hot, add egg and keep stirring until egg is absorbed and buckwheat groats are separated from each other. Add chicken broth, lower heat, and cover. Cook about 10–15 minutes, until liquid is absorbed.

6. Toss buckwheat with pasta and mushrooms and serve.

Nutritional information: 227.3 calories, 6.9 grams protein, 35.7 grams carbohydrates, 6.8 grams fat, 26.4 milligrams cholesterol, 648.8 milligrams sodium, 2.7 grams fiber, 16.1 milligrams calcium, 1.7 milligrams iron.

Tip: To reheat leftovers, place in a casserole dish, add a little additional gluten-free chicken broth, cover, and bake at 300 degrees F until hot.

** Allergy Tip: This recipe is GF, MF, SF, NF, PF, FF, SFF. To keep soy free, make sure the broth is soy free. To make egg free, use any gluten-free eggless egg substitute. To make vegetarian, use gluten-free vegetable broth. To make vegan, use a gluten-free eggless egg substitute and vegan vegetable broth.

Creamed Spinach   Serves 6

Creamed spinach is always a favorite, especially with a nice piece of steak and a baked potato.

16 oz fresh baby spinach
5 Tb butter
3 Tb finely chopped onion
1 small garlic clove, minced
1½ cups half-and-half (or see tip for other options)
1½ tsp sugar
5 Tb gluten-free instant mashed potato flakes
1 tsp salt
Pepper to taste
¼ tsp nutmeg

1. Cook onion and garlic in butter till golden.

2. Add the milk and sugar and stir until milk comes to slight boil.

3. Whisk in the instant mashed potato flakes. When sauce is smooth, add raw spinach.

4. Stir and cook 3 minutes until wilted down.

5. Season with salt, pepper, and nutmeg.

Nutritional information per serving: 190 calories, 3.9 grams protein, 7.3 grams carbohydrates, 16.6 grams fat, 1.9 grams fiber, 47 milligrams cholesterol, 557 milligrams sodium, 138 milligrams calcium, 2.5 milligrams iron.

Tip: Can substitute half-and-half with heavy cream, milk, or any combination of all three.

** Allergy Tip: This recipe is GF, EF, SF, NF, PF, FF, SFF, V. For soy free, double-check the potato flakes to make sure they are soy free. To make milk free and vegan, double-check that the potato flakes and use margarine and dairy-free milk in place of the half-and-half.

Sauces and Seasonings:

- Mango Chutney

- Yogurt Sauce

- Salsa

- Steak Sauce

- Barbecue Sauce

- Cream Sauce

** *See chapter 12 for additional easy-to-make sauces and seasonings.*

Mango Chutney   **Serves 4**

This is a great addition to many dishes. Papaya or peaches work well in place of the mango in this recipe.

1 (12-oz) bag frozen mango, or 2 cups cubed fresh mango
¼ cup golden raisins
½ cup cider vinegar
½ cup brown sugar
1 Tb garlic, minced
1 tsp fresh ginger, minced
¼ tsp cayenne pepper
¼ tsp black pepper
½ tsp salt

1. In a large skillet, bring all of the ingredients to a boil over medium heat.

2. Reduce heat to low and simmer, uncovered, for about 30 minutes, stirring constantly.

3. Remove from heat and cool before serving.

Nutritional information: 161.6 calories, less than 1 gram protein, 40.6 grams carbohydrates, less than 1 gram fat, 0 milligrams cholesterol, 300 milligrams sodium, 2 grams fiber, 33 milligrams calcium, less than 1 milligram iron.

Tip: This chutney can be stored in the refrigerator for up to a week.

** **Allergy Tip:** This recipe is GF, MF, EF, SF, NF, PF, FF, SFF, V, VG.

Yogurt Sauce   **Serves 4**

A terrific Middle Eastern sauce that is great with so many dishes.

2 Tb olive oil
½ tsp sugar
2 cups nonfat plain yogurt
1 tsp garlic powder
½ tsp salt
2 scallions, chopped, or ½ tsp onion powder
4 Tb lemon juice
½ cucumber, chopped (optional)
1 tsp dried mint

1. Mix all ingredients together.

2. Refrigerate until ready to use.

Nutritional information: 81.5 calories, 7.5 grams protein, 12.5 grams carbohydrates, less than 1 gram fat, 2.4 milligrams cholesterol, 242 milligrams sodium, less than 1 gram fiber, 256.7 milligrams calcium, less than 1 milligram iron.

Tip: Add extra garlic and lemon to taste. Great served with kebabs.

** Allergy Tip: This recipe is GF, EF, SF, NF, PF, FF, SFF, V.

Salsa   **Serves 4**

Salsa can be made from vegetables, fruits, and a variety of spices and seasoning agents. It is the perfect addition to almost any meal.

2 cups plum tomatoes, seeds and juice removed and chopped coarsely
½ jalapeno pepper, minced finely
½ cup red onions, finely chopped
½ cup cilantro, finely chopped
½ tsp salt
¼ tsp pepper

1. Combine all ingredients; chill until ready to serve.

Nutritional information: 25.5 calories, 1 gram protein, 5.6 grams carbohydrates, less than 1 gram fat, 0 milligrams cholesterol,

297 milligrams sodium, 1.5 grams fiber, 15.8 milligrams calcium, less than 1 milligram iron.

Tips: Salsa is great with chips or as a topping for fish or chicken. Try adding corn, chopped vegetables, fruits, and different spices to salsa to create your own signature variety.

** Allergy Tip: This recipe is GF, MF, EF, SF, NF, PF, FF, SFF, V, VG.

Steak Sauce   Serves 8

This sweet, savory steak sauce is a terrific addition to almost any meal.

¼ cup olive oil
⅓ cup gluten-free soy sauce (such as La Choy or San-J)
3 Tb brown sugar
3 Tb gluten-free Worcestershire sauce
2 Tb garlic, minced
½ tsp onion powder
½ tsp pepper

1. Whisk all the ingredients together; refrigerate until ready to use.

Nutritional information: 86.3 calories, less than 1 gram protein, 5.7 grams carbohydrates, 6.7 gram fat, 0 milligrams cholesterol, 750 milligrams sodium, less than 1 gram fiber, 7.5 milligrams calcium, less than 1 milligram iron.

Tip: This steak sauce is perfect as a topping choice for any barbecue.

** Allergy Tip: This recipe is GF, MF, EF, NF, PF, SFF.

Barbecue Sauce   Serves 12

Barbecue sauce is easy to make and delicious for using on your grilled recipes. Add your favorite spices until you get a flavor that is perfect for you.

2 Tb olive oil
½ small red onion, chopped
1 Tb garlic, minced
½ cup apricot preserves
½ cup ketchup
1 Tb molasses

1 Tb vinegar
1 tsp gluten-free hot sauce (more, if you like it hot)
2 Tb gluten-free Worcestershire sauce
⅛ tsp ground celery seeds
½ tsp salt
¼ tsp pepper

1. Heat olive oil and sauté onion until translucent. Add garlic and sauté for about 2–3 minutes more.

2. Add all other ingredients; simmer for about 5 minutes.

3. Taste and add extra seasoning if desired.

4. Refrigerate until ready to use.

Nutritional information: 73.3 calories, less than 1 gram protein, 13.7 grams carbohydrates, 2.3 grams fat, 0 milligrams cholesterol, 257.5 milligrams sodium, less than 1 gram fiber, 11.1 milligrams calcium, less than 1 milligram iron.

Tip: Any kind of preserves can be used in place of the apricot.

** Allergy Tip: This recipe is GF, MF, SF, EF, NF, PF, SFF. To make vegetarian, fish free, or vegan, omit Worcestershire sauce.

Cream Sauce   Serves 4

This is great to use as a base for a cream soup, or with any recipe that originally calls for a cream sauce.

2 Tb butter
2 Tb rice flour
1 cup half-and-half
½ tsp salt
⅛ tsp pepper

1. Melt butter in a sauce pan and stir in rice flour, stirring until it is a thick paste.

2. Slowly add half-and-half a little at a time, stirring until all half-and-half is added and the sauce begins to thicken and is smooth.

3. Add salt and pepper, heat for an additional 2–3 minutes, and serve.

Nutritional information: 147 calories, 2.2 grams protein, 6.4 grams carbohydrates, 12.7 grams fat, 37.4 milligrams cholesterol, 356.6 milligrams sodium, less than 1 gram fiber, 65.8 milligrams calcium, less than 1 milligram iron.

Tips: Add an egg yolk and shredded parmesan cheese and heat and stir until thickened for a terrific Alfredo sauce. To make a cheese sauce, substitute milk for the half-and-half and add some shredded cheddar cheese. Stir over a low heat until the cheese is melted.

** Allergy Tip: This recipe is GF, EF, SF, NF, PF, FF, SFF, V. To make milk free and vegan, substitute margarine (note that margarine often contains soy) for the butter and rice milk for the half-and-half and cook a little longer to thicken.

Sweets and Treats:

- Double Chocolate Chip Cookies

- Apple and Almond Tart

- Italian Ricotta Pie

- Apple and Cranberry Crumb Pie

- Strawberry Shortcake

- Chocolate Lava Cakes

- Cheesecake Bars

- Pumpkin Pie

- Linzer Tarts

- Cream Cheese Butter Cookies

- Chocolate Chip Coconut Meringue Cookies

- Oatmeal and Butterscotch Cookies

- Moist and Delicious Carrot Cake

- Yellow Cake

- Cream Filling

- Buttercream Frosting

- Almond Crust

- Rice Pudding

** See tip earlier in the chapter on how to convert savory crêpes to dessert crêpes.

Double Chocolate Chip Cookies   **Makes 48 Servings**

The ultimate chocolate chip cookie—no one would ever know they are gluten free!

2 cups gluten-free all-purpose flour blend (see chapter 5 or buy)
½ cup almond meal
2 tsp gluten-free baking soda
1 tsp gluten-free baking powder
1 tsp salt
1 tsp xanthan gum
2 sticks of butter
¾ cup white sugar
¾ cup brown sugar
2 eggs, slightly beaten
1 tsp vanilla extract
12 oz gluten-free semi-sweet chocolate chips
6 oz gluten-free semi-sweet chocolate chunks
Gluten-free cooking spray or olive oil

1. Preheat oven to 350 degrees F.

2. Combine all dry ingredients except sugar and chips.

3. Cream butter, then add sugar and beat until well-combined.

4. Add eggs and vanilla extract to the butter mixture and mix well.

5. Mix flour mixture into creamed mixture; if too wet, add a little extra flour blend or brown rice flour. Dough should be moist but hold together well.

6. Add ¾ of the chips, reserving the rest of the chips and chocolate chunks for topping. (See tips below for baking.)

7. Use a tablespoon scoop to place cookies on the baking sheet—spray scoop with cooking spray to keep the dough from sticking. Scoops that have a handle that pushes out the dough work best.

8. Spoon 3 cookies across on each row on the baking sheet to keep them from spreading into each other.

9. Top cookies with reserved chocolate chips and chunks, pushing in a little.

10. Bake cookies until they are just starting to brown but still a little light in the middle. Remove from oven, let sit for about 1–2 minutes, and remove from baking sheet to cool on aluminum foil or rack.

Nutritional information: 140 calories, 1.5 grams protein, 19.7 grams carbohydrates, 7.2 grams fat, 19 milligrams cholesterol, 141 milligrams sodium, less than 1 grams fiber, 13.6 milligrams calcium, less than 1 milligram iron.

Tips: Baking flour blends should be mixed and kept in containers, handy when all-purpose flour is called for in recipes. Also, note that nuts are also a great addition to these cookies. This recipe makes a soft, puffy cookie. If you like a crispy, flatter cookie, use a little less flour.

** Allergy Tip: This recipe is GF, FF, SFF, V. To make milk free, use margarine instead of butter and milk-free, gluten-free chocolate chips in place of the chips and chunks of chocolate. To make egg free, use any gluten-free eggless egg substitute.

Apple and Almond Tart   Serves 12

This decadent tart was adapted from a classic French tart often offered among dessert options at fine restaurants.

Crust

¾ cup all-purpose gluten-free flour blend (see chapter 5 or buy)
½ cup almond meal
1 tsp xanthan gum
¼ tsp salt
5 Tb cold, unsalted butter, cut into little pieces
1 egg yolk
3–4 Tb ice water
½ Tb unsalted butter, softened
9-inch tart pan

Filling

1 cup slivered almonds (or almond meal)
½ cup dark brown sugar
¼ cup gluten-free flour blend
½ tsp salt
1 tsp ground cinnamon
6 Tb unsalted butter, softened
2 eggs
2 Tb dark rum
3 golden delicious apples, cored, peeled, halved, and thinly sliced
½ cup dark brown sugar

1. Preheat oven to 400 degrees F.

2. By hand or in a food processor, blend together the flour blend, xanthan gum, salt, and 5 Tb butter until mixture resembles small peas.

3. Work in egg and ice water until the dough begins to hold together nicely (add more ice water if needed).

4. Wrap dough in plastic wrap and place in freezer for about 15 minutes.

5. On parchment paper, sprinkle a little of the leftover flour blend and then flatten out the dough. Sprinkle out the flour blend and then carefully roll out the dough until large enough to cover the inside of a tart pan.

6. Butter tart pan inside with ½ Tb butter.

7. Flip the dough into the tart pan and press into pan to fix nicely, reserving any pieces of extra dough for patching.

8. Bake tart dough for about 10–15 minutes, until it is dry to the touch and light brown.

9. If the crust has cracked at all, use leftover dough to patch insides. If no dough is left over, combine a little gluten-free flour with softened butter and spread over the crack.

10. Set crust aside.

11. In a food processor, pulse slivered almonds until they are chopped fine, and place them in a large bowl. (If using almond meal, skip this step.)

12. To the almonds add ½ cup brown sugar, ¼ cup gluten-free flour blend, ½ tsp salt and ½ tsp cinnamon and mix together.

13. Beat into the almond mixture 4 Tb of the soft butter, until well-blended.

14. Blend 2 eggs and rum into this mixture.

15. Spread creamed mixture into the baked shell.

16. Arrange the apples over the top of the tart in a flower design.

17. Melt remaining butter, pour over top of apples, sprinkle with brown sugar and remaining cinnamon.

18. Bake for about 1 hour, until apples are golden.

19. Let cool for about 30 minutes, until set; carefully remove from tart pan and place on a platter.

Nutritional information per serving: 308 calories, 4.7 grams protein, 35 grams carbohydrates, 17 grams fat, 82 milligrams cholesterol, 170 milligrams sodium, 2.4 grams fiber, 56.8 milligrams calcium, 1.1 milligrams iron.

Tip: This tart is yummy made with pears or peaches as well. Gluten-free tarts are easier to make then gluten-containing tarts and they come out perfect every time. Instead of a pie, try baking a tart with your favorite fillings.

** Allergy Tip: This recipe is GF, SF, PF, FF, SFF, V. Check the flour blend for soy or peanuts. Check the almond meal to make sure it is free from peanuts. To make milk free, use margarine in place of the butter (note that most margarine contains soy) and make sure the flour blend is milk free. To make egg free, use any gluten-free eggless egg substitute for the eggs and egg yolk. To make vegan, use margarine instead of butter and any vegan egg substitute (note that these may contain soy).

Italian Ricotta Pie   Serves 12

Don't be surprised when everyone asks for seconds of this delicious treat.

Crust

1⅔ cup gluten-free all-purpose flour blend (see chapter 5 or buy)
2 Tb sugar
½ tsp salt
½ tsp gluten-free baking powder
1 tsp xanthan gum
½ cup butter
2 eggs

Filling

15 oz part-skim ricotta cheese
1 cup sugar
1 Tb gluten-free flour blend
½ tsp grated lemon peel
Dash of salt
4 eggs
2 tsp vanilla extract
⅓ cup gluten-free semi-sweet chocolate chips
1 tsp orange extract
½ tsp cinnamon
Dash of nutmeg
9-inch pie pan

1. Combine gluten-free flour blend, sugar, salt, baking powder, and xanthan gum with butter; mix together with a fork or a food processor until the mixture resembles small crumbs.

2. Add eggs and work mixture until it holds together as a ball.

3. Wrap dough in plastic wrap and place in freezer for about 20 minutes.

4. Remove dough from freezer and place on parchment paper that has been dusted lightly with gluten-free flour, pressing dough down into a circle.

5. Sprinkle top of dough with gluten-free flour blend and carefully roll out into a large disk that will cover the inside of a pie pan.

6. Flip dough into pie pan and press into any cracks to make sure crust covers all areas of pie pan. Crimp edges.

7. Preheat oven to 350 degrees F.

8. In a large bowl, mix together ricotta, sugar, flour, lemon peel, and salt.

9. In a small bowl, beat eggs for about 3 minutes and fold into ricotta mixture.

10. Add all remaining ingredients and pour into prepared crust.

11. Bake for about 1 hour until just set; turn off oven, and let sit in warm oven another 15 minutes before removing and cooling.

Nutritional information: 334 calories, 8.9 grams protein, 43 grams carbohydrates, 14.8 grams fat, 137 milligrams cholesterol, 280 milligrams sodium, less than 1 gram fiber, 130 milligrams calcium, 1.3 milligrams iron.

Tips: This delicious pie freezes beautifully and can be cut and defrosted one piece at a time. Using a porcelain pie pan gives it a nice presentation.

** Allergy Tip: This recipe is GF, NF, FF, SFF, V. Make sure you check flour-blend ingredients for nuts. To make egg free, use any gluten-free eggless egg substitute.

Apple and Cranberry Crumb Pie   Serves 8

This pie can be made with many fruit fillings and is always perfect, especially topped with vanilla ice cream.

Crust

¼ cup potato starch
¼ cup tapioca starch
½ cup white rice flour
2 tsp granulated sugar
½ tsp xanthan gum
½ tsp gluten-free baking powder
½ sp salt
6 Tb unsalted cold butter
⅓ cup cold water
1 tsp cider vinegar

1. Sift all dry ingredients (flour through salt) into a large mixing bowl.

2. Add butter and use a pastry cutter or fork to work butter into the dry ingredients until they are well incorporated and mixture looks crumbly.

3. Mix together water and vinegar. Stir into the flour. The dough should be soft but hold together when squeezed. Wrap in plastic wrap and refrigerate while making filling.

Filling

3 large green apples
½ cup fresh cranberries
1 Tb lemon juice
2 Tb cornstarch
½ cup granulated sugar
1¼ tsp ground cinnamon
2 Tb unsalted butter, melted
¼ cup almond flour, finely ground
¼ cup white rice flour
2 Tb brown sugar

1. Peel and thinly slice the apples. Place in a medium mixing bowl. Add cranberries and lemon juice and stir gently to mix.

2. Add cornstarch, sugar, and 1 tsp of cinnamon. Stir until combined.

3. Mix butter, almond and rice flour, brown sugar, and remaining ¼ tsp cinnamon in a small bowl with a fork until mixed and crumbly.

4. Preheat oven to 375 degrees F.

5. Remove crust from refrigerator and plastic wrap. Place between 2 sheets of waxed paper and roll out into a 9-inch circle (use a little flour blend if dough is sticking to the wax paper).

6. Remove one sheet of waxed paper and invert crust into a 9-inch pie plate. Remove second sheet of waxed paper so pie crust fits nicely into the pan. Trim and crimp edges of the crust to make decorative border.

7. Pour apple mixture into crust. Sprinkle with crumb topping.

8. Bake for 40 minutes. If pie browns too quickly, cover with aluminum foil.

Nutritional information per serving: 286 calories, 1.6 grams protein, 44 grams carbohydrates, 12.5 grams fat, 32 milligrams cholesterol, 96 milligrams sodium, 2.5 grams fiber, 29 milligrams calcium, less than 1 milligram iron.

Tips: Use any kind of berry in this pie: blueberry, raspberry—the sky's the limit! Handle the crust as little as possible so that it will stay flaky.

** Allergy Tip: This recipe is GF, EF, SF, PF, FF, SFF, V. To keep peanut free, check almond meal and flour blend to make sure they do not contain peanuts. To make milk free and vegan, substitute margarine for butter (note that most margarine contains soy).

Strawberry Shortcake   Serves 4

In the spring and summer, when seasonally ripe berries are everywhere, this cake is a sure hit.

Gluten-free cooking spray or canola oil
½ cup brown rice flour
½ cup white rice flour
¼ cup tapioca starch
2 tsp gluten-free baking powder
½ tsp gluten-free baking soda
3 Tb sugar
¾ cup low-fat buttermilk
1 Tb raw turbinado sugar (white granulated sugar can also be used)
2 cups strawberries, sliced
⅓ cup gluten-free whipped cream

1. Preheat oven to 425 degrees F. Coat a cookie sheet with cooking spray.

2. In a large mixing bowl, mix brown rice flour, white rice flour, tapioca starch, baking powder, baking soda, and 2 Tb of sugar.

3. Add buttermilk; stir to combine.

4. Using two spoons, drop batter onto cookie sheet in four equal portions. Sprinkle with raw sugar.

5. Bake in preheated oven for 15 minutes, until golden brown.

6. Mix sliced strawberries with remaining 1 Tb sugar.

7. When biscuits have cooled, slice in half. Top one half with ½ cup strawberries and 1 Tb whipped cream; place other half of biscuit on top and serve.

Nutritional information per serving: 283 calories, 4.7 grams protein, 58 grams carbohydrates, 4.2 grams fat, 12 milligrams cholesterol, 330 milligrams sodium, 2.8 grams fiber, 113 milligrams calcium, less than 1 milligram iron.

Tip: Turbinado sugar or sugar in the raw is pure cane sugar; it is coarser and contains natural molasses.

** Allergy Tip: This recipe is GF, SF, EF, NF, PF, FF, SFF, V. To keep soy free, use a soy-free cooking spray or vegetable oil and double-check the whipped cream for soy. For milk free and vegan, use a dairy-free substitute for the buttermilk and whipped cream (note that this may contain soy).

Chocolate Lava Cakes   Serves 6

These gooey chocolate cakes are just perfect for the chocoholic in everyone.

Gluten-free cooking spray or canola oil
3 oz gluten-free semi-sweet chocolate
3 oz gluten-free bittersweet chocolate
3 Tb unsalted butter
4 egg yolks
5 Tb sugar
1 tsp vanilla extract
2 egg whites (room temperature)
½ tsp cream of tartar
1 Tb confectioner's sugar

1. Preheat oven to 425 degrees F. Coat the inside of six ¾-cup oven-safe custard cups with cooking spray. Place custard cups on a cookie sheet.

2. Combine chocolates and butter in top of a double boiler. Heat over simmering water until chocolate is melted, stirring frequently. Remove from heat and cool for 10 minutes (or microwave chocolate to melt it).

3. In a large bowl, beat egg yolks and sugar with an electric beater about 2 minutes, until thick and light in color. Fold in vanilla and chocolate.

4. Beat egg whites and cream of tartar in a separate clean bowl, until stiff peaks form. Gently fold into the chocolate mixture.

5. Divide batter evenly among 6 custard cups. Bake in preheated oven about 10 minutes, until cakes are puffed but still soft in the center.

6. Transfer cookie sheet to a rack. Let cool 1 minute.

7. Using a small knife, cut around sides of cakes to loosen. Remove cakes to a serving dish. Sprinkle with confectioner's sugar and serve.

Nutritional information per serving: 274 calories, 4 grams protein, 24 grams carbohydrates, 18 grams fat, 154 milligrams cholesterol, 24 milligrams sodium, 2 grams fiber, 28 milligrams calcium, 1.6 milligrams iron.

Tip: Serve with fresh raspberries or blueberries.

** Allergy Tip: This recipe is GF, NF, FF, SFF, V. For nut free, make sure the chocolate does not contain nuts. To make milk free, use milk-free bittersweet chocolate and margarine instead of butter with an additional 2 Tb of sugar (note most margarine contains soy).

Cheesecake Bars   **Makes 36 Servings (Serving Size, 1 Bar)**

These delicious bars are like miniature cheesecakes, perfect for an afternoon treat.

¾ cup crushed gluten-free graham crackers (such as Kinnikinnick or Schär gluten-free)
½ cup gluten-free all-purpose flour blend (see Chapter 5 or buy)
½ cup walnuts, chopped fine
¼ cup sugar
½ cup butter melted
8 oz cream cheese
⅓ cup sugar
1 egg
1 Tb lemon juice
½ tsp grated lemon peel

1. Preheat oven to 350 degrees F.

2. Stir together first four ingredients, except 2 Tb of the graham cracker crumbs. Add melted butter and combine.

3. Press into a 9 × 9-inch square nonstick baking pan.

4. Bake in a 350-degree oven for 12 minutes.

5. Cream together cream cheese and ⅓ cup sugar.

6. Add egg, lemon juice, and lemon peel; mix well.

7. Pour over baked layer, sprinkle with remaining gluten-free graham cracker crumbs, and bake for an additional 20–25 minutes.

8. Cool and cut into bars.

Nutritional information: 85 calories, 1.1 grams protein, 7 grams carbohydrates, 6 grams fat, 13.7 milligrams cholesterol, 54 milligrams sodium, less than 1 grams fiber, 7.8 milligrams calcium, less than 1 milligram iron.

Tip: If you prefer a taste besides lemon, why not use orange peel and orange juice in place of the lemon?

** Allergy Tip: This recipe is GF, FF, SFF, V.

Pumpkin Pie   Serves 8

There is no need for you to pass on the pumpkin pie on Thanksgiving—everyone will love this recipe.

9-inch Pie Crust

1⅔ cups gluten-free all-purpose flour blend (see chapter 5 or buy)
2 Tb sugar
½ tsp salt
½ tsp baking powder
1 tsp xanthan gum
½ cup butter
2 eggs

1. Combine gluten-free flour blend, sugar, salt, baking powder, and xanthan gum.

2. Work butter into the dry mixture with a fork or a food processor until the mixture resembles small crumbs.

3. Add eggs, and work mixture until it holds together as a ball.

4. Wrap in plastic wrap and place in freezer for about 20 minutes.

5. Remove dough from freezer and place on parchment paper that has been dusted lightly with gluten-free flour; press dough down into a circle.

6. Sprinkle top of dough with gluten-free flour blend and carefully roll out into a large disk that will fit into a pie pan.

7. Flip dough into pie pan and press into any cracks to make sure crust covers all sections of the pie pan.

8. Crimp edges to make a nice pie edge.

Filling

¾ cup dark brown sugar
1 tsp cinnamon
½ tsp salt
½ tsp ground ginger
¼ tsp ground cloves
2 eggs
1 tsp vanilla extract
15 oz pumpkin purée
12 oz evaporated milk

1. Preheat oven to 425 degrees F.

2. In a small bowl, mix together brown sugar, cinnamon, salt, ginger, and cloves.

3. In a large bowl, beat eggs, vanilla, pumpkin, and add into spice mixture. Fold in evaporated milk.

4. Pour pumpkin mixture into pie crust and bake for 15 minutes. Lower temperature to 350 degrees F and bake for an additional 50 minutes, until knife inserted in the center comes out clean.

5. Refrigerate until ready to serve.

6. Top with gluten-free whipped cream if desired.

Nutritional information per serving: 256 calories, 4.5 grams protein, 33.5 grams carbohydrates, 10 grams fat, 92 milligrams cholesterol, 302 milligrams sodium, 1.6 grams fiber, 120 milligrams calcium, 1.4 milligrams iron.

Tip: If you want to use homemade pumpkin purée, cut a small pumpkin in half and remove the seeds; place pumpkin halves cut-side down on a baking sheet and bake at 350 degrees F until pumpkin is soft and can be pierced with a fork. Scoop out pumpkin flesh; purée and strain. Refrigerate until ready to use.

** Allergy Tip: This recipe is GF, SF, NF, PF, FF, SFF, V. To keep soy free, make sure the whipped cream and flour blend do not contain soy. For nut free, check the flour blend for nuts. To make egg free, use any gluten-free eggless egg substitute.

Linzer Tarts   45 (3-in.) Tarts

These tarts are actually easier to roll than those made from gluten-containing flour. They are so light and delicious, you'll want to have them every day.

4 sticks unsalted butter
1½ cups sugar
4 egg yolks
2 tsp vanilla extract
6½–7½ cups all-purpose gluten-free flour blend (see below; if using a
    store-bought flour blend, for every 3 cups of flour blend, add ½ cup
    almond or hazelnut flour)
1½ cups almond flour
1 tsp salt
2 tsp xanthan gum
½ cup rice flour
½ cup powdered sugar
30 oz red raspberry preserves

Gluten-Free Flour Blend

(Makes 7 cups; store leftover blend in an airtight container as a gluten-free all-purpose flour.)

2¼ cups sorghum flour
2¼ cups potato starch or cornstarch

1½ cups tapioca flour

1 cup almond or hazelnut flour (nut flours give the best taste) or chick-pea or corn flour

1. In a large bowl, beat butter until creamy. Then cream sugar into butter, add egg yolks and vanilla, and blend together.

2. Combine 6½ cups all-purpose gluten-free flour blend with almond flour, salt, and xanthan gum. When well-combined, dough should be easy to shape with hands but not wet or sticky. If the dough is too wet, add gluten-free all-purpose blend or almond meal until you get the right consistency. Dough should be a little softer than Play-Doh.

3. Preheat oven to 350 degrees F.

4. On a work surface, spread a large piece of waxed paper and sprinkle with rice flour. Take a softball-sized piece of dough and shape into a ball; then flatten it out and flip so both sides have some rice flour on them.

5. Take a rolling pin and roll out to about ⅓-inch thick. If dough is too sticky, add a little more rice flour.

6. Take a cookie cutter about 3 inches across and cut out dough. You will need to cut 2 pieces for each tart. Take a smaller cookie cutter and cut a small design in the center of one of the cookies. I like to save the cutaway shapes to make smaller cookies (otherwise, just reincorporate it into the dough).

7. Bake the cookies for about 9–10 minutes, until cookies are set and just starting to turn golden in color.

8. Remove from tray with a spatula, and place on aluminum foil to cool. Sprinkle with powdered sugar.

9. When cookies are cool, spread about 1 Tb of preserves on each uncut cookie, and spread. Top with a cookie with a design cut out, and arrange cookies on a platter. Serve 1 tart per person.

Nutritional information per serving: 257 calories, 2.3 grams protein, 42 grams carbohydrates, 9.7 grams fat, 40.3 milligrams cholesterol, 59 milligrams sodium, less than 1 gram fiber, 12.8 milligrams calcium, less than 1 milligram iron.

Tips: If you would like to make smaller cookies without the cutout in the center, halve the recipe and cut 2 small cookies for each jam-filled cookie. Cookies can be kept in an airtight container for weeks or can be stored in the freezer and defrosted when ready to use. Dough can also be made ahead of time, then wrapped in plastic and refrigerated or frozen until ready to use. You can also make half the recipe if you are looking for a smaller batch of cookies.

** Allergy Tip: This recipe is GF, SF, PF, FF, SFF, V. To keep soy free, double-check the flour blend and almond meal for any soy. To keep peanut free, double-check the flour blend for peanuts. To make milk free, use margarine in place of butter (note that most margarine contains soy) and double-check the flour blend for any dairy.

Cream Cheese Butter Cookies   Makes 48 Servings

These cookies are simple to make and the perfect ultimate buttery cookie to dip into coffee. These cookies have been adapted from my mother-in-law Helen's famous cream cheese cookies.

1 cup (2 sticks) unsalted butter or margarine
3-oz package cream cheese, softened
1 cup granulated sugar
1 egg yolk
1 tsp vanilla extract
3½ cups all-purpose gluten-free blend (see chapter 5 or buy)
1 tsp salt
1 tsp xanthan gum
¼ cup powdered sugar

1. Preheat oven to 350 degrees F.

2. In a large bowl, cream together butter and cream cheese; add sugar and blend until smooth.

3. Add egg yolk and vanilla to butter mixture and mix to combine.

4. In a small bowl, combine flour blend, salt and xanthan gum.

5. Combine wet and dry ingredients until a nice dough forms.

6. Shape cookies into small balls and make a thumbprint in the center.

7. Place cookies on a cookie sheet and bake for 10–12 minutes, until they are just hinting at light gold.

8. Remove from cookie sheet and place on aluminum foil or rack to cool.

9. Sprinkle with powdered sugar; store in airtight container until ready to use.

Nutritional information per serving: 102.7 calories, less than 1 gram protein, 14.7 grams carbohydrates, 4.8 grams fat, 16.5 milligrams cholesterol, 58 milligrams sodium, less than 1 gram fiber, 9 milligrams calcium, less than 1 milligram iron.

Tips: Cookies can be kept in an airtight container for weeks or can be stored in the freezer and defrosted when ready to use. Dough can also be made ahead of time and wrapped in plastic and refrigerated or frozen until ready to use.

** Allergy Tip: This recipe is GF, SF, NF, PF, FF, SFF, V. Check the flour blend to make sure it is soy and nut free. To make egg free, use any gluten-free eggless egg substitute for the egg yolk.

Chocolate Chip Coconut Meringue Cookies   Serves 8

These delicious cookies will melt in your mouth.

2 egg whites (room temperature)
¼ tsp salt
⅛ tsp cream of tartar
⅔ cup granulated sugar
¼ cup cocoa powder
⅓ cup mini gluten-free chocolate chips
2 Tb dried cranberries
¼ cup shredded coconut
¼ cup walnuts, chopped
Gluten-free cooking spray or canola oil

1. Preheat oven to 300 degrees F.

2. In a mixer, beat egg whites with salt and cream of tartar until they start to peak.

3. Blend in sugar and cocoa powder 1 Tb at a time, until well-combined and stiff peaks are formed.

4. Fold in chocolate chips, cranberries, coconut, and walnuts.

5. Spray cookie sheet with cooking spray and cover with parchment paper.

6. Drop batter by the teaspoon onto parchment paper.

7. Bake for 30–40 minutes, until cookies are crisp.

8. Wait until cool before trying to remove from cookie sheet.

Nutritional information: 147 calories, 2.4 grams protein, 24.4 grams carbohydrates, 5.6 grams fat, 0 milligrams cholesterol, 88 milligrams sodium, 3.8 grams fiber, 9.1 milligrams calcium, less than 1 milligram iron.

Tip: Why not try dried blueberries, cherries, or chopped pecans in this recipe? Everything tastes great in a meringue. Let your imagination go wild!

** Allergy Tip: This recipe is GF, FF, SFF, V. To make milk free, use milk-free chocolate chips.

Oatmeal and Butterscotch Cookies   Makes 36 Cookies

These cookies make you feel like you are at a country picnic.

1 cup butter, softened
1 cup brown sugar
½ cup white granulated sugar
2 eggs
1 tsp vanilla extract
1¾ cups gluten-free all-purpose flour blend (see chapter 5 or buy)
1 tsp gluten-free baking soda
¼ tsp xanthan gum
½ tsp salt
2 tsp cinnamon
2½ cups gluten-free rolled oats
1 cup gluten-free butterscotch chips
½ cup sweetened coconut

1. Preheat oven to 350 degrees F. Line a cookie sheet with parchment paper.

2. In a large bowl, cream butter; then add brown and white sugar and beat until light and fluffy.

3. Add eggs and vanilla. Continue to beat until smooth.

4. Combine the gluten-free flour blend, gluten-free baking soda, xanthan gum, salt, and cinnamon. Stir into the sugar mixture.

5. Stir in the gluten-free oats, chips, and coconut.

6. Drop by rounded teaspoons onto prepared cookie sheet.

7. Bake for 10–12 minutes, until light and golden. Do not over bake. Let them cool for 1–2 minutes on cookie sheet. Set on aluminum foil or wire rack to cool completely.

8. Store in an airtight container or freeze until ready to use.

Nutritional information (per cookie): 165 calories, 1.6 grams protein, 21.6 grams carbohydrates, 8 grams fat, 25 milligrams cholesterol, 119 milligrams sodium, less than 1 grams fiber, 9.7 milligrams calcium, less than 1 milligrams iron.

Tip: Use chocolate chips or dried fruit in place of butterscotch chips if desired.

** Allergy Tip: This recipe is GF, FF, SFF, V. Check the flour blend to make sure it is nut free. Note that some people consider coconut a nut; check with your allergist to see if you can safely consume coconut.

Moist and Delicious Carrot Cake   Serves 16

Everyone loves this carrot cake. Cut it into squares, and it's a perfect dessert to go.

Gluten-free cooking spray or canola oil
2 cups gluten-free all-purpose flour blend (see chapter 5 or buy)
2 tsp gluten-free baking soda
1 tsp gluten-free baking powder
2 tsp cinnamon
½ tsp xanthan gum
½ tsp salt

½ tsp allspice
2 cups white granulated sugar
¾ cup canola or corn oil
2 Tb ground flaxseed
3 eggs
1 tsp vanilla extract
½ cup walnuts, chopped
1 (8-oz) can crushed pineapple
1½ cups finely grated carrot

Cream Cheese Frosting

1 (8-oz) package light cream cheese
1 lb confectioner's sugar
2 Tb butter, softened

1. Preheat oven to 350 degrees F. Spray two 9-in. round cake pans with cooking spray.

2. Sift together flour, baking soda, baking powder, cinnamon, xanthan gum, salt, and allspice.

3. In a large bowl, beat sugar, oil, and flaxseed until well-blended. Add the eggs, one at a time, beating well after each addition. Stir in the vanilla.

4. Stir flour mixture into wet ingredients until just blended. Do not over mix.

5. Fold in walnuts, pineapple, and carrots. Pour batter into prepared pans.

6. Bake for 30–35 minutes or until toothpick inserted in middle comes out clean. Remove from oven and cool cake.

7. While cake is cooling, prepare frosting by beating together frosting ingredients until light and creamy.

8. Cover cake with frosting and serve.

Nutritional information: 448 calories, 4.3 grams protein, 75 grams carbohydrates, 15.9 grams fat, 51.4 milligrams cholesterol, 32 milligrams sodium, 1.2 grams fiber, 44 milligrams calcium, 1 milligram iron.

Tip: For a festive touch, sprinkle cake with toasted coconut or finely ground walnuts.

** **Allergy Tip:** This recipe is GF, SF, PF, FF, SFF, V. Check the flour blend to make sure it is peanut free and soy free. To keep soy free, use a soy-free cooking spray or vegetable oil. To keep peanut free, double-check the nuts to make sure they do not include peanuts.

Yellow Cake   Serves 18
(One 12 in. × 9 in. × 3 in. Cake or 18 Cupcakes)

Spongy sweet and delicious.

1 stick butter, softened
¾ cup sugar
2 eggs
1 cup buttermilk
1 tsp vanilla extract
1 cup gluten-free all-purpose flour blend (see chapter 5 or buy)
⅔ cup tapioca starch
1 tsp xanthan gum
1 tsp salt
½ tsp baking powder
½ tsp baking soda
Gluten-free cooking spray or vegetable oil

1. Preheat oven to 375 degrees F.

2. Mix together butter and sugar. Add eggs, buttermilk, and vanilla extract.

3. Combine dry ingredients in mixing bowl. Slowly beat into wet ingredients for about 3 minutes until creamy.

4. Pour into cupcake cups and bake, or spray cake pan with cooking spray and pour batter in.

5. Bake cupcakes about 20 minutes until golden; bake cake about 35 minutes.

6. Cool then frost or stuff as desired.

Nutritional information per serving: 141 calories, 2 grams protein, 35 grams carbohydrates, 6.1 grams fat, 1.2 grams fiber, 35 milligrams cholesterol, 208 milligrams sodium, 41 milligrams calcium, less than 1 milligram iron.

** **Allergy Tip:** This recipe is GF, SF, NF, PF, FF, SFF, V. Check the flour blend to make sure it is nut free and peanut free. To keep soy free, use a soy-free cooking spray or vegetable oil and double-check flour blend. To make egg free, use any gluten-free eggless egg substitute. To make milk free, use margarine instead of butter (note that most margarine contains soy) and a milk substitute in place of the buttermilk.

Chocolate Cake Tips: For chocolate cake, after you blend wet ingredients from the yellow cake recipe, add ½ cup melted milk chocolate that has cooled to room temperature. To melt chocolate, put ½ cup of dark or milk chocolate chips in a small bowl and microwave for about a minute and then stir until creamy. If you like really chocolaty cake, add a few tablespoons of cocoa powder.

**Allergy Tip: Most chocolate chips will have milk, soy, and peanuts, and some may have gluten, so double-check the labels.

Cream Filling   30 Servings (2 Tb Each)

This recipe will bring back childhood memories.

5 Tb gluten-free all-purpose flour blend (see chapter 5 or buy)
1 cup skim milk
6 Tb powdered sugar
2 tsp vanilla extract
1 cup sugar
1 cup butter, softened

1. Heat gluten-free flour, skim milk and powdered sugar, continually stirring until pasty.

2. Beat together vanilla, sugar, and butter, add flour paste, and beat for about 5 to 10 minutes until thick white and creamy.

Nutritional information per serving: 95 calories, .4 grams protein, 10 grams carbohydrates, 6.2 grams fat, less than 1 gram fiber, 16.5 milligram cholesterol, 58 milligrams sodium, 11.8 milligrams calcium, less than 1 milligram iron.

Tips: Use in yellow or chocolate cake. To fill cupcakes, use a pastry bag and pipe into cake, or cut a small piece out of the top of the cake, spoon in 1–2 Tb of cream and put the top back on. Freeze on baking sheet, wrap in plastic wrap, and store in ziplock freezer bags. Defrost either in refrigerator, at room temperature, or in microwave for about 10 seconds.

** **Allergy Tip:** This cream filling is GF, EF, SF, NF, PF, FF, SFF, V. Double-check the flour blend to make sure it is free of soy, nuts, and peanuts. To make milk free and vegan, use margarine in place of butter (note that most margarine contains soy) and a milk substitute, such as rice milk, in place of milk. To make vegan, use margarine in place of the butter and a milk-free milk substitute.

Buttercream Frosting   Frosts 1 Layer Cake or 24 Cupcakes

Sweet, creamy, and easy to make. Flavor as desired and serve

4 cups powdered sugar
½ cup salted butter softened
3 Tb milk
1 tsp vanilla extract

1. Whip butter, slowly incorporating powdered sugar.

2. Add a little milk at a time, continually whipping until light and creamy

Nutritional information per serving: 100 calories, .1 grams protein, 167 grams carbohydrates, 3.9 grams fat, 0 gram fiber, 104 milligram cholesterol, 35 milligrams sodium, 3.5 milligrams calcium, 0 milligrams iron.

Tip: If you like chocolate frosting, whip in cocoa powder until you get the desired chocolate flavor.

** **Allergy Tip:** This recipe is GF, EF, SF, NF, PF, FF, SFF, V. To make milk free and vegan, use margarine in place of butter (note that most margarine contains soy) and dairy-free milk, such as rice milk, in place of milk.

Almond Crust   Serves 10 (Makes One Tart Sell)

This is a light flaky crust that works well with many recipes.

1 cup almond flour
⅓ cup gluten-free all-purpose flour blend (see chapter 5 or buy)
½ tsp sea salt
½ tsp baking soda
⅓ cup canola oil
1 tsp vanilla extra
3 Tb honey or maple syrup or agave

1. Mix all ingredients together, wrap in plastic, and chill in refrigerator for about 30 minutes.

2. Press into medium-sized tart pan, and bake in a 350-degree F oven for 10 minutes to set.

3. Fill with favorite fillings and bake until done.

Nutritional information per serving: 195 calories, 4.5 grams protein, 8.5 grams carbohydrates, 17 grams fat, 2.2 grams fiber, 0 milligrams cholesterol, 184 milligrams sodium, 45.2 milligrams calcium, 1 milligram iron.

Tip: Try with your favorite pie filling.

** Allergy Tip: This recipe is GF, MF, SF, EF, PF, FF, SFF, V, VG. Make sure you check the flour blend to be sure it is free from milk, soy, and peanuts.

Rice Pudding   Serves 6

This creamy, dreamy rice pudding is well worth the wait.

⅓ cup short grain rice
⅓ cup sugar
1 qt milk
2 egg yolks beaten with 1 tsp vanilla, at room temperature

1. Bring milk, rice, and sugar to a slight boil in a heavy pot.

2. Lower the heat to medium and bring to a low boil, stirring frequently.

3. If a skin forms, whisk it in.

4. Cook for approximately 45 minutes to one hour.

5. Remove pot from burner when rice is thick *and not sooner.* Immediately whisk the eggs briskly into the hot pudding to prevent eggs from scrambling.

6. Cool in an ice water bath. Pudding thickens somewhat as it cools. If it's too thick, it can always be thinned out with some half-and-half.

Nutritional information per serving: 190 calories, 6.7 grams protein, 26 grams carbohydrates, 6.9 grams fat, less than 1 gram fiber, 78 milligrams cholesterol, 73 milligrams sodium, 193 milligrams calcium, 6 milligrams iron.

Tips: For 12 servings, at least double the recipe (takes the same amount of time). Use pasteurized eggs, or Egg beaters, to reduce the risk of food-borne illness.

** Allergy Tip: This recipe is GF, SF, NF, PF, FF, SFF, V. To make milk free, egg free, and vegan, use a dairy-free milk such as rice, coconut, or soy milk, and a gluten-free eggless egg substitute for the eggs Or omit the eggs.

Creating Your Own Gluten-Free Recipes

Learning how to create gluten-free recipes allows you to easily prepare delicious, healthy meals every day. It also can save you a lot of money! Recipe development can be as simple or gourmet as you want it to be. Even if you haven't been much of a cook before, you'll find that taking it one step at a time will bring very satisfying results.

So How Do You Get Started?

Step 1: Pick up a basic all-purpose cookbook (I suggest one of the classics, such as *Fannie Farmer*, *The Joy of Cooking*, or *Good Housekeeping*). Any of these will give you a leg up in regard to basic techniques, cooking times, and so forth. You'll also find inspirations for combining different ingredients. Although typical cookbooks will include gluten-containing ingredients, the cooking methods will help you as you develop your own gluten-free recipes. Carol Fenster's book *1000 Gluten-Free Meals* is a great gluten-free addition to your cooking library that provides 1,000 gluten-free versions of classic recipes. Having a basic all-purpose cookbook and Carol's book can give you a lot of options and tips to choose from. As you get comfortable, you may want to add to this basic library other books on different types of cuisines.

    Step Two: Make a list of your favorite foods, whether you know how to make them or not. Add to your list other types of recipes you'd like to learn to prepare.

    Step Three: For your first attempts, start with simple recipes so that you will be successful from the beginning. You can build up to more challenging dishes from there.

Example

You love chicken and fruit, and you're looking to develop a recipe that includes both. You picked up some chicken thighs and pineapple at the supermarket, and you're ready to get started. Open your all-purpose cookbook to check cooking times and temperatures for the chicken. Decide which seasonings appeal to you, and be sure you have these on hand. Let's say that for the chicken you decide to use olive oil, garlic, onion powder, salt, and pepper. In addition, you have found a recipe for fruit salsa in your cookbook that you can alter a little, using your pineapple in place of the other fruit suggestions. Your dish will be "Baked Chicken with Pineapple Salsa," and on the side you've decided to serve rice and steamed broccoli. So the recipe would go as follows:

Baked Chicken with Pineapple Salsa   Serves 4

3 chicken thighs
1 Tb olive oil
¼ tsp garlic powder
¼ tsp onion powder
⅛ tsp pepper
¼ tsp salt

Pineapple Salsa   Serves 4

1 cup fresh pineapple, chopped
½ cup red onion, chopped
1 small jalapeno pepper, chopped
¼ tsp salt
Dash of pepper
½ cup cilantro, chopped
1 Tb olive oil
Juice of one lime

1. Preheat oven to 350 degrees F.

2. In a casserole dish place chicken, drizzle with olive oil, sprinkle with garlic, onion powder, salt, and pepper.

3. Roast chicken for about 30 to 40 minutes, until chicken is cooked through and golden brown.

4. While chicken is cooking, prepare salsa by combining all salsa ingredients in a medium bowl.

5. Serve salsa over baked chicken with a side of rice and steamed broccoli.

Gluten-Free Baking

These development techniques can be used for almost any recipe. Gluten-free baking can be a bit trickier, so it is best to take already-tested and successful gluten-free baking recipes and use them as your base. Pick gluten-free flour blends like those found in Chapter 5 to ensure a happy result.

If you bravely choose to develop your own gluten-free flour blends, it is important to understand how to combine flours in order to achieve the best results. Gluten-free flours generally produce denser breads, so adding a lighter starch to the blend can be helpful to obtain a desirable texture. Starches such as tapioca or potato starch work well when incorporated into the gluten-free flour blend to lighten things up. For improving texture, 1–2 tsp xanthan gum or expandex (usually about 1 tsp to every 2–3 cups of gluten-free flour blend) should be added to provide a better rise in your final product. Sometimes you'll need to adjust the amount of flour or modify the rising time of a recipe to get better results. Bread recipes work best when they include higher-protein selections (such as bean flours, eggs, milk, and cheese) that help provide an even better overall texture.

Dessert recipes usually work very well using the gluten-free flour combinations, but cakes usually require a little extra starch in the flour blend. The trick is starting with some basic skills, picking your favorite foods, and—above all—being creative and having fun.

Dining Out Gluten Free

Tips for Stress-Free Dining Out

Dining out is supposed to be an enjoyable experience. For the gluten-free diner it is also one of the greatest challenges; after all, this is when you have the least control over the food preparation and the least access to food labels for review. Because food is the basis of most social and business interactions, this is more than a little nuisance, and it is difficult to avoid. In order to make dining out easier for you, it is essential to have an understanding of how restaurants work.

Restaurants are usually busy places, and asking for special requests can be difficult or uncomfortable, especially when the staff is in a rush and have little time to listen to your questions. Some establishments don't make any provisions for those with special needs, and specific menus do not allow for any alterations or substitutes without tacking on an extra charge for each change or addition.

The fact is that most restaurants are afraid of people with food allergies or intolerances; the last thing that they want is for someone to get sick in their establishment. Also, restaurants often get confused since some people who are following gluten-free diets are doing so for nonmedical reasons, as a fad, and these individuals may be lax in their approach to gluten-free eating, making the restaurant's staff unsure if they really need to be careful with gluten-free choices. Many restaurants have also jumped into offering gluten-free options due to this increase in demand, without taking the time to learn about it or to train their staff. This makes it doubly important to let them know what you need to have a safe meal. Letting them know more helps reduce the chances of your food getting contaminated. Sometimes they may seem uncomfortable or overwhelmed by the restrictions involved, but don't allow that to interfere with your asking for what you need.

> **TIP**
>
> 1. Be proactive. Call ahead to the restaurant and ask if they have a gluten-free menu. Ask to speak to the manager and the chef. Inquire what gluten-free menu options they can safely provide for you.
> 2. Always be prepared; carry some crackers, nuts, or a meal replacement bar as a back-up plan.
>
> —Anne Lee, EdD(c), RD, LD
> Director of Nutritional Services, Dr. Schar USA, Inc.

Of course, all you are looking for is a delicious, safe meal. When placing your order, you are not looking to draw a lot of attention to yourself or to make a scene. You just want them to listen to your requests and bring back something amazing from the kitchen. Of course, this is less likely to happen in restaurants that have cooks with little experience or establishments that use mostly prepared broths, soups, sauces, and gravies.

In order to make sure you have a pleasant dining experience, try to call restaurants (or look them up online) prior to your visit and get a copy of their menu. When you call, ask to speak to the manager and be sure to call off-hours (for example, the middle of the afternoon, after the lunch rush and before dinner service); when they are not busy, and they will be able to talk to you without being rushed. Selecting your meal will always be easier if you have identified gluten-free foods prior to your arrival at the restaurant. A night out is supposed to be fun, and it shouldn't feel like a chore. Some restaurants are clearly more amenable to special requests than others, so try to choose those whenever you can. It's win–win when you give your business to establishments that make you feel most welcome.

It's a given that, at times, your restaurant experience will be rocky—be patient. And when you have a great meal, show the chef and waitstaff that you appreciate it by thanking them and tipping generously.

WHEN DINING OUT

- Check with local celiac support groups for restaurant suggestions.
- Select restaurants that have gluten-free menus; there are many listed in the resource section at the end of this book.
- Review the restaurant's menu ahead of time.
- Call ahead and speak to the manager or chef to find out whether they can provide you with safe and delicious selections. Call in the middle of the afternoon, when they are more likely to be slow and can answer all your questions.
- Try to avoid restaurants that may have a higher risk of cross-contamination, such as those that prepare bakery items in the same area where other foods are being made.
- It takes more care for a restaurant to prevent cross-contamination, so try to dine out when the restaurant is less busy, either early or late in the evening.
- Bring a copy of the gluten-free dining sheets found in this chapter, making it easier for the chef to provide you with safe selections.
- Explain to the server that you will become ill if particular care is not taken with your food.
- Send back food that has been contaminated with gluten, bread crumbs, croutons, and so forth. Let them know that removing or scraping off the problem food will not be enough to keep you from getting sick.

A Look Inside a Restaurant Kitchen

Even when a restaurant is trying to accommodate special requests, they may have equipment and space constraints that make it difficult to provide the level of safety you need.

First, some kitchens are very small, and all foods may be prepared within the same area. It may be impossible to separate pots and utensils, or even to find a separate safe counter area in order to prepare your food. On busy nights, chefs will be racing around so fast that the risk of cross-contamination will be huge. Even when they are trying to offer food choices that are not contaminated with gluten, it is easy to make a mistake.

Evaluate your restaurant choices carefully, and when it appears that space may be an issue during the food preparation, it is better to dine out during slow times when it is easier for the chef to keep your food isolated from gluten-containing ingredients and utensils that have been used in prepping unsafe foods.

Also, take into consideration the equipment used to prepare the food; a restaurant that cooks foods in individual sauté pans has more control over each dish served. Nevertheless, with a restaurant that uses premarinated meats and sauces, preparing everything on the same grill, with the same tongs, it is difficult to impossible for them to accommodate those who have food intolerances or allergy issues.

Chain restaurants often have specific operating procedures for every recipe, often using premixed seasoning blends and preprepped foods, so it could be difficult for them to make many adjustments to their selections. Try calling their corporate offices prior to your visit for additional support. In addition, when you visit a chain restaurant that has a gluten-free menu and find when you arrive that the waitstaff is uninformed about it, you should treat this restaurant just like one that doesn't have a gluten-free menu. After all, the menu can only be safe if those serving you are aware of cross-contamination issues.

Safe Choices to Order

Even if a restaurant has a gluten-free menu and knowledgeable staff, asking questions is necessary. Often, larger establishments have high staff turnovers, and they may not adequately train everyone equally in terms of their gluten-free offerings. In these types of situations, a mistake can be made. Double-check when each course is served, asking about toppings, sauces, sides, and garnishes to make sure something wasn't mistakenly added to your food. You may feel a little uncomfortable about doing this, but remember: you are out for an enjoyable experience, and you don't want to get sick.

Because wheat, flour, bread, soup bases, and soy sauce are where most gluten is lurking, it is sometimes easier to just say that you are allergic to wheat, and soy sauce (even though you are not) instead of explaining all the details about the gluten-free diet to those who have not heard of it. Remember that in restaurants barley is most commonly found in salad dressings and in desserts as malt, and rye is mostly found in bakery goods, so avoiding these items can make it possible to meet your needs without overwhelming the kitchen.

D's Dieting Dilemmas

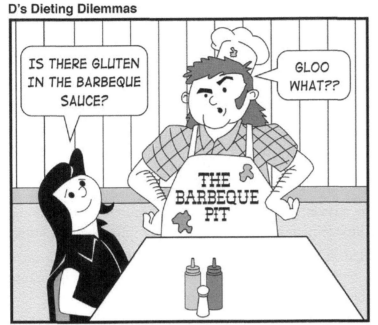

By M. Brown, Ken Brown, and Will Cypser ©

If you say, "I can't eat wheat, flour, bread, and soy sauce," and your waiter replies, "Do you mean gluten?" you know immediately that you are ahead of the game.

In general, when ordering from a typical menu, try to avoid prepared sauces, dressings, or broths that are not made completely from scratch (see below for some ways to dress up foods when there are no safe seasonings and sauces available at the restaurant). Generally, safe foods will include salads, plain veggies, meat, pork, chicken, and fish. Using the dining-out cards found in this chapter will help the chef understand what you can or can't eat. Sometimes just providing the information to the restaurant is enough for them to prepare many safe options for you. When you feel you are in an establishment that really isn't going to take your requests seriously, stick to plain food and jazz it up yourself.

Mixing Up Gluten-Free Sauces and Seasonings when Dining Out

When dining out, if you do not feel safe using the prepared salad dressings and barbecue sauces, why settle for eating your food plain?

Improvise! Mixing together available safe condiments can spice up your meal. Make sure you double-check that the side sauces are either individually sealed or safe from being cross-contaminated before you use them.

Always carry a gluten-free seasoning blend to spice up your food when needed. Store it in an old plastic spice jar, and keep it in a zip lock bag just in case it opens. Mix together garlic powder, onion powder, paprika, salt, pepper, and some dried herbs, such as basil, oregano, thyme, and parsley. At this time Lea & Perrins Worcestershire is only gluten free in the United States.

Barbeque Sauce: Mix together ketchup, mustard, vinegar, sugar, hot sauce, a little jelly or jam (if available), and spice blend to taste.

Cheese Sauce: Mix mayonnaise with a crumbly strong-flavored cheese (such as blue or feta), use milk to thin, add GF Worcestershire sauce, add a squeeze of lemon, and spice blend to taste.

Cranberry Glaze: Mix cranberry sauce with oil, vinegar, and spice blend to taste.

Fra Diavlo Sauce: Mix tomato sauce, hot sauce, and wine with spice blend to taste.

French Dressing: Mix ketchup, oil, vinegar, and sugar with GF Worcestershire.

Honey Mustard: Two parts mustard, one part honey; thin with water or apple juice. To make creamy honey mustard, add mayonnaise, plain yogurt, or sour cream until desired texture is achieved.

Lobster Sauce: Mix melted butter with spice blend and lemon.

Louis Sauce: Mix mayonnaise, ketchup, spice blend, chopped onion, and hot sauce to taste; use heavy cream to thin, and add a dash of salt and pepper and GF Worcestershire.

Mustard Sauce: Mix gluten-free Dijon mustard, vinegar, chopped onions or shallots, GF hot sauce, sugar mayonnaise, and spice blend to taste.

Olive Sauce: Mix chopped olives, onions, tomatoes, capers, olive oil, and spice blend to taste.

Salsa Topping: Ask for a side of tomatoes and onions, and chop it up. Add hot sauce or lime juice to taste (if fresh herbs like cilantro are available, that's just an added bonus!).

Steak Sauce: Mix ketchup, mustard, vinegar, gluten-free Worcestershire (use a safe choice like Lea & Perrins), salt, pepper, sugar, and a little bit of spice blend to taste.

Sweet-and-Sour Sauce: Mix vinegar, water, sugar, and spice blend to taste (or add mayonnaise to make it creamy).

Sweet-and-Spicy Sauce: Mix jam (apricot best), vinegar, and hot sauce to taste.

Tahini Sauce: Mix sesame seed paste, olive oil, garlic, lemon juice, water, and spice blend to taste.

Tartar Sauce: Mix mayonnaise, lemon juice, pickle relish, salt, and pepper to taste.

Thousand Island Salad Dressing: Mix ketchup and mayonnaise—add pickle relish if available.

Yogurt Sauce: Mix plain yogurt or sour cream with spice blend, lemon juice, and chopped onions

Mixing Up Gluten-Free Desserts when Dining Out

Most restaurants have ice cream, and most plain vanilla ice cream is gluten free. Unfortunately, it really seems pretty boring while everyone else is diving into a chocolate mud pie. Some yummy toppings or gluten-free cookies or bars can really jazz things up:

- Crushed gluten-free cookies swirled into ice cream

- Gluten-free chocolate bar broken into pieces and mixed into ice cream, with ordered liquor poured over the top

- Gluten-free brownie bar or M&Ms

- Chocolate-chip cookies dipped in single-serve peanut butter tubs along with your ice cream

- Individual gluten-free caramel sauce (available at restaurant supply stores)—a terrific ice cream topping

- Gluten-free fruit puree, or nut butter, or Nutella

- Mini ice cream sandwiches made from gluten-free cookies

The Gluten-Free Traveler

When traveling for business, it's likely you'll take part in meetings, group meals, or even buffets at which choices may be limited. In these cases, it is best to research ahead of time. If flying, call the airline and see whether they can provide gluten-free meals on long flights. Because most airlines now offer very few food options, always carry snacks with you. Even if the airline has promised you a gluten-free meal, you'll want to carry gluten-free snacks just in case. Good travel choices include gluten-free bars, trail mix, cereals, and individual cheese sticks. If you are taking a road trip, carry a cooler with salads, fresh fruit, gluten-free cereal, gluten-free wraps, and cold cuts. If possible, try to book a hotel that has a mini kitchen so you can stock up on favorites, making it easier to put together gluten-free meals. If a hotel with a mini kitchen is not available, ask if you can get a small refrigerator in your room. Let the hotel staff know it is for medical reasons—they will be more likely to accommodate you. For a list of dining and travel resources, see Chapter 12.

D's Dieting Dilemmas

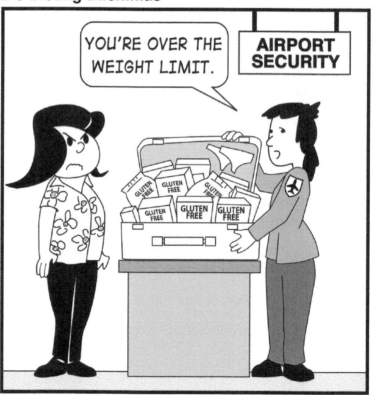

By M. Brown, Ken Brown, and Will Cypser ©

Find out what restaurant choices will be available in your hotel, and research gluten-free restaurants in the area. To find gluten-free restaurants in the United States, go to the many apps and sites that are available, such as Find Me Gluten Free and Yelp, or contact local celiac support groups for suggested choices in an area.

For business meetings, see if you can order special meals for your meetings prior to arrival. If you are unable to make any requests ahead of time and find that you are in an environment where you do not feel comfortable asking a lot of questions, request that your food be prepared as plain as possible, without sauces or marinades, and spice it up with some of the suggestions mentioned earlier in this chapter.

If travel is for pleasure, you'll likely have more flexibility. You might look into gluten-free tour groups—several are listed in the resource section at the end of this book. If traveling with a traditional tour group or cruise, I recommend that you not book your trip unless they can guarantee a gluten-free menu will be available at all your meals. This doesn't mean a buffet, or a preselected dinner, but a gluten-free menu. Some groups will say that the tour director will accommodate you, but this can mean anything from you getting a great meal to having the same choice over and over, to having no choice at all every time you dine out. Part of the enjoyment of traveling is sampling foods, especially in other countries. If you are paying the same money as everyone else, you should be taken care of properly.

In order to make it easier when traveling abroad, I have put together a listing of international celiac organizations that can help you find gluten-free choices wherever you go. It is delightful to discover that there are many gluten-free restaurants throughout the world.

International Celiac Organizations

Argentina: www.celiac.org.ar
Australia: (Coeliac Society of South Australia): www.coeliac.org.au
Australia: (The Coeliac Society of NSW): www.nswcoeliac.org.au
Australia: (The Queensland Coeliac Society): www.qld.coeliac.org.au
Austria: www.zoeliakie.or.at
Belgium: www.coeliakie.be; www.vcv.coeliakie.be
Bermuda: +1 441 232 0264
Brazil: www.acelbra.org.br
Canada: www.celiac.ca
French Canada: www.fqmc.org

Chile: www.coacel.cl
Croatia: www.celiac.inet.hr
Czech Republic: www.coeliac.cz
Denmark: www.coeliaki.dk
Finland: www.keliakia.org
France: www.afdiag.org
Germany: www.dzg-online.de
Greece: www.koiliokaki.com
Hungary: www.coeliac.hu
Ireland: www.coeliac.ie
Israel: www.celiac.org.il
Italy: www.celiachia.it
Luxembourg: www.alig.lu
Mexico: www.celiacosdemexico.com
Netherlands: www.coeliakievereniging.nl
New Zealand: www.coeliac.co.nz
Norway: www.ncf.no
Pakistan: www.celiac.com.pk
Portugal: www.celiacos.org.pt
Poland: www.celiakia.org.pl
Russia: www.celiac.spb.ru
Slovenia: www.drustvo-celiakija.si
Spain: www.celiacos.org
Spain: (S.M.A.P. Celiacs de Catalunya): www.celiacscatalunya.org
Sweden: www.celiaki.se
Switzerland: www.zoeliakie.ch; www.coeliakie.ch; www.celiachia.ch
United Kingdom: www.coeliac.co.uk
Uruguay: www.acelu.org

When Dining Out

In general, unless a restaurant has a gluten-free menu:

Avoid

- Anything that could be thickened with flour

- Breaded foods

- Casseroles

- Cream sauces

- Creamed soups

- Croutons

- Flour-coated food

- Gravies

- Imitation seafood

- Soups that have base added (unless the stock is 100 percent homemade)

Question

- Fried food (unless from a dedicated gluten-free fryer)

- Marinades and basting agents

- Salad dressings

- Sauces

Safe

- 100 percent dairy

- Fresh fruits and vegetables

- Meat, chicken, and fish (except self-basting, breaded, or marinated)

- Vegetable oils and added fat

- Wine, herbs, and pure spices such as garlic and onion powder

Dining Out Cards

In order to help chefs understand more about what is safe for you to eat, I have created dining-out cards in 14 different languages. They include lists of safe and unsafe food choices that are specific to each country. They can be copied directly from this book or downloaded and printed with a more extensive list of foods from www.glutenfreeeasy.com/facts/living/cards.asp.

Some establishments will be more willing than others to explore gluten-free choices with you, so there are two types of dining-out cards available. One is simple and to the point, and should be used in busy restaurants when you just want them to understand some of the basics about gluten-free eating. The second card available at the previous link is for those restaurants that are willing to put more effort into providing you with a special meal. These detailed dining cards provide different foods that are specific to that culture and are offered in both English and the native language. These cards can also help you to identify safe food choices for each cuisine, making it easier to select gluten-free selections when traveling.

Following are both simple and detailed cards in English and Spanish and simple quick-reference dining cards in Arabic, Mandarin, French, German, Greek, Hebrew, Indian (Hindi), Italian, Japanese, Polish, Thai, and Vietnamese. Detailed cards in these languages can be found on my website.

Gluten-Free Dining Out Card   English

To the Chef:

I am on a medically required diet and need special assistance with my meal. I cannot eat wheat and gluten (gluten is found in wheat, rye, and barley). Even the smallest amount of gluten can make me sick, and therefore I must avoid any food, sauce, or garnish containing gluten and any of its by-products, including wheat flour, oats, bread crumbs, soy sauce, bouillon cubes and purchased stocks, teriyaki sauce, commercial seasoning blends, marinades, and sauces (unless they are labeled gluten-free).

I can safely eat fruits, vegetables, rice, quinoa, buckwheat, amaranth, corn, potatoes, peas, legumes, millet, chicken, red meats, fish, eggs, dairy products, fats and oils, distilled vinegars, and homemade stocks and gravies, as long as they are not cooked with wheat flour, bread crumbs, or sauce.

Please prepare my food in a way that avoids cross-contamination with wheat. Use fresh water, separate oil, pots, pans, and utensils. If you are not sure about an ingredient that the food contains, please let me know and I may be able to give you more information.

Thank you for helping me to have a safe and pleasant dining experience.

Gluten-Free Dining Out Card   English

To the Chef:

I am on a medically required diet and need to know how my food is prepared. I cannot eat wheat and gluten (gluten is found in wheat, rye, and barley). Even the smallest amount of gluten can make me sick, and therefore I must avoid any food, sauce, or garnish containing gluten and any of its by-products. If you are not sure if a menu item, recipe, or ingredient contains gluten, please let me know and I may be able to give you more information.

Foods that I can safely eat include:
- Beef, fish, lamb, pork, duck, goose and other poultry, rabbit, seafood, tofu, and most soy products (except soy sauce made with wheat)
- Eggs
- 100% natural dairy products
- Fruits and juices, vegetables, including canned tomato products
- All beans, legumes, nuts, including peanut butter and nut butters
- Amaranth, buckwheat, corn, millet, certified gluten-free oats, potatoes, rice, quinoa, sorghum, and teff
- Homemade stocks and broths (without added wheat)
- Butter, margarine, and vegetable oils
- Pure spices and herbs, distilled vinegars that do not contain malt, wheat-free soy sauce
- Distilled alcohol, wine

Foods that I cannot safely eat (unless they have been checked to be gluten-free) include:
- Some luncheon and processed meats, self-basting poultry, artificial bacon bits, imitation crab meat
- Seasoning blends, modified wheat starch, soy sauce, teriyaki sauce, hydrolyzed vegetable protein, Worcestershire sauce
- Bouillon cubes, canned stocks and broth, packaged soup and soup bases, gravies, cream sauces, and some marinades
- Salad dressings and sauces that include malt or any gluten-containing by-product
- Barley, bread, bulgur, couscous, orzo, pasta, rye, semolina, spelt, stuffing, tabouli, wheat, wheat germ
- Beer

If a label says that a food product was made on equipment that processes wheat, rye, or barley, I cannot eat it. If the label lists malt or barley, I cannot eat it.

In the preparation of my food:

Please prepare my food in a safe way to avoid cross-contamination with wheat, rye, and barley. Use fresh water and separate oil, pots, pans, colanders, and utensils.

Thank you for preparing my meal in a creative way that includes safe foods so I can have a wonderful dining experience.

Gluten-Free Dining Out Card   Spanish

> To the Chef:
>   I am on a medically required diet and need special assistance with my meal. I cannot eat wheat and gluten (gluten is found in wheat, rye, and barley). Even the smallest amount of gluten can make me sick, and therefore I must avoid any food, sauce, or garnish containing gluten and any of its byproducts, including wheat flour, oats, bread crumbs, soy sauce, bouillon cubes and purchased stocks, teriyaki sauce, commercial seasoning blends, marinades, and sauces (unless they are labeled gluten-free).
>   I can safely eat fruits, vegetables, rice, quinoa, buckwheat, amaranth, corn, potatoes, peas, legumes, millet, chicken, red meats, fish, eggs, dairy products, fats and oils, distilled vinegars, and homemade stocks and gravies, as long as they are not cooked with wheat flour, bread crumbs, or sauce.
>   Please prepare my food in a way that avoids cross-contamination with wheat. Use fresh water, separate oil, pots, pans, and utensils. If you are not sure about an ingredient that the food contains, please let me know and I may be able to give you more information.
>   Thank you for helping me to have a safe and pleasant dining experience.

Español/Spanish

> Al cocinero:
>   Estoy en una dieta medicamente requerida y necesito ayuda especial con mi comida. No Puedo comer trigo y/o gluten (el gluten se encuentra en el trigo, centeno y cebada). Incluso la cantidad mas pequena de gluten puede hacer que me enferme y por lo tanto debo evitar cualquier alimento, salsa o adobo que contengan gluten y/o cualquiera de sus derivados, incluyendo harina de trigo, avena, migajas de pan, salsa de soya, cubos de caldo comprados almacenados, salsa teriyaki, mezclas de condimentos comerciales, adobos y las salsas (amenos que esten etiquetadas libres de gluten).
>   Puedo comer con seguridad frutas, vegetales, arroz, quinoa, alforfon, amaranto, maiz, patatas, guisantes, legumbres, mijo, sorgo, nueces, pollo, carnes rojas, pescado, huevos, productos lacteos, grasas, aceites, vinagre destilado, productos almacenados y salsas hechas en casa mientras no se cocinen con harina de trigo, migajas de pan o salsa.
>   Por favor prepare mi comida de una manera que evite la contaminacion cruzada con trigo. Utilice agua fresca, aceites separados, los potes, las cacerolas, y los utencilios. Si usted no esta seguro de un alimento o ingrediente que este contenga dejeme saber para darle mas informacion.
>   Gracias por ayudarme a tener una experiencia de cena mas segura y agradable.

Gluten-Free Dining Out Card   Spanish

To the Chef:

I am on a medically required diet and need to know how my food is prepared. I cannot eat wheat and gluten (gluten is found in wheat, rye, and barley). Even the smallest amount of gluten can make me sick, and therefore I must avoid any food, sauce, or garnish containing gluten and any of its byproducts. If you are not sure if a menu item, recipe, or ingredient contains gluten, please let me know and I may be able to give you more information.

Foods that I can safely eat include:
- Beef, fish, pork, poultry such as chicken and turkey, seafood, and most soy products
- Eggs
- Dairy products
- Fruits and juice, vegetables, canned tomato products, plantains
- All legumes, beans, nuts
- Corn tortillas, rice, potatoes
- Homemade stocks and broths (that do not contain wheat)
- Pure spices and herbs, distilled vinegars that do not contain malt
- Oils
- Distilled alcohol, wine

Foods that I cannot safely eat (unless they have been checked to be gluten-free) include:
- Any sauce that has been thickened with wheat flour such as mole, enchilada and salsa, and cheese dip
- Bread, churros, empanadas, flour tortillas
- Any soup or stew, including gazpacho that has been thickened with bread crumbs or wheat flour
- Tapas that contain bread or bread crumbs
- Spice and seasoning blends, seasoned rice mixes
- Bouillon cubes, canned stocks and broths, packaged soup mixes, some marinades, rice and malt vinegar, some barbecue sauces, food additives, salad dressing
- Beer
- Corn chips that have been fried in the same oil as flour tortillas or other gluten-containing products

If a label says that a food product was made on equipment that processes wheat, rye, or barley, I cannot eat it. If the label lists malt or barley, I cannot eat it.

In the preparation of my food:

Please prepare my food in a safe way to avoid cross-contamination with wheat, rye, or barley. Use fresh water and separate oil, pots, pans, colanders, and utensils.

Thank you for preparing my meal in a creative way that includes safe foods so I can have a wonderful dining experience.

Carta o Menu De Comida Libre De Gluten   Español/Spanish

Al cocinero

Estoy en una dieta medicamente requerida y necesito saber como esta preparada mi comida. No puedo comer trigo y/o gluten (el gluten se encuentra en el trigo, centeno y cebada). Incluso la cantidad mas pequeña de gluten puede hacer que me enferme, y por lo tanto debo evitar cualquier comida, salsa o adobo que contengan gluten o cualquiera de sus derivados. Si usted no esta seguro si un articulo del menu, receta o ingrediente contiene gluten, por favor dejeme saberlo para darle mas informacion.

Los Alimentos Que Puedo Comer Con Seguridad Son:
- Carne de vaca, pescado, cerdo, aves de corral tales como pollo, pavo, mariscos y la mayoria de los productos de la soya
- Huevos
- Productos lacteos
- Las frutas y jugos, vegetales, productos de tomate en lata, platanos
- Todos los legumbres, frijoles y nueces
- Tortillas de maiz, arroz y patatas
- Productos almacenados y caldos hechos en casa (que no contengan trigo)
- Especies puras y hierbas, vinagres destilados que no contienen malta
- Aceites
- Alcohol destilado y vino

Alimentos Que no Puedo Comer Con Seguridad (Amenos Que Sean Comprobados Libres De Gluten)
- Cualquier salsa que se haya espesado con harina de trigo tal como topo, enchilada, salsa e inmersion de queso
- Pan, churros, empanadas y tortillas de harina
- Cualquier sopa o guisado, incluyendo el gazpacho que se ha espesado con las migajas de pan o la harina de trigo
- Tapas que contiene el pan o las migajas de pan
- Mezclas de especies y condimentos, mezclas de arroz sasonados
- Cubos de caldos, productos y caldos conservados, mezclas de sopas empaquetadas, algunos adobos de vinagre, del arroz y de la malta, algunas salsas de barbacoa, comidas aditivas y salsas para ensaladas
- Cervesa
- Las virutas de maiz que hayan sido fritas en el mismo aceite que las tortillas de harina u otros productos con gluten

Si una etiqueta dice que un producto alimenticio fue hecho con el mismo equipo que procesa trigo, centeno o cebada, no puedo comerlo. Si la etiqueta dice malta o cebada, no puedo comerlo.

En La Preparacion De Mi Alimento:

Prepare por favor mi alimento de una manera segura y evite la contaminacion cruzada con trigo, centeno, y cebada. Utilice agua fresca, aceites separados, los potes, las cacerolas, los colanders y los utencilios.

Gracias por preparar mi comida de una manera creativa que incluya alimentos seguros para poder tener una experiencia maravillosa de cena.

Gluten-Free Dining Out Card   Arabic

إلى رئيس الطهاة:

انا أتبع نظام غذائيه مُوصى عليه طبياً و أحتاج مساعدة خاصة في وجباتي. أنا محظور عن تناول منتجات القمح والغلوتين (الغلوتين هي مادة بروتينية توجد في الدقيق و الشعير) حتى اقل آمية من الغلوتين تضرُّني صحياً و لذلك يجب علىٌ تجنُّب أي طعام أو مرقة أو توابل تحتوي على هذه المادة أو أياً من منتجاتها مثل دقيق الخبزأوالبليلة أوالشعير أوفتات الخبزأوصلصة الصويا أومكعبات مرقة الدجاج أوخلطة التوابل أومرق نقع قطع اللحم أو الخل (إلا إذا آان مطبوع عليها علامةخالي من الغلوتين) أستطيع آآل الفواآه والخضروات والأرز وحبة الحنطة والذرة والبطاطس والبازلاء والبقوليات والسرغوم والمكسرات والدواجن واللحوم والسمك والبيض ومنتجات الألبان والمواد الدهنية والزيوت ومرقة اللحم والشربة المنزلية طالما تم طبخها بدون دقيق أوفتات الخبزأوالصلصة. أرجوإعداد طعامي بما لا يدع مجالاً لخلط أي نوع من الدقيق. أرجوإستعمال ماء نقي وزيوت نقية وأدوات وأوعية معقمة. إن لم تكن متيقناً من محتويات أي من مقاديرالطعام أرجو أن تُخبرني فبإستطاعتي إعطاءك معلومات أآثر.
شكرآ لمساعدتي على تناول طعام صحٌّي وشهي.

Gluten-Free Dining Out Card   French

Pour la Cuisine:
   Je suis à un régime médicalement prié et ai besoin de l'aide spéciale avec mon repas. Je ne peux pas manger le blé et le gluten (du gluten est trouvé dans le blé, le seigle et l'orge). Même un peu de gluten peut me faire le malade et donc je moût éviter n'importe quelle nourriture, sauce ou garnis contenant le gluten et n'importe lequel de ses sous-produits comprenant la farine de blé, l'avoine, la chapelure, la sauce de soja, les cubes en bouillon et les stocks achetés, la sauce à teriyaki, les mélanges commerciaux d'assaisonnement, les marinades et les sauces (à moins qu'ils sont marqués gluten libre).
   Je peux sans risque manger des fruits, des légumes, riz, quinoa, sarrasin, amaranthe, maïs, des pommes de terre, des pois, des légumineuses, millet, sorgho et des écrous, poulet, des viandes rouges, des poissons, des oeufs, des produits laitiers, des graisses et des pétroles, des vinaigres distillés, et des stocks et des sauces au jus faits maison, tant que ils ne sont pas faits cuire avec la farine de blé, la chapelure ou la sauce.
   Veuillez préparer ma nourriture d'une manière dont évite la contamination transversale avec du blé. Utilisez l'eau doux, le pétrole séparé, les pots, les casseroles et les ustensiles. Si vous n'êtes pas sûr au sujet d'un ingrédient que la nourriture contient, faites-le moi savoir et je peux pouvoir te fournir plus d'information.
   Merci de m'aider à Avoir Une Expérience Dinante Sûre Et Plaisante

The English translation for each of these cards appears on p. 362

Gluten-Free Dining Out Card   German

Der Chef:

An den Kochlch ernähre mich nach einer medizinisch erforderlichen Diät und benötige spezielle Hilfe mit meiner Mahlzeit. Ich kann nicht Weizen und Gluten (Gluten wird im Weizen, im Roggen und in der Gerste gefunden) essen. Selbst eine kleine Menge an Gluten kann mich krank machen und folglich muß ich jede Nahrung, Soe oder Beilage die Gluten und ihre Nebenprodukte wie Weizenmehl, Hafer, Brotkrumen, Sojasoße, Brühwürfel und gekaufte Brühen, Teriyaki Soe, handelsübliche Gewürzmischungen, Marinaden und Soen enthält, meiden (es sei denn sie sind als Gluten-frei beschriftet).

Ich kann Früchte, Gemüse, Reis, Reismelde, Buchweizen, Amarant, Mais, Kartoffeln, Erbsen, Hülsenfrüchte, Hirse, Sorghum und Nüsse, Huhn, rotes Fleisch, Fisch, Eier, Milchprodukte, Fette und Öle, destillierten Essig und selbstgemachte Brühen und Soen sicher essen, solange sie nicht mit Weizenmehl, Brotkrumen oder Soe gekocht werden.

Bereiten Sie bitte meine Nahrung in einer Weise zu, die Querkontamination mit Weizen vermeidet. Benutzen Sie frisches Wasser und trennen Sie Öle, Töpfe, Pfannen und Küchenutensilien. Falls Sie sich nicht über eine Zutat sicher sind die in der Nahrung enthalten ist, fragen Sie mich bitte und ich kann Ihnen mehr Information geben.

Vielen Dank da_ sie mir dabei helfen, eine sichere und angenehme Mahlzeit zu geniessen.

Gluten-Free Dining Out Card   Greek

Προς τον μάγειρα / chef:

Βρίσκομαι σε μια αυστηρή ιατρική δίαιτα και χρειάζομαι ειδική βοήθεια όσον αφορά το γεύμα μου. Δεν μπορώ να φάω σιτάρι και γλουτένη (η γλουτένη βρίσκεται στο σιτάρι, στη σίκαλη και στο κριθάρι). Ακόμη και το μικρότερο ποσό γλουτένης μπορεί να με κάνει να αρρωστήσω και επομένως πρέπει να αποφύγω οποιαδήποτε φαγητό, σάλτσα ή γαρνίρισμα που περιέχει γλουτένη και οποιοδήποτε από τα υποπροϊόντα της, συμπεριλαμβανομένου του σιτάλευρου, της βρώμης, των τριμμένων φρυγανιών, της σάλτσας σόγιας, των κύβων σούπας και των αγορασμένων ζωμών, της σάλτσας τεριγιάκι, των εμπορικών μιγμάτων καρυκευμάτων, των μαρινάδων και των σαλτσών (εκτός κι αν αναγράφουν στην ετικέτα ότι δεν περιέχουν γλουτένη).

Μπορώ ακίνδυνα να φάω φρούτα, λαχανικά, ρύζι, κινόα, μπακαγουήτ, αμάραντο, καλαμπόκι, πατάτες, μπιζέλια, όσπρια, κεχρί, σόργο και καρύδια, κοτόπουλο, κόκκινα κρέατα, ψάρια, αυγά, γαλακτοκομικά προϊόντα, λίπη και έλαια, αποσταγμένο ξίδι, και τα σπιτικούς ζωμούς και τους ζωμούς, εφ' όσον δεν μαγειρεύονται με αλεύρι σίτου, τριμμένες φρυγανιές ή σάλτσα.

Παρακαλώ προετοιμάστε το γεύμα μου με τέτοιο τρόπο ώστε να αποφευχθεί η μόλυνση από το σιτάρι. Χρησιμοποιήστε καθαρό νερό, λάδι, δοχεία, τηγάνια και εργαλεία. Εάν δεν είστε βέβαιοι για ένα συστατικό που τα τρόφιμα περιέχουν, παρακαλώ ενημερώστε με και μπορώ να είμαι σε θέση να σας δώσω περισσότερες πληροφορίες.

Gluten-Free Dining Out Card   **Hebrew**

לכבוד השׁף

אני על דיאטה רפואית וצריכה עזרה בהכנת הארוחה. אין באפשרותי לאכל חיטה ועמילן (עמילן נימצא בחיטה, שיפון) גם הכמויות הקטנות הנימצאות בעמילן גורמות לי לחלות ולכן אינני יכולה לאכל עלי להימנע מכל מאכל המכיל עמילן וכל מוצרו כולל קמח לבן, שיבולת שועל, פרורי לחם, רוטב סויה, קוביות מרק צח, קופסאות שימורים, רוטב טריאקי תארובת תבלינים (אלה עם כן התווית מראה שלא נימצא עמילן)

אני יכולה לאכל פירות, ירקות, אורז, קינואה, כוסמת, חידע, תירס, תפוח אדמה, אפונה, קטניות, דוחן, אגוזים, עוף, בשר אדום, דגים, ביצים, דיברי חלב, שמן ושומנים, חומץ, רוטב ביתי ורוטב בשר כל עוד לא נעשו ובשלו עם קמח או פרורי לחם.

בבקשה להכין עבורי את האוכל ללא תערובת של חיטה להישתמש במים נקיים להפריד שמן מהמחבטים הסירים והמסינים. אם אתה לא בטוח בקשר למרכיב שהמזון מכיל תידע אותי ואני אוכל לתת לך יותר פרטים.

תודה רבה

Gluten-Free Dining Out Card   **Hindi**

रसोइये के लिए:

मैं एक चिकित्सकीय आवश्यक आहार पर हूँ और मुझे अपने भोजन के साथ विशेष सहायता की जरूरत है. मैं गेहूं और ग्लूटेन (लस) नहीं खा सकता/सकती (ग्लूटेन गेहूं, रागी और जौ में पाया जाता है). ग्लूटेन की थोड़ी सी मात्रा भी मुझे बीमार कर सकती है और इसलिए मुझे ग्लूटेन युक्त कोई भी भोजन, सॉस या सजावट की सामग्री और गेहूं का आटा, ओट्स (जई), ब्रेड के टुकड़े, सोया सॉस, शोरबे के क्यूब्स और खरीदे गए व्यंजन, तेरियाकी सॉस, वाणिज्यिक मसालों के मिश्रण, सिरके और सॉस (जब तक कि उन पर ग्लूटेन मुक्त होने के लेबल ना लगे हों) सहित ग्लूटेन के कोई उप-उत्पाद खाने से बचना चाहिए.

मैं फल, सब्जियाँ, चावल, कीन्वा [quinoa], बकव्हीट (कुट्टू), चौली, मक्का, आलू, मटर, फलीदार सब्जियाँ, बाजरा, ज्वार और मेवा, चिकन, लाल गोश्त, मछली, अंडे, डेयरी उत्पाद, वसा और तेल, आसुत सिरके, और घर के बने व्यंजन और शोरबे सुरक्षित रूप से खा सकता/सकती हूँ, जब तक कि वे गेहूं के आटे, ब्रेड के टुकड़ों या चटनी के साथ पकाए नहीं गए हों.

कृपया मेरा खाना इस प्रकार बनाएँ कि वह गेहूं से संदूषित होने से बचे. ताज़े पानी, अलग तेल, पतीलों, तवों और बर्तनों का इस्तेमाल करें. यदि आप भोजन में शामिल किसी भी सामग्री के बारे में निश्चित रूप से नहीं जानते हैं तो कृपया मुझे बताएँ, शायद मैं आपको और जानकारी दे सकूँ.

मुझे भोजन का एक सुरक्षित और सुखद अनुभव लेने में मदद करने के लिए धन्यवाद.

The English translation for each of these cards appears on p. 362

Gluten-Free Dining Out Card   Italian

Allo Chef:

Sono in una dieta medicamente richiesta e ho bisogno di una assistenza speciale per il mio pasto. Non posso mangiare il frumento ed il glutine (il glutine si trova nel frumento, nella segale e nell' orzo). Anche la più piccola quantità di glutine può farmi male e quindi devo evitare tutto l'alimento, e qualsiasi condimento contenente glutine e ogni suo relativo sottoprodotto, compresi la farina di frumento, avena, pangrattato, salsa di soia, estratti di brodo comprati, salsa di teriyaki, miscele commerciali di condimento, marinate e salse (a meno che siano identificati libero da glutine).

Posso mangiare con sicurezza gli ortofrutticoli, riso, quinoa, grano saraceno, amaranto, mais, patate, piselli, legumi, miglio, sorgo e nocciole, pollo, carni rosse, pesci, uova, latticini, grassi e olii, aceti distillati, brodi e sughi casalighi, purche non siano cucinati con la farina di frumento, il pangrattato o la salsa.

Per favore prepara il mio cibo in in modo da evitare la contaminazione trasversale con frumento. Utilizza acqua fresca, separare l'olio le pentole e gli utensili. Se non siete sicuri circa un ingrediente che l'alimento contiene, per favore fatemelo sapere cosi' posso darvi piu' informazioni.

Grazie per il vostro aiuto nel farmi avere una piacevole e sicura esperienza culinaria.

Gluten-Free Dining Out Card   Japanese

シェフの方へ

私は治療に必要な食事をしているので、その食事に対して特別な助けが必要です。私は小麦とグルテンが摂取できません。（グルテンは小麦、ライ麦、大麦に含まれています。）ほんの少量のグルテンでさえ症状がでてしまうので、グルテンを含む食べ物、ソース、付け合わせを避けなければなりません。グルテンが含まれていないと表示されていない限り、小麦粉、オート麦、パン粉、醤油、ブイヨン、市販のだし、照り焼きソース、そしてさらに市販のブレンド済みの調味料やマリーネード、ソースを含みます。

私は小麦粉やパン粉、ソースを使って調理されてない限り、差し支えなくフルーツ、野菜類、米、キノア、蕎麦、アマランス、とうもろこし、ジャガイモ、豆、豆類、キビ、モロコシ、ナッツ、鶏肉、赤い肉、魚、卵、乳製品、油脂、蒸留酢、自家製のだしやグレービーソースは食べる事ができます。

どうか小麦を使わないで私の食事を作ってください。新鮮な水を使い、油や鍋、フライパンや調理器具も別にしてください。もし、材料の中身が確かでないときは、私にお知らせください。もう少し情報を提供できるかもしれません。

安全で快適な食事の為にご協力いただきありがとうございます。

Gluten-Free Dining Out Card   Mandarin

致廚師：

在醫學上，我被指定遵循特殊的飲食需要和幫助。我不能食用麥類和麩類的食物 (小麥，黑麥和大麥含有麩類)。既使是最小量的麩類也會使我惡心，因此我不得不避免任 何含有麩類的食品，湯

及配料，任何可能含有麩類的副產品包括麥粉，燕麥，面包屑，醬油，牛肉和雞肉湯, 及各种湯料，腌和醬食品(除非他們是標明不含麩類食品)。

對我安全的食物有：水果，蔬菜，大米，黎，喬麥，莧菜，玉米，馬鈴薯，豌豆，豆類， 小米，高粱和堅果，雞肉，紅肉類，魚，蛋，乳制品，脂肪和油類，蒸餾水，自制湯料和 鹵汁。只要上述食物不与小麥面粉，面包屑，湯汁同煮即可。

在准備我的食物時，請避免与小麥產品及副產品接触。請用淡水，單獨的烹調油，平底鍋 ，盤及餐具。如果你對任何食物的所含原料不确定，請告訴我。我可以提供更多的信息給 你。

感謝你為我提供一個既安全又愉快的用餐經歷。

Gluten-Free Dining Out Card   Polish

Szef Kuchni:

Jestem na diecie i lekarskie potrzebuję szczególnej pomocy ze swoim posiłkiem. Nie mogę jeść glutenu (glutenu występuje w pszenicy, żyta i jęczmienia) . Nawet najmniejsze ilości glutenu może mnie zrobic chore i dlatego należy unikać wszelkich żywności, sos lub dekorować zawierające gluten i wszystkich jej byproducts w tym mąki pszennej, owsa, sos sojowy kostki i zakupionych zapasów, handlowych przypraw mieszanek, marynat i sosów (chyba że są one odpowiednio oznaczone bezglutenowy) .

Mogę bezpiecznie jeść owoce, warzywa, ryż, quinoa, gryki, amarant, kukurydza, ziemniaki, groch, rośliny strączkowe, proso, sorgo i orzechy, kurczak, czerwonych mięs, ryb, jaj, nabiału, tłuszczów i olejów, destylowanego octu i domowych zapasów i gravies, tak długo jak nie są one gotowane z mąki pszennej, lub sos.

Proszę przygotować moje żywności w taki sposób, aby uniknąć zanieczyszczeń krzyżowych z pszenicy. Używać świezą vodę, oddzielne olej, garnki, patelnie i naczyńia. Jeśli nie jesteś pewien jaki składnik, środek spożywczy zawiera, proszę dać mi znać i mogą być w stanie podać więcej informacji.

Dziękujemy za pomoc mi będę miał bezpieczne i przyjemne odżywianie.

The English translation for each of these cards appears on p. 362

Gluten-Free Dining Out Card   Thai

ถึง พ่อครัว/แม่ครัว:

     ฉันมีความจำเป็นทางการแพทย์ที่จะต้องควบคุมอาหารบางอย่าง และต้องการความช่วยเหลือเป็นพิเศษในการเตรียมอาหารของฉัน ฉันทานข้าวสาลีและกลูเท็นไม่ได้ (กลูเท็นเป็นโปรตีนที่อยู่ในข้าวสาลี ข้าวไรย์ และข้าวบาร์เลย์) ถ้าฉันทานกลูเท็นแม้แต่เพียงนิดเดียวก็ตาม จะทำให้ฉันป่วย ดังนั้นฉันจึงต้องหลีกเลี่ยงอาหาร ซอส หรือของแต่งหน้าทุกชนิดที่มีกลูเท็นเป็นส่วนประกอบ ตลอดจนผลผลิตพลอยได้ทั้งหมดของสิ่งเหล่านี้ ซึ่งได้แก่แป้งสาลี ข้าวโอ๊ต ขนมปังป่น ซอสถั่วเหลือง ซุปก้อน และน้ำซุปที่ซื้อมา ซอสเทอริยากิ ผงปรุงรสต่างๆ ที่จำหน่ายในห้องตลาด ซอสสำหรับหมัก และซอสต่างๆ (เว้นเสียแต่ว่าจะระบุบนฉลากสินค้าว่า "ปลอดกลูเท็น")

     ฉันทานผลไม้ ผัก ข้าว ข้าวคีนัว บัควีท ผักโขม ข้าวโพด มันฝรั่ง พืชตระกูลถั่ว พืชผักตระกูลถั่ว ข้าวเดือย ข้าวฟ่างและถั่วต่างๆ ไก่ เนื้อแดง ปลา ไข่ ผลิตภัณฑ์ที่ทำจากนม ไขมันและน้ำมัน น้ำส้มสายชูกลั่น และซุปและน้ำเกรวีที่ทำเองได้ ตราบเท่าที่ไม่ใช้แป้งสาลี ขนมปังป่น หรือซอสในการปรุงอาหารเหล่านี้

     กรุณาเตรียมอาหารของฉันโดยไม่ให้มีการปนเปื้อนกับข้าวสาลีเลย ขอให้ใช้น้ำใหม่ และใช้น้ำมัน หม้อ กะทะ และเครื่องมือเครื่องใช้ในการปรุงอาหารแยกต่างหาก ถ้าคุณไม่แน่ใจเกี่ยวกับส่วนผสมในอาหารชนิดหนึ่งๆ กรุณาบอกให้ฉันรู้ เพราะฉันอาจให้ข้อมูลเพิ่มเติมแก่คุณได้

     ขอบคุณมากที่ช่วยให้ฉันเพลิดเพลินกับการรับประทานอาหารที่ปลอดภัย

Gluten-Free Dining Out Card   Vietnamese

Kính gỹi quí vỹ ỹỹu bỹp:

Do nhu cỹu sỹc khỹe, tôi ỹỹỹc yêu cỹu ỹn uỹng theo mỹt chỹ ỹỹ ỹỹc biỹt và cỹn sỹ giúp ỹỹ cỹa bỹn ỹỹi vỹi thỹc ỹỹn cỹa tôi. Tôi không thỹ ỹn lúa mì và gluten* (có trong lúa mì, lúa mỹch ỹen và lúa mỹch). Ngay cỹ vỹi mỹt lỹỹng gluten nhỹ nhỹt cỹng có thỹ làm cho tôi bỹ bỹnh và vì vỹy tôi phỹi tránh bỹt kỹ thỹc ỹn, xỹt, hay các lỹai thỹo mỹc dùng ỹỹ trang trí trên thỹc ỹn có chỹa gluten và các sỹn phỹm phỹ cỹa nó bao gỹm bỹt mì, yỹn mỹch, ruỹt bánh mì, tỹỹng, bỹt nêm súp cô ỹỹc và nỹỹc súp hỹp, xỹt teriyaki, bỹt nêm tỹng hỹp, xỹt ỹỹp gia vỹ và các lỹai xỹt khác (ngỹai trỹ sỹn phỹm có nhãn không chỹa chỹt gluten)
Tôi có thỹ ỹn trái cây, rau cỹi, gỹo, quinoa, bỹt kiỹu mỹch, giỹng rau dỹn, bỹp, khoai tây, ỹỹu, các lỹai rau ỹỹu, hỹt kê, cây và hỹt bo bo, gà, các lỹai thỹt ỹỹ, cá, trỹng, bỹ sỹa, chỹt béo và dỹu ỹn, dỹm cỹt, nỹỹc súp nỹu, và nỹỹc cỹt thỹt làm xỹt, nỹu nhỹ các thỹc ỹn này không nỹu chung vỹi bỹt mì, ruỹt bánh mì hoỹc các lỹai xỹt.
Xin vui lòng chuỹn bỹ thỹc ỹn cỹa tôi theo phỹỹng thỹc tránh liên hỹ vỹi lúa mì. Sỹ dỹng nỹỹc sỹch, dỹu, nỹi, chỹo và muỹng nỹa riêng biỹt. Nỹu nhỹ bỹn không chỹc chỹn vỹ các chỹt chỹa trong thỹc phỹm, xin vui lòng cho tôi biỹt, tôi có thỹ cung cỹp thêm vỹ thông tin này. Xin cỹm ỹn bỹn giúp tôi thỹỹng thỹc mỹt bỹa ỹn ngon miỹng và an tòan cho sỹc khỹe.

(*Gluten la hon hop dam co tinh dinh (nhu nhua), con lai sau khi loc tinh bot. Chat nay co chua trong lua mi va lua mach den, giu mot vai tro quan trong trong viec lam banh mi. Khi nhoi voi nuoc, gluten tro nen dinh va giu duoc khong khi de tao thanh bot nhoi. Tre em nhay cam voi chat nay se bi benh tang phu.)

The English translation for each of these cards appears on p. 362

Gluten-Free, Hassle-Free Entertaining

Some people love entertaining and preparing foods for friends and family; others prefer to cater their parties relying on the professionals to cover all the details. If you eat gluten there are lots of caterers to choose from, but if you are gluten free the choices are limited. Even though nowadays there are more and more gluten-free restaurants and caterers popping up, some clearly do not know to prevent cross-contamination (they are completely clueless). If you want to have a great party and eliminate most of the risks associated with cross-contamination it is safer to prepare your own foods, or at least be able to oversee most of the food production yourself.

Don't let these obstacles stop you from entertaining—and showing off your delicious gluten-free dishes to your friends and family. The tips in this chapter will help you throw a fun, safe event.

The Basics

When planning a party, I like to work around a specific cuisine or theme (a *Gone with the Wind* or roaring '20s party), or holiday (big or small, such as Thanksgiving, Christmas, Derby Day, Cinco de Mayo, or National Ice Cream Month) to tie every element of the event together. The possibilities are endless because, let's face it, any time is a good time to celebrate. Once you've picked a theme, make a list:

- What is your budget?

- Who do you want to invite?

- When do you want to have the event and how many hours will it run?

- Where do you want to have it—at your home or another location?

- If the location is outside, what will you do if the weather is poor?

- How do you want chairs and tables to be set up? Paper or china?

- Will you need help?

- What kind of beverages will you serve?

- Should you include any games or special things do?

- Do you want to have live music, dancing, or other entertainment?

- Do your guests have any special dietary preferences or allergies? Be sure to ask!

After you have the general plan for your party, the best way to go gluten free is to make the whole party gluten free. This is the easiest way to prevent cross-contamination, which is the biggest concern at any event.

If it isn't possible to go completely gluten free you will need to take special precautions in order to ensure the gluten-free choices stay gluten free. No matter what, make sure there are gluten-free options for all courses, and plan how to separate the foods to minimize the risk of cross-contamination.

Preventing Cross-Contamination

Most gluten-containing foods aren't off limits because of the bread; it is more likely that there are other problem ingredients such as regular soy sauce or other gluten-containing sauces, thickening agents, or instant broths used during preparation. These can be easily substituted for gluten-free products, reducing much of the gluten in the meal.

Regular crackers, foods boiled in beer, a shared fryer, and breading are the other major causes of gluten contamination. To be safe use only gluten-free crackers, beer, and bread crumbs and a dedicated gluten-free fryer.

Taking these steps will eliminate the main culprits of contamination. Here are some additional suggestions to avoid cross-contamination:

- Make as much of the menu as possible safe for all.

- Greet your guests and let them know how you have indicated safe foods. Make special mention that you were careful about cross-contamination, and assure them that you checked the salad dressings and condiments so they won't feel hesitant to eat.

- Keep regular food and gluten-free food as separate as possible.

For a small event, label food items as "gluten free; please don't cross-contaminate" and place them on different tables or far away from each other on the same table may be safe enough.

For larger events, labels are important, but it's essential to keep gluten-free items on a unique table, far away from the gluten-containing food.

- Do not place regular crackers or bread anywhere near gluten-free spreads and dips, to prevent someone from dunking a piece of gluten-containing bread directly into them.

- Never place a regular food near a gluten-free food on a buffet. People are impatient and it's highly likely they will cross-contaminate the food by using the serving spoon for one food item to serve themselves another food item.

- The dessert area can be particularly dangerous. Be sure to place gluten-free desserts on a side table or area away from regular desserts, and make sure each item has its own appropriate utensil so someone doesn't break a cookie over the gluten-free item or use a knife from a cake to cut a gluten-free brownie. If you are offering flavored coffee, make sure it is gluten free.

Implementing these precautions will ensure that everyone enjoys your event.

TIP   When it comes to entertaining and coordinating your own party, these tips will help make any event a success.

- Plan, plan, and plan. Eliminate last-minute running around.
- Don't leave *anything* until the day of the event; do as much ahead of time as possible.
- Try to make food that requires little to no extra work once served, such as kabobs, or a casserole, or a platter with appetizers that don't need to be heated. Simplicity is the key to great entertaining.
- Bring in extra help if needed.
- Stay within your budget (this means setting a budget ahead of time).
- Put out food that you are proud to serve.
- Enjoy the party! Never let playing hostess prevent you from experiencing the event.

Menu Plans

The following options are great gluten-free menus taken from the recipes in this book. For a large party you will need several choices for each course; for smaller parties there can be one choice or more at each course, but you should tie the courses together so they complement each other.

Completely Gluten Free for a Large Party

First Course

Eggplant Dip with Gluten-Free Crackers (p. 258)
Chicken Satay (p. 260)
Shrimp Scampi Wrapped in Bacon (p. 266)

Second Course

Garlic Knots (p. 248)
Pear, Gorgonzola Cheese, and Walnut Mixed Green Salad (p. 278)

Main Course

Crescent-Shaped Ravioli with Red Sauce (p. 291)
Chicken in Vodka Sauce with Mushrooms (p. 116)
Escarole and White Beans (p. 313)
Eggplant Rollatini (p. 119)

Desserts

Chocolate-Covered Peanut Butter Balls (p. 125)
Cheesecake Bars (p. 333)
Apple and Almond Tart with Vanilla Ice Cream (p. 325)

Completely Gluten Free for a Small Party

First Course

Grilled Stacked Eggplant and Mozzarella Tower (p. 267)

Second Course

French Onion Soup (p. 273)

Main Course

Chicken and Spinach–Stuffed Crêpes (p. 299)

Dessert

Strawberry Shortcake (p. 331)

Completely Gluten Free for a Holiday Party

First Course

Hot Crab meat Dip with Gluten-Free Crackers (p. 107)
Black Bean and Mango Salsa with Corn Chips (p. 103)
Beets with Blue Cheese (p. 262)
Shrimp Cocktail with Gluten-Free Cocktail Sauce

Second Course

Butternut Squash and Apple Soup (p. 280)
Gluten-Free, Dairy-Free Biscuits (p. 99)

Main Course

For ham: Prior to purchasing, contact the manufacturer to confirm the ham and seasoning packet are gluten free.

For turkey: Make sure it is not a self-basting turkey (the self-basting agent can have gluten in it). If you add broth to the pan, make sure it is gluten free.

Sides:

Apple Cranberry Quinoa Salad (p. 101) or a large green salad with gluten-free dressing.

Mashed Potatoes: any favorite family recipe will do.

Stuffing: Use gluten-free bread and follow your favorite recipe. If broth is used make sure it is gluten free.

Gravy: Thicken with any gluten-free flour or starch and use gluten-free chicken broth.

Vegetables: Add a steamed veggie such as green beans with almond slivers

Dessert

Chocolate Lava Cakes (p. 332)
Moist and Delicious Carrot Cake (p. 341)
Pumpkin Pie (p. 334)

Completely Gluten-Free Party for Children

First Course

Pigs in a Blanket (p. 248)
Cheese Puffs (p. 248)
Chicken Fingers (p. 264) with Gluten-Free Barbecue Sauce (p. 321)
Gluten-Free Store Bought Chips

Main Course

Pizza (Mediterranean p. 246, Italian p. 249)
Cheddar Quesadillas (p. 113)

Desserts

Yellow Cake or Cupcakes with Cream Filling (pp. 343–44)
Gluten-Free Frosted Cupcakes (or Birthday Cake). Use a store bought gluten-free mix and make homemade gluten-free Buttercream Frosting (p. 345)
Ice Cream with Gluten-Free Toppings

Quick and Easy (and Budget-Friendly) Gluten-Free Appetizers and Entrees

Remember, naturally gluten-free items are the easiest to prepare and usually the least-expensive.

Appetizers

Appetizers are usually the best part of most meals. Sometimes it is more fun to pick on appetizers than to sit down for a whole meal, and they encourage conversations. Try some of these at your next event:

- A variety of dips. They are inexpensive, can be made ahead of time, and are perfect for a large group (much less fussing).

- Use gluten-free chips instead of gluten-free crackers for a budget-friendlier option. Or make the Socca flat breads found in our quick-and-easy recipe section (p. 97).

- Cold veggies with creamy gluten-free salad dressing

- An assortment of cheeses or mozzarella with sliced tomato or roasted peppers

- Cherry tomatoes stuffed with tuna, crab, or egg salad

- Grilled veggies drizzled with olive oil and shavings of parmesan cheese.

- Baked brie stuffed with apples and caramel served with gluten-free crackers.

- Wrap slices of prosciutto around honeydew melon or around Schär gluten-free bread sticks.

TIP   **THE PERFECT PARTY DIPS**

Blue Cheese Mousse

In a food processer with a steel blade, place 1 cup of blue cheese (or Stilton, Maytag, Danish) with 1 cup of cream cheese. Blend well and serve at room temperature over toasted slices of a crusty gluten-free baguette or Belgian endive spears. Garnish with a grape or pecan.

Salmon Mousse

Blend equal parts of smoked salmon and cream cheese in a food processor until smooth. Save some money by buying containers of smoked salmon ends, often available at the fish store or counter. We like to pipe the mousse through a pastry bag with a star tip into a kiss on one of our gluten-free baguette rounds. Garnish with a spring of dill or parsley, a few capers, a slice of gherkin pickle, and a sliver of red onion.

—Bruce and Pedro at Everybody Eats

- Baked clams or stuffed mushrooms with gluten-free bread crumbs
- Chicken fingers wrapped in bacon
- Chicken kabobs with gluten-free dipping sauces
- Prepared snacks like olives and pickled veggies, gluten-free nuts, and dried fruits

Use your imagination; the choices are endless!

Entrees

Quick and easy entrees are the ones you can serve and then sit with your guests: fajitas, pepper steak, risotto, paella, lasagna, baked ziti, eggplant parmesan, short ribs, souvlaki, and chicken marsala. Dishes like these only require a veggie, a starch, or a salad to make it a complete meal. So when you are entertaining and you put out one of these dishes on the table, there is no up and down and running around. Also, since most of these dishes can be prepared ahead, you can relax and enjoy the event—and a clean kitchen.

STEP III: RESOLVING COMPLICATIONS

Making It Easy for Family, Friends, and You

Telling Others about Your Gluten Sensitivity

Most people who change their diet for medical reasons are able to vary their food choices during special events such as a birthday, wedding, or vacation. However, for those with celiac disease or non-celiac gluten sensitivity this is not the case. Cheating is never allowed—this is the most difficult thing to get others to understand. After all, "a little taste can't hurt once in a while, can it?" And you will need to explain to them that it will.

You are following a gluten-free diet because gluten will make you ill, and as long as you follow this diet strictly, you won't get sick. Even if you are symptom free, celiac disease is an autoimmune condition and even the smallest amount of gluten will cause a negative autoimmune response. You are not choosing this diet because it's the latest fad; you need to follow this diet. And you probably don't like it any more than your friends and family do. It is important to convey to them what gluten is, how it is added to many foods, and that even the smallest amount can hurt you.

Encourage family, friends, and coworkers to read about it, and explain to them that this is not your choice, but something that is medically required. Most importantly, stress the difficulties of cross-contamination. Be understanding. It is a hard concept to grasp. After all, they probably have seen you eating gluten in the past; how can it be such a big problem all of a sudden? Remember how difficult and confusing it was for you, too, when you first heard about it.

It will be hard for them to learn what is safe to eat when they are not living with it every day. They will be as shocked as you were that soups, salad dressings, and seasonings may have gluten added to them. They may even try to prepare special meals for you only to find out you can't have the salad because of the croutons, or the turkey because they didn't realize that self-basting turkeys could contain gluten. Some may even make a special effort to make things easier for you by searching out gluten-free restaurants. These are the acts of a caring, supportive friend or relative.

Of course, some individuals are more supportive than others. There are those who just don't get it, or they don't want to get it. These people won't even try to understand. They may think that you are just being picky and are making a big deal out of nothing. This is especially true when you have not been officially labeled or diagnosed with celiac disease and are saying that you have a non-celiac gluten sensitivity. In these situations, expect little support: you are on your own, and they may not go out of their way to accommodate you.

Most of us know both types of people, so instead of trying to explain why you are following a gluten-free diet, start out by giving them a copy of: "Getting Started Living Gluten Free," in this chapter and print them out a copy of the dining-out cards found in chapter 12 or at www. glutenfreeeasy.com/facts/living/cards.asp to make it easier for them to understand which foods are gluten free and which are not.

GETTING STARTED LIVING GLUTEN FREE

Living with someone who cannot eat gluten can be hard. But as hard as it is for you, it is ten times harder for them, because they have to deal with it every single time they need to eat.

Celiac disease and non-celiac gluten sensitivity are conditions in which a person can never eat gluten without getting sick. Gluten is a protein found in wheat, rye, and barley. The biggest difficulty in avoiding gluten is that it is often added to foods where you wouldn't expect to find it. It can turn up in seasonings, sauces, dressings, and condiments, and it can be used in fillers, thickeners, and binders. That's why people who need to live gluten free need to question every single food that they put into their mouth.

Celiac disease and non-celiac gluten sensitivity never goes away. Even eating the smallest amount of gluten will start a whole array of negative reactions within their body. Crazy as it sounds, if a crouton gets put on a salad and it is later removed, those few crouton crumbs may contain enough gluten to make them ill.

When someone is unable to eat gluten, they can't even use a toaster that has previously toasted any gluten-containing product—or mayonnaise where someone might have spread some of it on a piece of gluten-containing bread and then put the knife back into the jar.

Unlike other health problems that might allow occasional exceptions to their diets, people who have celiac disease can never make exceptions. Each exposure to gluten may cause an autoimmune attack. That's why they may seem absurdly careful—and why they'll be so adamant about never eating the slightest bit of gluten, even on a special occasion like their birthday.

Untreated celiac disease can be related to other disorders, such as:

- Thyroid disease
- Cancer
- Type 1 diabetes
- Anemia
- Osteoporosis
- Autoimmune liver failure
- Lupus
- Rheumatoid arthritis
- Severe gastrointestinal problems
- Frequent infections
- Skin problems

   * *Additional health problems can be found in chapter 1.*

So when someone in your life suffers from gluten sensitivity, take it seriously.

How Not to Be a Party Pooper

Going to a party is all about having fun, seeing family and friends, mingling, and catching up. The last thing you want is to have a bad reaction to the gluten in the food and need to leave early. But going around and asking a million questions about the food, or telling everyone that you cannot eat anything is bound to make you and others feel bad. So what to do?

Call the host ahead and find out about the menu. Offer to bring a dish and a dessert—this way, you'll know there will be some safe choices for you. If it is a set menu, explain that you are on a medically required diet and ask if it is okay to just bring a separate dish of food for you. This will be especially helpful when it is a large party and the host is already overwhelmed. In some cases, the host may ask what you can have and offer to prepare items in a way that will be safe for you. Each situation is unique and should be handled as you think will work best.

Sometimes you may not know the host well enough to call ahead about the menu. In this case, find out what you can, have a little something before you go to the party, and always bring something with you to complement any meal, such as an appetizer or dessert. If you are not a great cook, prepare one of the simple recipes in this book, pick up something at a gluten-free restaurant, or make up a cold antipasti platter—always a great option. Don't make the party just about the food. It's about having a good time, but make sure you take care of your needs!

Making Social Events Easier for Everyone

If you are following a gluten-free diet, being prepared will make social events easier for everyone. Always carry snacks with you so that when everyone stops to grab something at the local hot dog/pretzel stand, you can have something, too. Look up lists of gluten-free restaurants, or call ahead of time so you can evaluate what will be available for you. There are many smartphone apps that may make things easier, such as Find Me Gluten Free, which can help you locate nearby restaurants that have gluten-free choices. When you are confident about what you can have, it is much more enjoyable. Planning ahead makes it better for everyone. The trick is to find ways to enjoy every situation. Bring gluten-free candy or popcorn to the movie theater, bring your favorite gluten-free cookies to a birthday party, and bring a show-stopping appetizer to a barbecue.

You should never have to feel deprived—social events are made to be social, and they should be enjoyed.

Making It Easy for Yourself

Tips for Everyday Gluten-Free Eating

There are many foods that are naturally gluten free; it is only when we start combining and mixing foods that gluten secretly creeps in. Although wheat has been used as the base of many recipes, it does not have to be. When it comes to our foods, we really shouldn't have to refer to our gluten-free foods as gluten free—they are just foods. But since gluten is added to so many food choices, we need to be careful.

Today, the world is starting to discover the importance of having gluten-free selections, and every day it is becoming easier and easier to live gluten free. For now, in order for us to find safe food choices, stick with these simple tips:

- Pick foods that are naturally gluten free.

- Learn how to read labels to identify gluten-free products.

- Call manufacturers when you are in doubt (many times you can find out this information on a manufacturer's website as well).

It is important to stay on track with gluten-free eating. Even if you don't feel ill when you eat gluten, many people have silent celiac disease. Having even the smallest amounts of gluten can cause damage to their health even though they feel well. Knowing how to deal with a gluten-contaminated world is essential to protecting your health. Here are some easy tips:

- carry toaster-safe bags to make it possible to toast up your gluten-free breads when using shared toasters

- look up gluten-free restaurants for safe selections

- carry safe foods and seasoning agents with you

- join local celiac organizations to benefit from the research that other people have done

- when in doubt, reach for one of your safe snack options.

Easy-to-Carry Gluten-Free Snacks

Snacks are an important part of everybody's day. Most people don't plan ahead, they just grab snacks while they are on the run. Since gluten-free snacks may not be available everywhere you go, it is important to know what to pack so that you will always be prepared. The following are some gluten-free snacks:

- Dried fruits (double-check labels to make sure your dried fruit isn't dusted with wheat or oat flour)

- Dried vegetables (check labels)

- Fresh fruit or fruit cups

- Gluten-free crackers, cheese puffs, crisps, or chips

- Unseasoned nuts, cheese sticks, and peanut butter (available in individual single servings)

- Individual gluten-free puddings, canned fruit, and gelatin

- Gluten-free yogurt or yogurt shakes

- Gluten-free pretzels

- Gluten-free popcorn, potato chips, apple chips, or corn chips

- Gluten-free fruit roll-ups

- Gluten-free cereal blends

- Gluten-free rice cakes

- Gluten-free energy bars and cookies

- Gluten-free shakes such as Boost, Ensure, or Glucerna

- Fruit juices

Gluten-Free Eating in Unexpected Situations

No matter how carefully you try to plan, there will inevitably be situations when you will need to just wing it. Imagine that

- You are on a cruise to an exotic island, it is 100 degrees, and the buffet meal is being served by individuals who don't speak English.

- You are on a three-day scuba diving and boating trip.

- You are at a ski resort, and all your gluten-free supplies are back at the cabin.

- You have gotten last-minute tickets to a baseball game and didn't have time to pick up your supplies.

- You are in a business meeting where you are low in the chain of command, and it is a three-day meeting, 9 a.m. to 9 p.m., with all meals being catered in.

We live in the real world, and we can't account for every situation. It is important to try to make the most appropriate choices whenever possible. There will be times when you just have to do what you can, so learning as much as you can about gluten-free living and cooking techniques makes you better prepared to deal with each situation as it comes up. Although it may not be easy to carry snacks with you everywhere, or to call ahead to evaluate menus for each restaurant, following these guidelines makes it possible for you to have the best experience you can.

Making It Easy for Children

As difficult as it is for adults to follow a gluten-free diet, it is so much harder for children. When a child who has been diagnosed with celiac disease is very young it is hard to explain to them why they can't eat like the other kids. Often when it comes to meals and snacks there could be many different adults looking after them, such as babysitters, daycare workers, and teachers. It is difficult for those who are not living a gluten-free lifestyle to understand the diet, especially all the cross-contamination restrictions. People with good intentions frequently offer food to children as a treat, even when they have been told not to (especially if you have a child that doesn't exhibit immediate symptoms). They don't think they are hurting the child; they just think it would be a special treat that the child doesn't always get. Even if you have made every effort to inform caretakers about your child's dietary restrictions, it is always a possibility that someone doesn't really understand the instructions you have provided. Also, let's not forget that children often share their food with their friends, so the source of the gluten-containing food could be another child.

Having a good plan is essential to successful gluten-free living. Start by taking the extra steps as needed to ensure safety:

- In your house, keep gluten-free foods within reach for your children and unsafe foods out of sight and out of reach.

- Create a quick list of safe and unsafe foods to give to each caregiver.

- Involve your child in label-reading and meal planning as soon as possible so he or she can better understand what is safe to eat. chapters 4 and 11 offer lots of simple and delicious gluten-free recipe choices.

- Help teenagers discover safe choices that are available at fast food restaurants and on the go so that they can hang out with their friends without feeling as if they don't fit in (see some suggestions in chapter 6).

- If the stress of staying on track is difficult to manage, chapter 7 provides suggestions for helping your child through it.

The easier and more enjoyable you can make gluten-free living, the better it will be for both you and your children.

Cross-Contamination Tips

It is important to explain cross-contamination. Teach your children about not sharing food, washing their hands before eating, and wiping off surfaces before putting their food down. Teach them to ask questions about cooking liquids for gluten-free pasta, or shared fryers when it comes to

D's Dieting Dilemmas

By M. Brown, Ken Brown, and Will Cypser ©

French fries. Teaching your children what to look out for is the most important step to successful cooperation between you and your child. Empowering your child to make informed choices will make them feel less helpless about their intolerance.

At School

- Write a note to your child's school and teachers explaining the seriousness of your child's dietary needs. Children with celiac disease now fall under the Individuals with Disabilities Education Act (IDEA), which makes it a requirement for schools to provide gluten-free selections that are similar to their daily menu (of course, although this is a law, in many cases it is an uphill battle to get full compliance).

- Bring in an assortment of safe snacks that are similar to those the school will be giving out to make sure your child doesn't feel left out. Make it clear that you do not want your child sitting there watching other children having cupcakes while they can't have anything. You need to be informed ahead of time about parties, contests, rewards, treats, and special events so you can arrange for special treats for your child (and this doesn't mean the night before the event). It is always a good idea to make delicious frosted gluten-free cupcakes in batches and freeze them so all you need to do is take them out of the freezer whenever a quick gluten-free treat is needed.

- Make sure you pack fun lunches.

Field Trips and Picnics

It takes more time to plan for special events, but planning ahead will make it so much better for your child. If when you are researching an event and a busy teacher or restaurant manager tries to hurry you off by telling you not to worry—don't accept that; you need specifics so you can cover all the possibilities. Many people will *yes* you, telling you there are no worries, when they really don't know what gluten-free for health issues entails. Make sure you ask these types of questions:

- Are they offering snacks, cookies, or treats on the bus ride? If your child is very young and the teacher will be giving out the food, make sure you send hand wipes and instructions so they deglutenize their hands before touching your child's food.

- Are they stopping for bagels, heroes, pizza, on the route?

- If stopping and you provide a frozen meal, pizza, soup, or so on, will the restaurant be able and willing to heat it for your child?

- Is there a meal included, and if so, what are the gluten-free options?

- Is it possible for your child to get his or her food at the exact time as everyone else so he or she doesn't need to sit there with nothing in front of them when everyone else is served?

- Will there be more than one bus and parent helper on the trip? Can you go? If not, print out instructions for each bus and ask if your child can be on a bus with someone who has been instructed on safe gluten-free meals. Note that you don't want your child pulled off the bus with their friends and moved to another bus; you just want to make sure a knowledgeable person is on the bus, or with your child's group.

> Since much eating is social (i.e., school and birthday parties), dietary restriction can be difficult. But due the increased prevalence of food allergies as well as awareness of gluten, it has become a bit easier for parents than in years past.
>
> —Benjamin Lebwohl, MD, MS, Assistant Professor of
> Clinical Medicine and Epidemiology
> The Celiac Disease Center at Columbia University

Holidays and Family Events

Make sure holidays and special occasions are just as special for your child as they are for others. Make most holiday choices gluten free so everyone can have the same meal with less chance of cross-contamination.

Some family members will bend over backwards to offer great gluten-free options for your child. Others may not really believe the risks associated with cross-contamination or eating just a little gluten, so they may not take you seriously and they may make it difficult for you. Having a little gluten with celiac disease isn't like a diabetic having a little sugar; it is something that will trigger an immune system response even with the smallest amount. Don't go head-to-head with a difficult person; get allies and have them support you when someone isn't taking this need seriously. Do the things you can do, which includes everything you can to make it a fabulous event for your child. Don't let your child know about the difficulties; just make things happen.

Make sure there is a gluten-free choice that is similar to all the child's favorites, such as gluten-free stuffing (same as your family's recipe just use gluten-free bread), gluten-free gravy (thicken with rice flour or cornstarch and use gluten-free broth), and gluten-free desserts.

For religious events such as Passover, order gluten-free matzo ahead of time since it may not be available in local stores. For the church, buy gluten-free communion wafers (some churches allow these to be blessed and used and others do not, so it's best to check). Note that Catholic churches require that the wafers have some wheat in them to be used. The Benedictine Sisters make a communion wafer that contains wheat but falls below 10 parts per million—within the safe levels for someone who has celiac disease. It is important that the wafers are kept in a safe gluten-free container and not mixed with other wafers at the church or handled right after a regular communion wafer. Also, while this product is safe for those on a gluten-free diet it is not safe for those who have a wheat allergy. If you are having difficulties with a local church, go to the bishop who can help let them know the changes you are asking for have been okayed.

The goal is for your child to have a happy family memory and to feel as much a part of things as everyone else.

Parties

When it comes to parties, it is absolutely necessary to call the host or hostess ahead of time to find out about the plans for the day and the menu. Don't just show up for the party and try to wing it. Let them know that your child can't have any gluten and that you want to help provide gluten-free options for the menu. Prepare choices that are similar to those that the other children will be having. The last thing you want is for your child to feel like he or she is missing something. Try to bring foods that will be appealing to everyone so that the gluten-free food seems like a special treat, not a penalty.

If the party is at a restaurant with burgers, fries, or pizza, find out what the restaurant has to offer and if you can supply foods that they will heat for you. Make sure you can contact the restaurant and talk to the person in charge the day of the event so your child doesn't have to go to there on their own and request food.

Find out what kind of cake or dessert they are having so you can provide something similar for your child. Even if you have food brought to the party it is a good idea to also supply a bag of snacks for your child in case there is a delay or any mishaps with their gluten-free meal. If other parents are going to the party, it is even better if you can be there, too.

Camp

Sending your children away to camp, especially sleep-away camp, is stressful for most parents. For children that have food sensitivities or allergies the prospect can be terrifying for all. Following these tips can make it less stressful for the parents and more enjoyable for the child.

- Find out if your child wants to go to camp and address any of their thoughts and concerns.

- Call ahead and talk to the camp director and ask how they usually manage children with allergies and food intolerances. If they just say no problem, ask for details; their idea of no problems could be the same lunch every day for your child.

- Do they have an allergy policy, menu, gluten-free menu, or training information they can share with you?

- If your child is old enough, make sure he or she is able to read a food label.

- Can you review the menus ahead of time?

- Do they offer gluten-free bread, cereals, pancakes, French toast, waffles, rolls, pasta, and pizza, or do they just omit foods from your child's menu? What do they do to prevent cross-contamination of food?

- Will it be easy for your child to contact you if there are any issues with the food?

- Is there a dedicated fryer, toaster, and work area for preparing gluten-free foods?

- Do they have dedicated condiments and spreads for those on gluten-free diets?

- Can you send food for your child, and how will they be stored at camp? Make sure your child will be served at the same time as everyone at the table.

- How many children who are gluten free usually go to this camp?

- Do they have a registered dietitian and nurse on-site? If so, are they trained on gluten-free diets? If not, who is trained on the diet and where did they get their training?

- What types of excursions do they have at camp, and what types of snacks and meals are provided at these events? What do they have for children who cannot consume gluten?

Finding camps that specialize in working with children who have celiac disease and food allergies makes things easier. There are many more options available now than ever before. Type "gluten-free summer camp" into any search engine for numerous possibilities. I've listed two resources below.

Celiac Disease Foundation runs an annual camp for kids
www.celiac.org

National Foundation for Celiac Awareness lists numerous camps in their Resources section
www.celiaccentral.org

Eating on the Go

It is important for everyone to be able to enjoy spontaneous moments; this is especially important for children and teenagers. Stopping at a theme park, going biking, taking a swim in the lake, staying out at the picnic grounds, and going tubing are just some examples; life is full of exciting moments. If you plan ahead with on-the-go gluten-free foods your child can enjoy all the moments as they present themselves.

- Always carry gluten-free bars, chips, crackers, and fruit roll-ups.

- Keep gluten-free hot dog and hamburger buns in the freezer. When going out for an event, take two with you for a fast sandwich.

- Keep gluten-related apps on your phone (such as Find Me Gluten Free) so you can easily search for gluten-free restaurants wherever you may be.

- Keep a cooler in your car stocked with gluten-free yogurts, puddings, cold cuts, fresh fruit, cheese sticks, and more.

- Call ahead to theme parks to see if they have any gluten-free options.

- Check out which ice cream trucks are in your neighborhood and find out which choices are gluten free.

- Ices are always a great treat, just watch out for places where they might be cross-contaminated, or companies that add gluten to any of their flavors.

- Carry gluten-safe toaster bags with you so you can always heat your gluten-free bread safely.

Gluten-Free Snacks

It is especially important for kids to have similar snacks as their friends. Again, the key here is to have an action plan in place so there will always be choices. And fresh fruits and vegetables are naturally gluten free!

- Keep gluten-free candy and chocolate bars such as M&Ms and Hershey's milk chocolate bars available.

- Try the gluten-free peanut butter balls, truffles, gelatin jigglers, and gluten-free cream filled cakes listed in this book.

- Know which pizza places in your area have gluten-free pizza (if safe from cross-contamination), and keep some in your freezer as well.

- Keep gluten-free muffins, cupcakes, and brownies in the freezer. It's just 10 seconds in the microwave for a quick defrost.

- Keep gluten-free cookies in the freezer, or gluten-free cookie dough for an easy way to scoop and bake fresh cookies.

> If you have regular and gluten-free products in the house and are worried about your child grabbing the wrong thing, put the gluten-containing items on shelves that would make it difficult for your child to reach for them.
>
> —Suzanne Simpson, RD
> Celiac Disease Center at Columbia University

Throwing Together Treats

- Bake or buy gluten-free cookies and fill with ice cream, freeze on a cookie sheet, and store in a ziplock freezer bag until ready to use as a mini ice cream sandwich.

- Puree fruit and freeze in ice cube trays with a lollipop stick in them.

- Make up trail mixes with popcorn, dried fruit, and plain roasted nuts.

- Pack low-fat cheese sticks for a nice treat.

- Gluten-free pudding is always a satisfying choice.

- Pack baby carrots and mini containers of hummus.

- Fruit in its own juice packs well.

- Dried 100% fruit roll-ups

- Half of a peanut butter or almond butter sandwich is always a favorite.

- Serve gluten-free brownies with toppings such as ice cream, M&Ms, coconut, mini chocolate chips, nuts, marshmallow cream, and peanut butter.

- Layer pudding and whipped cream with gluten-free candy, gluten-free chocolate syrup, and gluten-free brownies in a glass bowl (a gluten-free "Death by Chocolate").

- Make a gluten-free chocolate cake and partially freeze. Slice in half, frost between the two layers with whipped cream, and place back in freezer. Slice, wrap, and store each slice in the freezer until needed. Defrost in a refrigerator.

- Mix ricotta cheese with powdered sugar, and mini chocolate chips and serve with gluten-free cookies.

- Buy a frozen gluten-free pie crust and bake it, then fill with pudding, whipped cream, and sliced bananas.

- Keep gluten-free cupcakes in the freezer (see recipes in chapter 11).

- Make gluten-free yellow cake, or a store-bought boxed cake, sprinkle in chocolate chips, and bake.

- Make a gluten-free cookie batter and freeze in a freezer-safe plastic container. When a child wants fresh cookies, scoop, top with favorite topping (peanut butter or chocolate chips, coconut flakes, M&Ms, nuts, raisins) and bake.

- Sandwich a roasted marshmallow and piece of Hershey's milk chocolate between two gluten-free graham crackers for a yummy S'more.

Nonfood-Related Issues

Although it may not be as important for adults to buy gluten-free shampoo, bubble bath, soap, and hand cream, since adults don't eat these things, *kids* sometimes do. Buying gluten-free choices for very young children might be something to consider. Also buy gluten-free alternatives to Play-Doh or anything that could be put in a child's mouth (Play-Doh contains gluten). You might ask your kids not to put these things in their mouths, but unfortunately, *yes, they do!*

Don't forget to check things such as vitamins, medications, candy, and anything that might possibly have gluten added too. There was an issue with a child who got sick after he had braces put on and the rubber bands for the braces were dusted with flour at the manufacturer so the rubber bands wouldn't stick.

In addition, before meals or snacks, make sure kids' hands are washed and surfaces wiped down in case there is any trace of gluten remaining. Make sure adults wash their hands if they handle any gluten-containing foods or products prior to preparing your child's foods. If they do wash their hands, explain to them that they should dry their hands with a paper towel, not a dish towel, since a dish towel is a

---

MORE TREATMENT CENTERS FOR CHILDREN

Centers for children are opening up throughout the country. One such facility just opened at Stony Brook University, in New York. Dr. Chawla and her team at Stony Brook believe that their biggest challenge in opening a pediatric celiac center will be overcoming the myths regarding gluten allergy, gluten intolerance, and celiac disease. Dr. Chawla states, "By launching our celiac center we hope to also help those who are unsure of their diagnosis, and those who have self-diagnosed or may have not yet been diagnosed."

source of possible cross-contamination. Planning ahead can assure a safe gluten-free environment.

Zero Tolerance to Bullying

It has been shown that some children use food allergies as a way to bully other children. When your child is away at school or camp you need to be sure that the teachers or counselors are going to be on the lookout for this type of behavior and that they will be ready to step in at the first sign of any bullying. Since contamination of a problematic food can cause such a huge reaction, it is not a situation that can just be ignored or taken lightly. It is therefore necessary to work with the schools and camps to discuss what is usually done in these types of situations so they can implement a zero tolerance policy for bullying. It needs to be emphasized at the highest level since this type of behavior poses a serious health risk to your child and any such problem needs to be addressed. Many times in camps, teenagers are used as counselors. That is why you need to find out as much as possible. Note that because celiac disease is now considered a disability, you can utilize this as leverage if you find it difficult to get cooperation.

The Bottom Line on Losing Weight on a Gluten-Free Diet

16

Follow a gluten-free diet and lose weight! This topic has been getting a lot of press lately, and although I would love to find such a simple way to lose weight, this statement is riddled with error. For many people gluten antagonizes their immune system, leading to inflammation that can cause numerous problems. In the case of celiac disease the response is an autoimmune one attacking different body systems, including the villi in the small intestines. Therefore, for some individuals gluten damages their small intestines and interferes with absorption of nutrients; for others, gluten may cause autoimmune issues and disease states. Many who have a gluten-related disorder will suffer with gastrointestinal problems or difficulties in either gaining or losing weight. Each person will have a different set of symptoms that will affect them in a unique and specific way. Therefore, it is difficult to make any one-size-fits-all type of statement about gluten.

If you don't suffer with a gluten-related disorder, then gluten in itself will not be the magical food that will change your weight. Gluten is found in wheat, rye, and barley and most people get their gluten from the cereal, breads, bagels, pizzas, pastas, cakes, cookies, and pies that they eat. These foods are usually high in calories. What would happen if they just gave all those higher calorie foods up? What I mean is, what if they gave up breads, pizza, pasta, and most desserts, and replaced these high-fat, high-calorie, starchy choices with fruits, veggies, lean proteins, and low-fat dairy products? Would they lose weight? Most likely yes, unless they were out of control with their portion sizes. But this weight loss wouldn't be attributable to giving up gluten, it would be a result of having given up highly processed, high-calorie foods, and replacing them with healthful, nutrient rich, lower calorie foods.

Don't get me wrong. The inflammatory response to gluten may negatively affect many people's health and weight; however, the recent diet craze that is driving people to go gluten free to lose weight is a *fad*, not a realistic weight-loss plan.

If you do not have a gluten-related disorder, reducing or eliminating gluten, which is a large, almost impossible to digest protein, likely won't hurt you and may help you feel healthier, but doing so just to lose weight is misguided. There is no scientific evidence to support a gluten-free diet as a weight-loss program.

If you are one of the people who are underweight from a gluten-related disorder (such as someone who is malnourished from celiac disease), going on a gluten-free diet will most likely help you to gain the weight back. But what if you need to be on a gluten-free diet and you are already overweight? If you simply replace gluten-containing bread, pancakes, and pies for gluten-free bread, pancakes, and pies, you will not lose weight. In fact, you will probably gain weight. Most packaged gluten-free foods that are starch options, have more fat, calories, and sodium than their gluten-containing counterparts. This is because in order to create a product that is light and crispy, starches and fats are added to give that gluten-like texture. Most people who go gluten free will gain weight if their dietary choices are not planned properly. If you want to lose weight consider this: What type of diet would you need? Where would you start and how do you develop a meal plan that will work for you? These tips and meal plans may help you on your way.

Losing Weight on a Gluten-Free Diet

First, follow the basic guidelines of any successful weight-loss plan:

- **Evaluate your health**, especially if you had been run down from celiac disease. Have a physical, and ask your doctor and registered dietitian if you have any specific limitations or health issues that will require you to include, or exclude specific foods. For example, some blood pressure and heart medications require a higher potassium intake while others require a lower intake; some diabetes medications require additional carbohydrates to prevent low blood sugar. In some cases your medication or health issues may require additional or reduced amounts of sodium. Each person is an individual with specific requirements. If you don't give your body what it needs you can do more harm than good, so it is always important to be aware of these issues and to make accommodations for them.

- **Set Goals:** Make a realistic list of goals you'd like to achieve. Setting manageable benchmarks for yourself is key. Instead of writing, "I want to lose 60 pounds in the next two months," try, "I want to lose 60 pounds over the next year, ideally about 1 to 3 pounds a week." And think beyond the scale to measure your success. Consider:

  - I want to look and feel better.
  - I want to have more energy.
  - I want to improve my health.
  - I want to have a good nutritional balance.

By setting positive, realistic goals, you are more likely to achieve them and feel good about each lifestyle change you make.

- **Acknowledge Problem Areas:** Make a list of your challenges: sweets, starches, times of the day that you overeat, lack of exercise, and so on. We all have our problem areas. It is important to discover *and admit to them* in order to develop strategies to overcome them.

- **Exercise:** Plan a minimum of 30 to 40 minutes of exercise a day. If it seems like too much at one time, it's okay to split the exercise throughout the day, such as 15 minutes in the morning and 15 minutes in the afternoon or evening. If you can, exercise for an additional 30 minutes two to four times a week. Make exercise a part of your daily routine and only skip exercise on a day if you are not feeling well. Try to stretch before and after exercise and always take the time to warm up and cool down. If you have any physical issues, such as a bad back, it pays to consult a physical therapist to find the safest ways for you to exercise.

- **Plan Meals:** Plan three meals and two to three snacks a day, evenly spaced. Have at least four to eight predetermined choices to select from at each meal and snack. It is hard enough to find healthful gluten-free choices when you want them. If you wait until you are hungry to think about what you want to eat, you are almost certain to make a poor choice.

- **Include Favorite Foods:** Make a list of your favorite foods and make an effort to include them into your meal plan. This will help to make it easier for you to stay on track, and easier to stay satisfied.

- **Time Meals and Snacks:** Try to plan your meals and snacks so you have something every two to three hours. This way your appetite stays under your control. When you wait too long to eat you not only get hungry but your blood sugar may dip, making you feel so hungry that your appetite gets out of control. This is especially important on a gluten-free diet because gluten-free foods may not always be available, and many skip meals only to overeat later.

- **Keep a Food Journal:** Okay, everyone hates journaling, but study after study has shown that people lose more weight and make better choices when they maintain a food journal. It is a form of self-accountability. Try to review your journal on a regular basis; you may be surprised when you review it and see what you actually eat!

- **Eliminate Your Trigger Foods:** Plan on keeping trigger foods out of your house. If in the past whenever you brought in gluten-free crackers or cupcakes you couldn't stop eating them, don't keep these foods in your house. We both know you are going to eat them. Never go shopping hungry or you will have less control and will be more likely to buy these trigger foods.

- **Prepare for Dining Out:** Review menus from your favorite gluten-free restaurants to select things that you feel will fit into your weight-loss plan. Whenever you go there, don't even give yourself the opportunity to be distracted by looking at the menu. Order from the items you have predetermined are good choices.

- **Give Yourself a Break:** Have at least one meal a week that is off-plan but still gluten free as a treat. This will help you to stay comfortably on track, and you will be more successful over the long term.

- **Reduce Stress:** Plan at least one relaxing activity each week, and make sure you have at least 30 minutes of downtime each day. Work on including stress-reducing activities such as yoga, tai chi, Pilates, meditation, daily walks or swims, dancing, or anything else that centers you and helps you relax.

A Gluten-Free Weight-Loss Plan

> Always check with your health care provider or registered dietitian before beginning a diet or exercise plan. Make sure that this plan will work in conjunction with your medications and health issues.

Always read labels, and try to do the following every day:

- **Sodium:** Keep main meals to less than 350 to 400 mg sodium, and snacks to less than 200 mg sodium.

- **Carbohydrates:** Keep main meals to about 25 to 40 grams of total carbohydrate, snacks to less than 20 grams of carbohydrate (carbohydrates include fruits, vegetables, and low-fat dairy, not just starches).

- **Fats:** Keep main meals to less than 12 grams of total fat, snacks to less than 7 grams of total fat. Try to avoid trans fats and saturated fats whenever possible.

- **Supplements:** Have your health care provider or registered dietitian help you to select which supplements will meet your needs, and always make sure they are gluten free.

- **Hydrate:** Have a minimum of eight glasses of water each day.

Sample Weight Loss Plan Without Gluten-Free Packaged Foods

Some possible options:

Breakfast Choices

- **Egg White Omelet:** 6 egg whites (about ½ cup) with sautéed vegetables (onions, zucchini, tomato, cooked in nonstick pan with 1 tsp vegetable oil and a dash of sea salt and pepper). Serve with 1 cup sliced melon.

- **Cottage Cheese and Fruit:** 1 cup 1% cottage cheese and 1 cup mixed fruit.

- **Yogurt Smoothie**: Blend 1 cup lite vanilla yogurt, 1 Tb almond butter, ½ banana, and 1 Tb of ground flax meal. Serve cold with a straw.

- **Ricotta Parfait:** ⅔ cup fat-free ricotta cheese layered with 3 Tb apple butter, 2 Tb chopped walnuts, and cinnamon.

- **Fruit and Vegetable Smoothie:** Blend 1 cup vanilla unsweetened almond milk, 1 cup strawberries, ½ banana, and ½ cup kale. Add some stevia if additional sweetness is desired.

Lunch Choices

- **Grilled Chicken Plate**: 3 oz grilled sliced chicken breast with ½ cup cherry tomatoes and 2 slices red onion over spinach greens, tossed with ½ cup sliced grapes, 1 Tb almond slivers, 2 tsp olive oil and balsamic vinegar.

- **Bean Salad:** 1 cup cooked white beans mixed with 2 tsp minced garlic, 1 tsp olive oil, 1 Tb lemon juice, ¼ cup minced sweet onions, 1 chopped stalk of celery, 2 chopped carrots, served over 2 cups Bibb lettuce.

- **Italian Tuna Salad:** 3 oz cooked fresh tuna (or 3 oz gluten-free solid tuna in water, rinsed), ¼ cup chopped onions, 1 cup gluten-free pickled veggies such as cauliflower, carrots, and broccoli (or chopped fresh veggies), 1 quartered tomato, and 1 sliced cucumber served over 2 cups soft baby greens tossed with 1 Tb lite gluten-free Italian dressing and 1 Tb lemon juice, or 2 tsp olive oil and lemon juice. Top with a dash of sea salt, pepper, garlic, and onion powder.

- **Tofu Griller:** Marinate ½ pound firm tofu sliced into 1-in. slices in gluten-free low sodium teriyaki sauce. Grill tofu and 4 slices of pineapple. Serve with other grilled vegetables such as zucchini, mushrooms, onions, and tomatoes.

Dinner Choices

- **Kabobs:** Cut 4 oz of chicken, firm fish, or pork loin into 1-inch chunks and alternate on skewers with pieces of onion, zucchini, pepper, tomato, and mushroom. Marinate in herbs and 1 Tb gluten-free salad dressing and grill. Serve with ⅔ cup cooked brown rice or quinoa.

- **Roasted Chicken:** Cut 4 oz of boneless skinless chicken into 2-in. chunks, wrap in aluminum foil with garlic cloves, onions, grape tomatoes, sliced carrots, and green beans, with 2 tsp of olive oil, lemon, and select spices, and roast.

- **Pan Seared Fish:** Spray and heat the pan. Season a piece of 4 oz red snapper filet with a dash of sea salt and pepper and pan sauté in a nonstick pan coated with gluten-free cooking spray until brown on both sides and cooked through. Serve with a small sweet potato and steamed green beans.

- **Turkey Avocado Burger:** Cook a 4 oz pattie of ground turkey breast that has been seasoned with garlic and onion powder. In a pan coated with gluten-free cooking spray, sautée spinach with garlic. Place turkey burger on top of spinach. Slice ⅓ of an avocado and arrange over burger. Serve with ½ cup cooked black beans.

Snack Choices

Space snacks between meals and only have one item below at each snack time. Otherwise these healthful choices will add up to a lot of extra calories.

- 1 small apple, pear, peach, plum, or orange

- 1 cup chopped melon, or 1 cup mixed berries

- ½ banana, or ½ cup cherries, or pineapple slices

- 10 nuts

- 1 piece of string cheese

- Gluten-free lite yogurt, or low-fat plain yogurt with ½ cup berries (top yogurt with 2 tsp of either ground flax, chopped nuts, or chia seeds)

- 1 cup air-popped popcorn

- 1 cup fresh vegetables with 2 Tb of hummus

- ½ cup bean salad (listed for lunch previously)

- 1 kabob (listed with dinner choices previously)

- Mixed green salad with 1 tsp of olive oil and vinegar

 TIP If you increase your daily exercise, drink lots of water, take appropriate supplements, provide your body what it needs, eat healthy gluten-free foods, and reduce your calorie intake, you will lose weight. For lasting success, create the healthiest weight-loss plan possible for yourself.

Sample Weight-Loss Plan Using Gluten-Free Packaged Foods

Breakfast Choices

- **Gluten-Free Waffle:** One gluten-free waffle with 2 tsp of peanut butter and 1 Tb raisins, served with 1 cup unsweetened almond milk.

- **Gluten-Free Cereal**: One cup gluten-free cereal, such as Chex, with ½ cup skim milk.

- **Gluten-Free Egg Sandwich:** One toasted gluten-free roll stuffed with a scrambled egg.

- **Gluten-Free Oatmeal**: One package, instant gluten-free oatmeal.

Lunch Choices

- **Sandwich:** 2 oz of gluten-free sliced turkey or roast beef on 2 slices of gluten-free bread with mustard and a side salad with 1 Tb light gluten-free salad dressing.

- **Salad Plate:** Large salad with veggies, 3 oz sliced grilled chicken, 2 Tb fat-free gluten-free salad dressing, ½ cup chick peas, and 5 gluten-free whole grain crackers.

- **Open Faced Grilled Cheese:** Place 2 slices reduced-fat cheddar cheese on 2 slices whole grain gluten-free bread (which has already been toasted in a gluten-safe toaster) with some sliced tomato and place it under the broiler until cheese is melted.

- **Gluten-Free Quesadilla:** Fill four small warmed corn tortillas, each with a quarter of the following ingredients: 2 oz slices grilled chicken, ¼ cup fat-free cheddar cheese, ¼ cup salsa, 2 Tb plain 0% fat Greek yogurt with lettuce and tomato.

Dinner Choices

- **Pasta and Mixed Vegetables:** 1 cup cooked quinoa pasta with 2 cups mixed vegetables tossed with 2 tsp olive oil and garlic powder, and 1 Tb Parmesan cheese. Served with a side salad with 1 Tb gluten-free fat-free salad dressing.

- **Stuffed Potato:** Medium baked potato stuffed with broccoli and topped with 2 slices gluten-free reduced-fat melted cheese. Serve with a steamed or roasted vegetable platter.

- **Grilled Chicken Cutlet Parmesan:** 3 oz grilled chicken tenderloin, topped with ½ cup tomato sauce, and ¼ cup sliced skim mozzarella. Heat in a microwave to melt. Serve sliced over ½ cup cooked brown rice pasta with steamed vegetables.

- **Barbequed Pork Loin:** 3 oz grilled pork loin topped with 1 Tb gluten-free barbecue sauce. Serve with ½ cup or 1 ear of corn and steamed green beans.

Snack Choices

Space snacks between meals and only have one item below at each snack time. Otherwise these healthful choices will add up to a lot of extra calories.

Any snacks listed previously as well as these additions. Please note only one snack at each snack break.

- 80–120 calorie gluten-free bar

- 100 calorie gluten-free ice cream

- 5 gluten-free crackers
- 1 large gluten-free rice cake with 1 tsp of peanut butter or jam
- Fat-free, sugar-free, gluten-free pudding
- Jell-0
- Sugar-free ice pop
- 60–80 calorie gluten-free fruit roll up
- 100 calorie gluten-free nut pack
- 1 gluten-free cookie (that has 80 calories or less)

Learning More about Gluten and Your Health

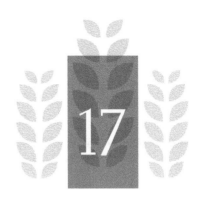

The Hidden Faces of Celiac Disease

The dangers of untreated or undiagnosed celiac disease may have many consequences. In this section, we will explore some of the dangers and some of the other issues that can arise when gluten is not eliminated from the diet.

Vitamin and Mineral Deficiencies

Untreated celiac disease often leads to vitamin and mineral deficiencies, which may lead to conditions such as anemia and osteoporosis. The deficiencies might not be obvious, as is the case with calcium and vitamin D (causing osteoporosis). It is a cycle where continued consumption of gluten will continue to negatively affect the absorption of these key vitamins and minerals. Even if someone is diagnosed with celiac disease and is 100 percent compliant with their diet, it can take years for their villi to heal. Since celiac disease usually causes deficiencies, supplementation may be beneficial to get them stable.

Neurological Disorders

Another common problem found with untreated celiac disease is neurological disorders. These nervous system disorders can lead to problems such as ataxia, seizures, and neuropathy. Ataxia is a lack of coordination. It can occur in your muscles or in your ability to speak. It can be also affect the inner ear. This means that you can suffer from vertigo and dizziness. If it affects your eyes, you might have poor hand-eye coordination.

Seizures are changes in behavior that occur from abnormal electrical activity in the brain. Seizures can be very mild or severe. The mild forms could lead to simple changes in feelings, such as a sudden feeling of fear or changes in vision. The most severe types can cause unconsciousness or altered consciousness and terrible body twitching. Neuropathy is a broad term that means problems with your nerves. It can present as pain, numbness, weakness, or tingling commonly seen in hands and feet. Some people may even feel an extreme sensitivity to touch.

The Dangers of Untreated Celiac Disease

Some other complications that may occur from untreated celiac disease can range from things as simple as lactose intolerance to dangerous conditions such as primary biliary cirrhosis (which in severe cases may require a liver transplant). In some cases, illnesses may be reversed by switching to a gluten-free diet; in other cases, the damage is irreversible; that is why rapid diagnosis is essential. The list of health issues that may be related to celiac disease is so extensive that it is hard to believe; many of them are listed in chapter 1, the reasons for these connections are being researched. Some of the more common problems associated with celiac disease include, infertility, osteoporosis, gastrointestinal problems, anemia, and thyroid disease.

It is important to understand that even though the treatment for celiac disease is only a change in diet, not changing your diet could be life-threatening in some instances.

Cancers

Cancer is one of the more serious risks of untreated celiac disease. Most frequently, cancer would be located in the intestinal tract, which includes the esophagus (the tube that brings food from your mouth to your stomach), the stomach, and small intestine. Other cancers that might occur include thyroid or lymphoma (specifically, non-Hodgkin's lymphoma). Since cancer cannot be reversed by just switching to a gluten-free diet, prevention by diagnosing and treating celiac disease is the most important course of action.

Infertility

Infertility is defined as an inability to have a baby either through not getting pregnant or because of miscarriages. When celiac disease is untreated, there is a higher rate of infertility; the cause is not very well understood at this time. Some suggest that it is related to the nutritional deficiencies seen with the illness, another possibility may be related to the celiac disease leading to miscarriages. Other possibilities include a problem with the reproductive cycle in women (shorter periods and earlier menopause) and gonadal dysfunction in men (problems making sperm).

Autoimmune Diseases

Because celiac disease is an autoimmune disease, when it goes undiagnosed there is an increased risk of other autoimmune diseases compromising an individual. Autoimmune diseases occur when our immune system attacks cells in our own body. The following diseases have been associated with celiac disease:

Type 1 Diabetes: An autoimmune disease that causes your body to stop making the hormone insulin by damaging the cells of the pancreas that make the hormone. The insulin is needed to move the sugar from your blood into your cells. Without it, your body cells cannot get the energy (sugar) from the foods you eat, and the amount of sugar in your blood becomes very high, causing damage to the eyes, kidneys, nerves, and blood vessels.

Grave's Disease and Hashimoto's Thyroiditis: The thyroid is the organ that regulates your metabolism. It also determines how many calories a day you need. There are two autoimmune diseases of the thyroid: Grave's disease and Hashimoto's thyroiditis. In Grave's disease, the metabolism runs too quickly. Someone with Grave's disease loses weight, has frequent bowel movements, feels irritable, loses sleep, and has bulging eyes. Palpitations, increased blood pressure, and tremor may also occur. The thyroid grows and may need to be removed. In Hashimoto's thyroiditis, conversely, the metabolism runs too slowly. Those with this disease will gain weight, are sensitive to cold, and have constipation, depression, migraines, muscle cramps, and infertility. If left untreated, it can cause failure of the muscles—including failure of the heart, which may lead to death. The disease is treated with thyroid hormone taken in a pill form.

Systemic Lupus Erythematosus (SLE), Rheumatoid Arthritis, Scleroderma, and Sjögren's Syndrome: Connective tissue is a tissue in the body that is fibrous. It is what holds our organs in place, makes up the ligaments and tendons surrounding our joints, and forms the lymphoid tissues in the body, the fatty tissue, and the elastic tissue. The connective tissue diseases we often see in untreated celiac disease include systemic lupus erythematosus (SLE), rheumatoid arthritis, scleroderma, and Sjögren's syndrome. Let's look at each of these.

- **SLE** is a disease that leads to an inflammation of the connective tissue in the body; thus, it can affect many areas in the body. The name comes from the typical appearance of a red rash on the face. The rash looks like a butterfly as it spreads over the nose from one cheek to the other. People with the disease will have times of remission (no inflammation) and other times with flares (with inflammation). It is a difficult disease to diagnose because of its complexity.

- **Rheumatoid arthritis** is different from regular arthritis—which is really called osteoarthritis. Osteoarthritis is caused by damage to the joint, leading to inflammation. However, in rheumatoid arthritis, your immune system attacks the membrane surrounding the joints. It causes severe pain in the joints, as well as deformity. Rheumatoid arthritis can affect many organs, including the heart, lungs, and eyes.

- **Scleroderma** is a disease that causes the development of scar tissue in the skin, internal organs, and small blood vessels. It causes these tissues to harden. There are two kinds: a localized kind known as morphea and a generalized kind known as systemic sclerosis. The localized disorder causes hardening of tissues and leads to disability. The systemic type can damage the heart, lungs, kidneys, and intestine, any of which may be fatal.

- **Sjögren's disease** is also called Sjögren's syndrome. It causes damage to the exocrine glands. Exocrine glands are the glands that secrete products into ducts (versus endocrine glands, which secrete products into the bloodstream). The exocrine glands in our body are the ones that produce sweat, tears, breast milk, digestive enzymes (the proteins we need to break down food), and hormones. The symptoms, as you may have already guessed, are dry mouth and eyes. Besides the dryness of these areas, often there is dry skin, nose, and, in women, vagina. This disorder very often occurs with other autoimmune disorders such as rheumatoid arthritis and scleroderma.

Gluten Sensitivities and Autism

Autism spectrum disorders are a set of conditions that affect the brain and development. People with this disorder have a difficult time with social interaction and communication. They often have symptoms that include sensory integration problems, repetitive behaviors, and muscle weakness. Many people with autism are unable to make eye contact. They can have restrictive interests—for instance, focusing only on trains.

Little is known about what causes this disorder. Many people have formulated their own theories; for example, some people believe that it occurs after the start of vaccinations. Other causes could be heavy metal toxins, disruptions to immune development, and inborn errors of metabolism. It is thought to have a genetic link. Most likely, someone is genetically predisposed to the disorder but does not develop it unless it is triggered by something else.

Some people with autism have gastrointestinal problems. These problems cause constipation, diarrhea, and vomiting. There is also a greater incidence of allergies in a person with autism. Food allergies and intolerances are more common. Some get relief from their stomach problems by eliminating gluten, casein (a protein found in milk), and, less frequently, soy protein.

However, there are some who do not have stomach problems or a clear intolerance to gluten and yet are still reported to respond favorably when they stop consuming it. One theory as to why this happens, which is still unproven, is based on intestinal permeability. What we do know is that the gluten and casein proteins are so large that they are not completely broken down in the stomach. These larger proteins normally should not get into the body without being broken down, but the theory is that the gut can be permeable, letting things in. Therefore the gluten and casein may get into the body through the intestinal permeability and may act like opiates, similar to drugs such as morphine, codeine, and opium. The opiate-like proteins, like these drugs, cause neurological disturbances. Another theory is that these proteins cause an unusual immune reaction in the body. There is also research looking at amylase trypsin inhibitors (ATIs) which are sort of natural insecticides found in wheat and their possible connection to behavior disorders.

Therefore, some believe that by removing the gluten and casein from the diet, these proteins cannot cause their damage or the immune response. Some parents of children with autism have reported improvements in many areas when they remove gluten and casein (dairy) from the diet, but this information is based on subjective observations by the parents. The improvements vary from decreases in sensory-seeking behavior (like hand-flapping and toe-walking) to improvement in eye contact and verbal communication. Not all children on this diet see improvement, and studies at this point are inconclusive since its success varies from one case to the next.

It is suggested for those that want to experiment with the diet that they should do so for six months with 100 percent compliance. If behavior changes are noted, continue for another six months. At the one-year mark, it is a good idea to challenge the child to see if it was really the proteins, not some other therapy, that made the difference. Reintroduce each of the proteins, gluten and casein. If the behaviors do not return, the child can be taken off the diet. If they do return, eliminate them for good. Some people can have a sensitivity to casein and not gluten, others gluten and not casein. Some may not have gluten, casein, or soy sensitivities.

Neither of these theories are substantiated by significant research at this time, although work is ongoing.

Other Behavior Disorders

There are many unanswered questions when it comes to gluten's possible involvement in many issues pertaining to physical and mental health and behavior. Further research is needed to yield a clearer picture about the role of gluten. For example, at Johns Hopkins University (laboratory of Dr. Robert H. Yolken) and Columbia University (laboratory of Dr. Armin Alaedini), investigators are exploring a potential link between gluten and schizophrenia. Only with continued research will we fully understand the impact of gluten and its relationship to different disorders.

Resources for Gluten-Free Living

Celiac Organizations and Research Centers

American Celiac Disease Alliance (ACDA)
Alexandria, VA
1 (703) 622-3331
info@americanceliac.org
http://americanceliac.org/

Academy of Nutrition and Dietetics, Nutrition Evidence Analysis Project
"Gluten Intolerance/Celiac Disease"
www.andevidencelibrary.com/topic.cfm?cat=1403

Canadian Celiac Association (CCA)
Mississauga, ON
1 (800) 363-7296
info@celiac.ca
www.celiac.ca

Celiac Disease Clinic, Department of Internal Medicine,
Gastroenterology
University of Iowa
Iowa City, IA
1 (319) 356-1616
www.uihealthcare.org/

Celiac Disease Foundation (CDF)
Woodland Hills, CA
1 (818) 716-15131
1 (818) 267-5577 (fax)
www.celiac.org

Celiac Disease Program at Boston Children's Hospital, Gastroenterology
and Nutrition Division
Boston, MA
1 (617) 355-6058
www.childrenshospital.org/clinicalservices/Site2166/
mainpageS2166P0.html

Celiac Sprue Association (CSA)
Omaha, NE
1 (877) CSA-4-CSA [1 (877) 272-4272]
1 (402) 558-0600
www.csaceliacs.info

Center for Celiac Research & Treatment, Yawkey Center for
Outpatient Care
Boston, MA
1 (617) 726-8705
1 (617) 643-2384 (fax)
www.celiaccenter.org

Gluten-Free Certification Organization (GFCO)
Auburn, WA
1 (253) 833-6655
www.gfco.org
customerservice@gluten.net

Gluten Intolerance Group (GIG) of North America
Auburn, WA
1 (253) 833-6655
1 (253) 833-6675 (fax)
www.gluten.net
customerService@gluten.net

National Foundation for Celiac Awareness (NFCA)
1 (215) 325-1306
1 (215) 643-1707 (fax)
www.celiaccentral.org/
info@celiaccentral.org

National Institute of Digestive Diseases Information Clearinghouse:
Celiac Disease
www.digestive.niddk.nih.gov/ddiseases/pubs/celiac/
nddic@info.niddk.nih.gov

National Institutes of Health (NIH) Celiac Disease Awareness Campaign
Bethesda, MD
1 (800) 891-5389
1 (866) 569-1162 (TTY)
1 (703) 738-4929 (fax)
www.celiac.nih.gov
celiac@info.niddk.nih.gov

North American Society for Pediatric Gastroenterology, Hepatology, and
Nutrition
Flourtown, PA
1 (215) 233-0808
www.naspghan.org/wmspage.cfm?parm1=642
naspghan@naspghan.org

U.S. Department of Health and Human Services/National Institutes
of Health
Bethesda, MD
301-496-4000
NIHinfo@od.nih.gov
www.nih.gov

Educational Institutions

American College of Gastroenterology: Digestive Health SmartBrief
www2.smartbrief.com/dhsb/index.jsp?campaign=acg

Celiac Center at Beth Israel Deaconess Medical Center, Harvard Medical
School
Boston, MA
1 (617) 667-1272
www.celiacnow.org

Celiac Disease Center at Columbia University
New York, NY
1 (212) 305-5590
www.celiacdiseasecenter.columbia.edu

Celiac Disease Clinic at Mayo Clinic
1 (507) 284-2511 (Rochester, MN)
1 (480) 301-8000 (Scottsdale, AZ)
1 (904) 953-2000 (Jacksonville, FL)
www.mayoclinic.org/celiac-disease

Celiac Group at University of Virginia Health System, Digestive Health
Center of Excellence
Charlottesville, VA
(434) 924-2959
www.medicine.virginia.edu/clinical/departments/medicine/divisions/
digestive-health 1

The Culinary Institute of America
Hyde Park,
NY St. Helena, CA San Antonio, TX
1 (800) 888-7850
http://enthusiasts.ciachef.edu/cooking-and-baking-classes

Mayo Clinic
1 (800) 446-2279 (Arizona)
1 (904) 953-0853 (Florida)
1 (507) 538-3270 (Minnesota)
www.mayoclinic.com

The Natural Gourmet Cooking School, Natural Food Cooking School
New York, NY
1 (212) 645-5170
www.naturalgourmetschool.com

Simon Fraser University's Nutrition Blog: The Dish
http://blogs.sfu.ca/services/thedish/

Stanford Celiac Sprue Management Clinic, Stanford Medical Center
Stanford, CA
1 (650) 723-6961
http://stafordhospital.org/clinicsmedServices/clinics/
gastroenterology/celiacSprue.html

St. Johns University
New York, NY
www.stjohns.edu/

University of Chicago Celiac: Disease Program
Chicago, IL
1 (773) 702-7593
1 (773) 702-0666 (fax)
www.cureceliacdisease.org/

University of Virginia, School of Medicine, Division of Gastroenterology
& Hepatology Charlottesville, Virginia
434-924-2959
www.medicine.virginia.edu/clinical/departments/medicine/
divisions/digestive-health

William K. Warren Medical Research Center for Celiac Disease and the
Clinical Center for Celiac Disease at the University of California
San Diego, CA
1 (858) 822-1022
http://celiaccenter.ucsd.edu
celiaccenter@ucsd.edu

Autism-Related Websites

Autism Research Institute
www.autism.com

Autism Society of America
www.autism-society.org

Autism Speaks
www.autismspeaks.org

National Institute of Child Health and Human Development
http://nichd.nih.gov/health/topics/autism/Pages/default.aspx

General Gluten-Free Information

Academy of Nutrition and Dietetics
www.eatright.org
www.adajournal.org
www.nutritioncaremanual.org

Dr. Schär Institute (for professional research information and travel tips)
www.drschaer-institute.com

CarolFenster
www.savorypalate.com

Celiac.com
www.Celiac.com

Celiacs, Inc.
www.e-celiacs.org

Celiac Frequently Asked Questions (FAQ)
www.enabling.org/ia/celiac/faq.html

Find Me Gluten Free (for finding gluten-free restaurants)
www.findmeglutenfree.com

Finer Health & Nutrition
www.finerhealth.com

Gfree Cuisine (GF recipes and menus)
www.gfreecuisine.com

Glutenfreeda Online Cooking Magazine
www.glutenfreeda.com

The Gluten-Free Page: Celiac Disease/Gluten Intolerance Websites
http://gflinks.com

Karina's Kitchen (gluten-free recipes)
www.glutenfreegoddess.blogspot.com

Marlisa Brown's Website and Blog
Website: www.glutenfreeeasy.com
Blog: www.glutenfreeez.com

Meijer Stores (posts gluten-free products available at their locations)
www.meijermealbox.com/healthy-living

National Foundation for Celiac Awareness, Celiac Central
www.celiaccentral.org

Shelly Case's Gluten-Free Website
http://glutenfreediet.ca

Tricia Thompson's Website
www.glutenfreedietitian.com

Food Labeling Resources

United States, New FDA gluten-free labeling law links:

www.tinyurl.com/q6zezf7

www.gpo.gov/fdsvs/pkg/FR-2013-08-05/pdf/2013-18813.pdf

http://www.fda.gov/Food/GuidanceRegulation/
GuidanceDocumentsRegulatoryInformation/LabelingNutrition/
ucm053455.htm

http://www.fda.gov/Food/GuidanceRegulation/
GuidanceDocumentsRegulatoryInformation/LabelingNutrition/
ucm053455.htm

Information regarding the Food Allergen Labeling and Consumer Protection Act of 2004:
www.fda.gov/Food/GuidanceRegulation/
GuidanceDocumentsRegulatoryInformation/Allergens/ucm106187.htm

U.S. Department of Health and Human Services Dietary Guidelines:
www.health.gov/DietaryGuidelines

U.S. Department of Agriculture Food Safety and Inspection Service:
www.fsis.usda.gov/wps/portal/fsis/home

Canada

Information regarding the food allergen labeling amendments:
www.hc-sc.gc.ca/fn-an/label-etiquet/allergen/index-eng.php

Questions and answers on the labeling of food allergens:
www.hc-sc.gc.ca/fn-an/label-etiquet/allergen/project_
1220_qa_qr-eng.php

Europe

European Starch Industry Association, EU allergen labeling of wheat starch derivatives and of gluten-free food:
www.aaf-eu.org/communication-on-eu-allergen-labelling-of-wheat-
starch-derivatives-and-their-use-in-gluten-free-food/

Labs

Kimball Genetics (DNA testing)
1 (800) 320-1807
www.kimballgenetics.com

Prometheus Labs (celiac diagnostic testing)
1 (888) 423-5227 Opt. #3
www.prometheuslabs.com

Medications and Supplements

Gluten-Free Drugs
www.glutenfreedrugs.com

Other

Alternative Cook (gluten-free cooking DVDs)
www.alternativecook.com

Dietary Guidelines
www.health.gov/dietaryguidelines

Toaster bags
www.toastitbags.com

To find a registered dietitian in your area:
www.glutenfreedietitian.com/newsletter/?page_id=14

Whole Grains Council (information on whole grains)
www.wholegrainscouncil.org

Allergy-Friendly Foods

Allergaroo
Allergy Friendly Foods
P.O. Box 790
Springfield, MO 65801
(417) 799-1875
(417) 863-0402 (fax)
www.allergaroo.com

Allergyfree Foods
310 West Hightower Drive
Dawsonville, GA 30534
1 (706) 265-1317 ext. 111
1 (706) 265-1281
info@allergyfreefoods.com
www.allergyfreefoods.com

Dining Out and Travel

AIC (Italian Celiac Association)
www.celiachia.it/home/HomePage.aspx

Bob and Ruth's Gluten-Free Dining and Travel Club (traveling gluten-free)
1 (410) 939-3218
info@bobandruths.com
www.bobandruths.com

Celiac Travel
www.celiactravel.com

Dining Info Service from Coeliac UK (gluten-free travel information)
www.gluten-free-onthego.com

GIG Gluten Intolerance Group (restaurants with gluten-free restaurants)
www.gluten.net

GF Culinary Productions, Inc., Gluten-Free Culinary Summit
www.theglutenfreelifestyle.com

Gluten-Free Delights (lists of gluten-free restaurants)
www.GFDelights.com

The Gluten-Free Guide to Italy, by Maria Ann Roglieri, PhD
www.gfguideitaly.com

The Gluten-Free Guide to New York (also Spain, France, Italy, and Washington, D.C.)
www.gfguideny.com

Gluten-Free Passport (booklets on gluten-free travel)
www.glutenfreepassport.com

Gluten-Free on the Go (lists of gluten-free restaurants)
www.Glutenfreeonthego.com

Gluten-Free Restaurant Awareness Program (GFRAP) (lists of gluten-free restaurants)
www.glutenfreerestaurants.org

Gluten-Free Travel Site (gluten-free travel information)
www.glutenfreetravelsite.com

Living with Cards
www.livingwithout.com/catalog/-7-1.html

Triumph Dining: The Essential Gluten-Free Restaurant Guide and Dining Cards
www.triumphdining.com/products/gluten-free-restaurant-guide

Gluten-Free Books

1000 Gluten-Free Recipes, Carol Fenster

American Dietetic Association's Easy Gluten-Free, Marlisa Brown and Tricia Thompson

Celiac Disease Nutrition Guide, Tricia Thompson

Canadian Celiac Association Pocket Dictionary: Ingredients for the Gluten-Free Diet

Celiac Disease: A Hidden Epidemic, Dr. Peter Green and Rory Jones

Celiac Disease: A Guide to Living with Gluten Intolerance, Sylvia Llewelyn Bower, Mary Kay Sharrett, and Steve Plogsted

The Complete Idiot's Guide to Gluten-Free Eating, Eve Adamson and Tricia Thompson

Cooking Free, Carol Fenster

The Essential Gluten-Free Restaurant Guide, Triumph Dining

Gluten-Free 101, Carol Fenster

Gluten-Free Baking with the Culinary Institute of America, Richard J. Coppedge, Jr., and George Chookazian.

The Gluten-Free Bible, Jax Peters Lowell

Gluten-Free Cooking for Dummies, Dana Korn and Connie Sarros

Gluten-Free Diet: A Comprehensive Resource Guide, Shelley Case

Gluten-Free Girl: How I Found the Food That Loves Me Back and How You Can, Too, Shauna James Ahern

Gluten-Free Everyday Cookbook, Robert M. Landolphi

The Gluten-Free Gourmet Cooks Comfort Foods: Creating Old Favorites with New Favorites, Bette Hagman

The Gluten-Free Gourmet Cooks Fast and Healthy: Wheat-Free and Gluten-Free with Less Fuss and Less Fat, Bette Hagman

The Gluten-Free Gourmet Bakes Bread, Bette Hagman

Gluten-Free Grocery Shopping Guide, Matison and Matison

The Gluten-Free Nutrition Guide, Tricia Thompson

The Gluten-Free Vegan, Susan O'Brien

The Gluten-Free Vegetarian Kitchen, Donna Klein

Going Gluten-Free, Chris Ford and Rodney Ford

Guidelines for a Gluten-Free Lifestyle, Celiac Disease Foundation

Living with Celiac Disease: Abundance beyond Wheat and Gluten, Claudine Crangle

Living Gluten-Free for Dummies, Danna Korn

Living Gluten-Free Answer Book, Suzanne Bowland

Serving People with Food Allergies: Kitchen Management and Menu Creation, Joel J. Schaefer

Tell Me What to Eat If I Have Celiac Disease, Kimberly A. Tessmer

The Wheat-Free Cook, Jacqueline Mallorca

Wheat-Free Gluten-Free Cookbook for Kids and Busy Adults, Connie Sarros

Wheat-Free Gluten-Free Dessert Cookbook, Connie Sarros

Wheat-Free Recipes and Menus, Carol Fenster

Publications

Delight Gluten Free magazine
www.delightglutenfree.com

Gluten-Free Living
www.glutenfreeliving.com Info@glutenfreeliving.com

Glutenfreeda (online cooking magazine)
www.glutenfreeda.com

Living Without magazine
1 (847) 480-8810
www.livingwithout.com

Shopping Guides

Gluten-Free Diet Guide for People with Newly Diagnosed Celiac Disease
www.ext.colostate.edu/pubs/foodnut/09375.html

Gluten-Free Grocery Shopping Guide, Matison & Matison
www.ceceliasmarketplace.com

Guide to Gluten-Free Shopping
http://central-market.com/health-and-wellness/gluten-free-guide

Recipe Directory with Allergy Information

Use this directory as a quick reference to find pertinent allergy information and potential modifications for all of the recipes in this book.

The codes are: QE = quick and easy, GF = gluten free, MF = milk free, SF = soy free, EF = egg free, NF = nut free, PF = peanut free, FF = fish free, SFF = shellfish free, V = vegetarian, VG = vegan.

X = allergen omitted from recipe
P = it is possible to adapt the recipe to omit this allergen

I have utilized current resources to provide allergy recommendations. Since ingredients often change, always read labels and call manufacturers on any questionable products.

Breakfast	QE	GF	MF	SF	EF	NF	PF	FF	SFF	V	VG
Bread, Banana Chocolate Chip (p. 241)		X			P	P		X	X	X	
Breakfast Cakes, Cornmeal (p. 91)	X	X	P	X	P	X	X	X	X	X	P
Cinnamon sticks, toasty (p. 92)	X	X	P	X	P	X	X	X	X	X	P
Corncakes, Blueberry Buckwheat (p. 242)		X	X	X	X	P	X	X	X	X	X

(continued)

Breakfast (continued)	QE	GF	MF	SF	EF	NF	PF	FF	SFF	V	VG
Frittata, Italian (p. 239)		X	P	X		X	X	X	X	X	
Granola, Amaranth and Apricot (p. 235)		X	X	X	X	P	X	X	X	X	X
Muffins, Blueberry Crumb (p. 238)		X	P	X	P		X	X	X	X	P
Muffins, Corn (p. 243)		X	P	X	P	X	X	X	X	X	P
Omelet, Eggs and Salsa, in a Corn Tortilla (p. 93)	X	X	X	X		X	X	X	X	X	
Pancakes, Banana (p. 89)	X	X	P	X	P	X	X	X	X	X	P
Pancakes, Quick-and-Easy, Coconut (p. 90)	X	X	P	X	P	X	X	X	X	X	P
Pancakes/Waffles, Pumpkin (p. 236)		X	P	X	P	X	X	X	X	X	P
Pancakes with Cream Cheese Filling (p. 240)		X		X	P	X	X	X	X	X	
Ricotta Surprise (p. 94)	X	X		X	X	X	X	X	X	X	
Yogurt Parfait (p. 95)	X	X		X	X	X	X	X	X	X	

Breads

	QE	GF	MF	SF	EF	NF	PF	FF	SFF	V	VG
Challah (p. 255)		X	P	X		X	X	X	X	X	
Arepas, Stuffed (p. 98)	X	X	P	X	X	X	X	X	X	X	P

(continued)

Breads (continued)	QE	GF	MF	SF	EF	NF	PF	FF	SFF	V	VG
Biscuits, Gluten-Free, Dairy-Free (p. 99)	X	X	X	X	P		X	X	X	X	P
Calzones, Broccoli and Cheese (p. 245)		X		X	P	X	X	X	X	X	
Crêpes, Basic (p. 253)		X	P	X		X	X	X	X	X	P
Flat Bread, Potato (p. 247)		X	P	X	P	X	X	X	X	X	P
Muffins, English (p. 254)		X		X	P	X	X	X	X	X	
Pizza, Italian (p. 249)		X	P	X	X	X	X	X	X	X	P
Pizza, Mediterranean (p. 246)		X		X		X	X	X	X	X	
Popovers (p. 96)	X	X	P	X		X	X	X	X	X	
Pretzel Nuggets, (p. 252)		X	P	X	X	X	X	X	X	X	P
Rolls, Hamburger (p. 250)		X		X	P	X	X	X	X	X	
Socca (p. 97)	X	X	X	X	X	X	X	X	X	X	X

Starters and Small Plates

	QE	GF	MF	SF	EF	NF	PF	FF	SFF	V	VG
Beets with Blue Cheese (p. 262)		X		X	X	X	X	X	X	X	
Burgers, Portabella Mushroom (p. 111)	X	X	X	X	X	X	X	X	X	X	X

(continued)

Starters and Small Plates (continued)	QE	GF	MF	SF	EF	NF	PF	FF	SFF	V	VG
Capellini Fritti, Gluten Free (p. 271)		X		X		X	X	X	X		
Cheese Puffs (p. 248)		X		X	P	X	X	X	X	X	
Chicken Fingers with Apricot Sauce (p. 264)		X	X	P	P		X	X	X		
Chicken Satay (p. 260)		X	X		X	X		X	X		
Chicken Tenders, Cornmeal Crusted (p. 106)	X	X	X	X	P	X	X	X	X		
Chicken, Wings, Buffalo (p. 268)		X		X		X	X	X	X		
Chicken Wings, Honey–Soy Glazed (p. 269)		X	X		X	X	X	X	X		
Dip, Artichoke and Cheese (p. 102)	X	X	P	P		X	X	X	X	X	P
Dip, Baked Vidalia Onion (p. 102)	X	X	P	P		X	X	X	X	X	P
Dip, Black Bean with Corn Chips (p. 104)	X	X	X	X	X	X	X	X	X	X	X
Dip, Crabmeat, Hot (p. 107)	X	X	P	P	P	X	X	X			
Dip, Eggplant (p. 258)		X	P	X	X	X	X	X	X	X	P
Dip, Layered Taco (p. 108)	X	X	P	X	X	X	X	X	X	X	P

(continued)

Starters and Small Plates (continued)	QE	GF	MF	SF	EF	NF	PF	FF	SFF	V	VG
Dip, Super Bean (p. 259)		X	X	X	X	X	X	X	X	X	X
Eggplant, Grilled, stacked with mozzarella (p. 267)		X		P	X	X	X	X	X	X	
Fries, Parsnip and Carrot (p. 109)	X	X	P	X	X	X	X	X	X	X	P
Garlic Knots (p. 248)		X	P	X	P	X	X	X	X	X	P
Hushpuppies (p. 265)		X	P	X	P	X	X	X	X	X	P
Kinishes, Mini (p. 248)		X	P	X	P	X	X	X	X	X	P
Meatballs, Albanian (Quofte) (p. 263)		X	X	X	P	X	X	X	X		
Noodles, Sesame (p. 105)	X	X	X	P	X	X	X	X	X	X	X
Pigs in a Blanket (p. 248)		X	P	P	P	X	X	X	X	X	P
Polenta Cups with Avocado and Mango Salsa (p. 270)		X	X	X	X	X	X	X	X	X	X
Quesadillas, Cheddar (p. 113)	X	X	P	X	X	X	X	X	X	X	P
Salad, Salmon (p. 260)		X	P	P	P	X	X		X		
Salsa, Black Bean and Mango (p. 103)	X	X	X	X	X	X	X	X	X	X	X

(continued)

Starters and Small Plates (continued)	QE	GF	MF	SF	EF	NF	PF	FF	SFF	V	VG
Shrimp Scampi Wrapped in Bacon (p. 266)		X	P	X	X	X	X	X			
Shrimp Salad–Stuffed Tomato (p. 111)		X	P	X	P	X	X	X			

Soups, Salads, and Sandwiches

	QE	GF	MF	SF	EF	NF	PF	FF	SFF	V	VG
Bisque, Gluten-Free Butternut (p. 281)		X		X	X	X	X	X	X	X	
Salad, Crispy Chicken, Chopped (p. 277)		X	P	X	P	X	X	X	X		
Salad, Italian Tuna (p. 110)	X	X	X	X	X	X	X		X		
Salad, Mixed Green, with Pear, Gorgonzola Cheese, and Walnut (p. 278)		X	P	X	X	P	X	X	X	X	P
Salad, Quinoa and Cranberry (p. 273)		X	X	X	X	P	X	X	X	P	P
Salad, Roasted Peppers and Tomato (p. 115)	X	X	X	X	X	X	X	X	X	X	X
Salad, Sautéed Spinach (p. 279)		X	P	X	P	X	X	X	X	X	P
Sandwich Melt, Turkey Avocado (p. 114)	X	X	P	P		X	X	X	X	P	P
Soup, Butternut Squash and Apple (p. 280)		X		X	X	X	X	X	X	X	
Soup, Easy Chicken and Rice (p. 112)	X	X	X	X	X	X	X	X	X	P	P

(continued)

Soups, Salads, and Sandwiches (continued)	QE	GF	MF	SF	EF	NF	PF	FF	SFF	V	VG
Soup, French Onion (p. 273)		X	P	X	X	X	X	X	X	P	P
Soup, Swiss Chard and White Bean (p. 276)		X	P	X	X	X	X	X	X	P	P
Stew, Beef (p. 275)		X	X	X	X	X	X	X	X		
Quinoa Salad, with Apple and Cranberry (p. 101)	X	X	P	X	X	X	X	X	X	X	P

Entrees

	QE	GF	MF	SF	EF	NF	PF	FF	SFF	V	VG
Cabbage, Unstuffed (p. 305)		X	X	X	P	X	X	X	X		
Chicken Breasts, Walnut Crusted with Mustard Sauce (p. 295)		X	P	X	P		X	X	X		
Chicken Cutlet Francese (p. 287)		X	X	X	P	X	X	X	X		
Chicken Cutlet Parmesan (p. 304)		X	P	X	P	X	X	X	X		
Chicken Enchiladas (p. 292)		X		X	X	X	X	X	X	P	
Chicken, Roasted Breasts of, with Carmelized Onions (p. 284)		X	X	X	X	X	X	X	X		
Chicken in Vodka Sauce with Mushrooms (p. 116)	X	X	P	P	X	X	X	X	X	P	P

(continued)

Entrees (continued)	QE	GF	MF	SF	EF	NF	PF	FF	SFF	V	VG
Chicken Vegetable Curry with Mango Chutney (p. 297)		X	P	X	X	X	X	X	X		
Chili (p. 302)		X	X	X	X	X	X	X	X	P	P
Chili, Gluten-Free White Bean and Turkey (p. 303)		X	X	P	X	X	X	X	X		
Crêpes, Chicken and Spinach–Stuffed (p. 299)		X	P	X	P	X	X	X	X		
Eggplant Rollatini (p. 119)	X	X		X	X	X	X	X	X	X	P
Flank Steak, Asian Rubbed (p. 118)	X	X	X		X	X	X	X	X		
Gnocchi, Parmesan (p. 296)		X	P	X	P	X	X	X	X	X	P
Grouper Piccata (p. 294)		X	P	X	X	X	X		X		
Lasagna (p. 288)		X		X	X	X	X	X	X	P	
Mahi Mahi, Blackened (p. 117)	X	X	P	X	X	X	X		X		
Pasta Gluten-Free Fresh (p. 290)		X	X	X	P	X	X	X	X	X	P
Pepper Steak, Annie Brown's Sweet and Sour (p. 308)		X	X		X	X	X	X	X		
Pie, Spinach and Feta (p. 306)		X		X	P	X	X	X	X	X	
Pierogies with Potato Cheese Filling (p. 300)		X	P	X	P	X	X	X	X	X	

(continued)

Entrees (continued)	QE	GF	MF	SF	EF	NF	PF	FF	SFF	V	VG
Ravioli, Crescent-Shaped (p. 291)		X		X	P	X	X	X	X	X	
Shrimp, Beer Battered (p. 283)		X	X	X	P	X	X	X			
Shrimp Teriyaki (p. 286)		X	X		X	X	X	X			
Stir Fry, Vegetarian (p. 285)		X	X	P	X	X	X	X	X	X	X

Sides

	QE	GF	MF	SF	EF	NF	PF	FF	SFF	V	VG
Black Beans and Rice (p. 309)		X	X	X	X	X	X	X	X	X	X
Broccoli, Steamed in Garlic Sauce (p. 311)		X	P	X	X	X	X	X	X	X	P
Escarole and White Beans (p. 313)		X	X	X	X	X	X	X	X	X	X
Fries, Spicy Baked Sweet Potato (p. 314)		X	X	X	X	X	X	X	X	X	X
Kasha Varnishkes (p. 316)		X	X	X	P	X	X	X	X	P	P
Pilaf, Wild Rice and Pecan (p. 313)		X	X	X	X	P	X	X	X	X	X
Quinoa with Sautéed Onions and Lima Beans (p. 312)		X	X	X	X	X	X	X	X	X	X
Red Potatoes and Bacon (P. 310)		X	X	X	X	X	X	X	X	P	P
Spinach, Creamed (p. 318)		X	P	X	X	X	X	X	X	X	P

(continued)

Sides (continued)	QE	GF	MF	SF	EF	NF	PF	FF	SFF	V	VG
Tomatoes, Stuffed (p. 315)		X	P	X	X	X	X	X	X	X	P

Sauces and Seasonings

	QE	GF	MF	SF	EF	NF	PF	FF	SFF	V	VG
Chutney, Mango (p. 319)		X	X	X	X	X	X	X	X	X	X
Salsa (p. 320)		X	X	X	X	X	X	X	X	X	X
Sauce, Barbecue (p. 321)		X	X	X	X	X	X		X	P	P
Sauce, Cream (p. 322)		X	P	X	X	X	X	X	X	X	P
Sauce, Steak (p. 321)		X	X		X	X	X		X		
Sauce, Yogurt (p. 320)		X		X	X	X	X	X	X	X	

Desserts

	QE	GF	MF	SF	EF	NF	PF	FF	SFF	V	VG
Bananas Foster (p. 123)	X	X		X		X	X	X	X	X	
Blancmange (p. 128)	X	X	P	X	X	X	X	X	X	X	P
Brownies, Gluten Free (p. 126)	X	X	P	X	P	P	P	X	X	X	P
Cake, Carrot, Moist and Delicious (p. 341)		X		X			X	X	X	X	
Cake, Chocolate (p. 344)		X	P		P	X	X	X	X	X	
Cake, Quick-and-Easy Cheesecake (p. 121)	X	X	P		P	P	X	X	X	X	

(continued)

Desserts (continued)	QE	GF	MF	SF	EF	NF	PF	FF	SFF	V	VG
Cake, Stawberry Shortcake (p. 331)		X	P	X	X	X	X	X	X	X	P
Cake, Yellow (p. 343)		X	P	X	P	X	X	X	X	X	
Cakes, Chocolate Lava (p. 332)		X	P			X		X	X	X	
Cheesecake Bars (p. 333)		X						X	X	X	
Chocolate Dream Treats (p. 122)	X	X			X	X	X	X	X	X	
Cookies, Chocolate Chip Coconut Meringue (p. 339)		X	P					X	X	X	
Cookies, Cream Cheese Butter (p. 338)		X		X	P	X	X	X	X	X	
Cookies, Double Chocolate Chip (p. 324)		X	P		P			X	X	X	
Cookies, Oatmeal and Butterscotch (p. 340)		X						X	X	X	
Cookie Truffles, Quick-and-Easy (p. 125)	X	X		P				X	X	X	
Crust, Almond (p. 345)		X	X	X	X		X	X	X	X	X
Filling, Cream (p. 344)		X	P	X	X	X	X	X	X	X	P
Frosting, Buttercream (p. 345)		X	P	X	X	X	X	X	X	X	P

(continued)

Desserts (continued)	QE	GF	MF	SF	EF	NF	PF	FF	SFF	V	VG
Frozen Banana Cream (p. 124)	X	X	X	X	X	X	X	X	X	X	X
Gelatin Chews (p. 128)	X	X	X	X	X	X	X	X	X		
Peanut Butter Balls, Chocolate Covered (p. 125)	X	X	P	P	X			X	X	X	
Pie, Apple and Cranberry Crumb (p. 329)		X	P	X	X			X	X	X	P
Pie, Italian Ricotta (p. 328)		X			P	X	X	X	X	X	
Pie, Pumpkin (p. 334)		X		X	P	X	X	X	X	X	
Pie, Yogurt (p. 121)	X	X			X	X	X	X	X	X	
Pudding, Rice (p. 346)		X	P	X	P	X	X	X	X	X	P
Tart, Apple and Almond (p. 325)		X	P	X	P		X	X	X	X	P
Tarts, Linzer (p. 336)		X	P	X			X	X	X	X	

Index

Step-by step recipe items are listed in bold type

About the Author

Marlisa Brown, MS, RD, CDE, CDN, is a registered dietitian, certified diabetes educator, chef, author, and international speaker. She has served as president of Total Wellness Inc., for over 20 years, and is co-owner of MC Seminars. Brown works as a nutritional consultant specializing in diabetes education, celiac disease, gastrointestinal disorders, cardiovascular disease, sports nutrition, culinary programs, and corporate wellness.

She is the author of *American Dietetic Association Easy Gluten-Free* (with Tricia Thompson, MS, RD), and has contributed to many dietary programs and books, including Richard Simmons's *The Food Mover* program, Jorge Cruise's cookbook *The 3 Hour Diet*, Leslie Sansone's *Walk Away the Pounds*, and Kathy Smith's *Project: YOU! Type 2*.

With over 30 years' culinary experience, she has been featured in over 50 cooking shows for the American Heart Association on International Cooking. Brown is on the Board of Directors of the Long Island chapter for The Gluten-Intolerance Group of North America and is chair of The International Association of Culinary Professionals nutrition section. She is also on the advisory panel for *Today's Dietitian* as a gluten expert. She has served as the past president of the New York State Dietetic Association and nominating chair for Dietitians for Integrative and Functional Medicine.

Brown has been the recipient of the following awards: "2011 Diabetes Educator of the Year" from The American Dietetic Association's Diabetes Care DPG; "1996 Emerging Dietetic Leader" from The American Dietetic Association; "2008 Dietetic of the Year" from The Long Island Dietetic Association; "Best Nutritionist" 2008/2009/2010/2011 from *The Long Island Press*; and "1994 The Community Service Award" from CW Post Long Island University.

Brown has a BS in Marketing and MS in Nutrition from CW Post Long Island University and is currently listed on the university's website as an outstanding alumna. She has also studied at the Culinary Institute of America.

For more information on celiac disease and gluten-free living, visit her website, www.glutenfreeeasy.com, and blog, www.glutenfreeez.com.